Foreword

It is with pleasure that I write the foreword for this book by Bobbee Terrill. Although written by an Australian author, it reflects the holistic principles and concepts of renal nursing which are comparable throughout the UK. Australian data quoted within the book is referenced against similar UK data. This book will not only complement, but also provide a beneficial contribution to, the limited number of renal nursing books available. It will undoubtedly be used as a reference for general nurses caring for patients with impaired renal function, to assist in the development of novice renal nurses and as a resource for experienced nurses to update their knowledge. The book lays the foundation on which nurses can build their evidence-based practice and knowledge skills to enhance patient care. Although written primarily for nurses, other healthcare professionals interested in nephrology will find the book a valuable resource.

The aim of this book is to provide a practical holistic guide for nurses to the skills and knowledge required by them to care for their patients. It covers the renal patients' experiences both physically and psychologically, incorporating the dialysis therapies of acute and chronic failure, on to renal transplantation. It describes the nurse's role in relation to the different treatment modalities. The section on paediatric nephrology offers an insight into the complexity of care required by this patient group.

Nursing renal patients within an acute hospital setting, a chronic dialysis unit or a satellite unit places many challenges on the nurse caring for them today. With the age of the dialysis population and co-morbid factors ever-increasing, so too are the knowledge and skills needed by the nurse to deliver quality care to an ever-changing population group.

I hope therefore that this book will provide the knowledge needed by those working in the field of renal nursing and that it will be used as a resource in renal units throughout the UK.

Avril Redmond
Chair of RCN Nephrology Nurses Forum

Acknowledgements

A special thank you to Yogarani (Yogi) Jeyakumar for her help with writing Section 6: Paediatric renal failure. Yogi has been involved in the care of children for ten years and specialised in the care of children with compromised renal function since 1992. Yogi generously shared her vast knowledge of the special needs of children with renal failure, especially those requiring renal replacement therapies. I am indebted to her for providing me with the opportunity to share her knowledge with those who read this book.

Thank you also to Margaret Morris for her patient proof reading of the book and to my editor Trisha Dunning for her encouragement and assistance with the editorial and publication process.

I am grateful to Rosie Heintz for drawing Figures 1, 2 and 3 in Chapter 1.3, Section 2, D G Oreopoulos MD, Professor of Medicine at Toronto Western Hospital for permission to use the Peritoneal Catheter Exit Site Classification Guide and Baxter Healthcare Corporation for permission to reproduce the information presented in Appendix A.

Many people contributed to my education over the years. While it is not possible to acknowledge them all individually, they include my nursing colleagues, the nephrologists with whom I have worked and the many allied health personnel who shared their collective wisdom with me. However, I suspect that I learned the most from my patients, and it is to them that I owe special acknowledgement; I am grateful to them for sharing their courage, hopes and fears and their anger and frustration. It is from the honesty of these patients and their families that I have begun to understand what it is to live with a life threatening illness. I have a special fondness for the World War II end stage renal disease Veteran population on whom I 'cut my teeth'. They are all gone now, but I still remember the camaraderie that was shared, and the fun times that were had.

Radcliffe Medical Press

Radcliffe Medical Press Ltd
18 Marcham Road
Abingdon
Oxon OX14 1AA
United Kingdom

www.radcliffe-oxford.com
The Radcliffe Medical Press electronic catalogue and online order facility.
Direct sales to anywhere in the world.

This book was originally published in Melbourne, Australia by Ausmed Publications Pty Ltd.

British Library Cataloguing in Publication Data

A catalogue record for this book is available from the British Library.

ISBN 1 85775 838 2

Typeset by Egan-Reid Ltd, Auckland, New Zealand.
Printed and bound by T J International Ltd, Padstow, Cornwall, UK.
Cover cartoon by Jock McNeish, Strategic Images Pty Ltd.

Table of Contents

SECTION 7 COMPLEMENTARY THERAPIES

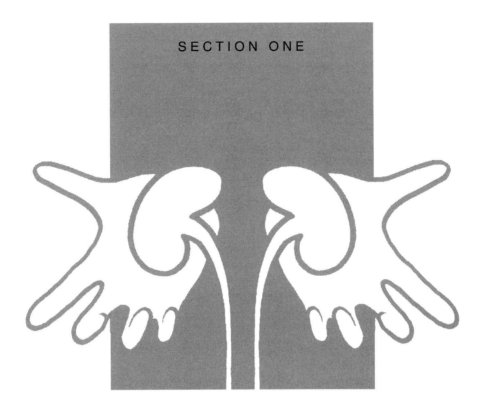

SECTION ONE

Chronic renal failure

Introduction

The incidence of chronic renal failure (CRF), and its consequence, end stage renal disease (ESRD), is increasing throughout both the western and developing worlds. As economies develop there is a corresponding increase in access to, and demand for, health care and health care technologies. The World Foundation for Renal Care estimated that by the year 2020 over 1 million people would be required to provide care for the approximate 1.4 million people receiving dialysis, and the approximate 1.2 million with functioning transplants. A daunting proposition!

As renal function declines, the person with CRF or ESRD eventually experiences involvement of all body systems. Quality of life is altered and major adjustment in physical, social and psychological aspects of life are required. Nurses face a variety of challenges when caring for these patients whether the person chooses to undergo treatment or to allow the natural progression of the disease to cause their death.

1.1 Pathophysiology: renal impairment

Terminology

Errors are frequently made when using the terms 'chronic renal failure' and 'end stage renal disease'. While one follows the other, the two are not interchangeable. Chronic renal failure refers to the progressive decline in function that follows injury to either glomerular or tubular structures within the nephron, and that continues until the kidneys can no longer maintain homeostatic function. End stage renal failure is the term used when the abnormalities of homeostasis have reached a stage where survival requires the use of renal replacement therapy. Renal replacement therapy refers to dialysis and transplantation that are used to sustain life in the presence of end stage renal failure.

The term 'uraemia' is used to describe the clinical syndrome that develops when the kidneys are no longer able to perform their normal excretory functions, and toxic products accumulate within body organs. The signs and symptoms of the uraemic syndrome include:

- The development of deep sighing respirations (Kussmaul respirations) that represent the pulmonary compensatory response to metabolic acidosis.

- Confusion and disorientation that indicates cerebral swelling that can lead to seizures and coma, known collectively as uraemic encephalopathy.

- Uraemic fetor and an odour of ammonia that represent an enzymatic response to increased serum urea.

- Deposition of urea crystals in the skin, known as uraemic frost.

- Laboratory findings include low haemoglobin, decreased serum bicarbonate, abnormal calcium phosphate balance and elevated serum potassium.

- Death is usually the result of cardiac arrhythmia.

Disease progression

CRF is usually considered to be an irreversible condition that will eventually progress to end stage disease (Finkel and DuBose 1997, p 151). The progression may take many years or it may follow within weeks or months of diagnosis. Renal disease has been described as 'progressing along a continuum from diminished renal reserve to end stage renal disease' (Crandall 1989, p 62). Early diagnosis, and where appropriate, aggressive treatment, may retard the progression of the disease and delay the need for replacement therapy if this is the chosen option.

Diminished renal reserve is a sub-clinical condition and is not usually diagnosed unless pre-existing factors such as congenital disease indicate that follow up of renal function is desirable. Diminished renal reserve usually lasts until up to 70% of nephron function has been lost, and may only be detected when a decrease in the creatinine clearance is recorded. Serum biochemistry and haematology are usually normal due to the 'intact nephron hypothesis'; a hypothesis that suggests that remaining functioning nephrons will hypertrophy in an attempt to retain normal regulatory function for as long as possible (Crandall 1989, p 62).

As more nephrons are lost, 'renal insufficiency' becomes apparent. Biochemical and haematological data are recognisable as outside normal parameters, although the person who is affected may not feel unwell. Diagnosis at this stage usually follows routine investigation for an apparently unrelated problem, unless it was made at the stage of diminished renal reserve.

Renal failure follows over a period of months or years, with the person exhibiting pallor, exercise intolerance and chest pain, which are associated with anaemia. Fluid retention leads to sacral, leg and periorbital oedema and, shortness of breath. Hypertension can cause headaches. As serum biochemistry worsens, and the symptoms commonly associated with the uraemic syndrome become apparent, the person needs to commence dialysis, or to receive a transplant in order to survive.

Causes of End Stage Renal Disease

Australia has one of the world's most extensive registries of the incidence, treatment and complications of end stage renal disease (ESRD). It is known as the Australian and New Zealand Dialysis and Transplant Registry (ANZDATA), and is available to all renal units. A total of 1708 new patients were recorded on this registry between 1997 and 1998. The annual rates of the individual causes of ESRD in Australia during this period were:

Glomerulonephritis	519 new cases	(30%)
1. Diabetic nephropathy	420 new cases	(25%)
2. Hypertension	182 new cases	(11%)
3. Polycystic kidney disease	115 new cases	(7%)
4. Analgesic nephropathy	97 new cases	(6%)
5. Reflux nephropathy	75 new cases	(4%)
6. Miscellaneous	174 new cases	(10%)
7. Uncertain	128 new cases	(7%)

ANZDATA 1999

In the UK similar data is available through the UK Renal Registry annual reports.

'Miscellaneous' includes the rarely encountered causes such as interstitial nephritis, lead nephropathy and renal tuberculosis. The 'uncertain' group consists primarily of patients who present late, and on whom no biopsy was performed, or for whom biopsy findings were inconclusive because of the extensive damage that was observed.

Clinical presentation and treatment options

There are four valid treatment options for the patient with end stage renal failure. They are listed below and will be discussed in full in subsequent chapters:

1. Haemodialysis (or any of its accepted variants)

2. Peritoneal dialysis

3. Transplantation

4. No treatment.

According to Dawborn (1990, p 367) knowledge about renal replacement therapies within the Australian community is such that most people will begin to enquire about active treatment when their health declines to the point where their quality of life is compromised. While knowledge of available treatment exists, there is seldom a corresponding knowledge about the degree of commitment that is required if treatment is to be successful.

Ideally, a competent patient, with a comprehensive understanding of the facts relating to their illness, and a reasonable guide to their prognosis, makes an autonomous choice as to whether to accept treatment or not. If treatment is chosen, then the patient, assisted by nursing and medical advice, chooses a therapy that will best suit their lifestyle.

Unfortunately, the ideal situation seldom arises. Family members may pressure patients into treatment, or they may have unrealistic expectations of the goals of treatment. Comorbid conditions can be present that makes attempting treatment unlikely to be beneficial, or treatment preference may simply not be available. Possibly even more difficult are the following scenarios:

1. The patient may be compromised in their decision-making capacity.

2. The physician, health care workers, and patient (or family) may be in conflict.

3. There may be conflict between the personal and professional values held by members of the health care team causing additional confusion for the patient.

Consider the following scenario and the advice that you would provide:

Geoffrey is 62 years old and has been suffering ongoing chronic ill health for many years. Chronic renal failure (CRF) was diagnosed five years previously and Geoffrey decided not to undergo any form of treatment at the time. He now has ESRD and finds himself in some difficulty with his original decision. He still does not want dialysis and has been told that transplantation is not an option, a decision with which he agrees. He comes to you for advice, outlining his dilemma as follows:

1. His daughter is suffering from severe schizophrenia and has been told that her children will be placed in protective care if both she and her children cannot continue to live under the close supervision of her parents.

2. Geoffrey does not believe that his wife is capable of providing the help that their daughter needs without his support.

3. Geoffrey's wife supports his original decision in principle, but feels that he should consider the needs of their grandchildren, at least until they are 'a little older'.

Scenarios with complexities such as this are not uncommon when considering treatment options for people with end stage renal failure, and for this reason, a multidisciplinary approach to decision-making is often taken.

1.2 Pathophysiology: a system review

Where the problems start

Regardless of the initiating event renal failure commences in one of two ways:

1. Failure to filtrate:

This is a glomerular dysfunction and results in the progressive retention of electrolytes that rely on filtration for removal. The serum levels of such electrolytes rise, as do metabolic waste products such as urea and creatinine.

There is often a corresponding increase in the permeability of the glomerular basement membrane that results in the appearance of substances such as blood and protein in the urine.

Fluid *retention* occurs with hy*per*tension, oedema and difficulties with respiration.

2. Failure to secrete and to selectively reabsorb:

This is a tubular dysfunction and begins early in primary medullary diseases. The ability to conserve water is lost and urinary concentrating ability falls.

Fluid and salt *loss* occurs, with dehydration and hy*po*tension.

While most patients suffer from problems related to fluid and electrolyte retention, some retain minimal filtration function and, because tubular function has been lost, they excrete all that has been filtered and may need fluid and sodium replacement.

What happens to the systems involved?

Body fluids

Salt and water: It is important to differentiate between the patient who needs salt and fluid restriction, and the one who needs salt and fluid replacement, because glomerular and tubular function may decline at different rates. Nursing interventions involve recognising that fluid intake should be 500 mls plus the previous day's output. Fluid intake includes all foods that are liquid at room temperature (jellies and ice creams) and, as these differences are often difficult for patients to understand, be sure to explain to each patient why they are different from the patient in the next bed!

Electrolytes: Sodium restrictions are usually limited to 'no added salt' and a caution against using prepackaged/tinned foods, unless the patient is a 'salt loser'. Salt loser is a term applied to a person whose renal dysfunction originates in the renal medulla, the part of the kidney primarily responsible for selective reabsorption of water and solute that was non-selectively filtered at the glomerular level. Such people require additional salt and water in their diets.

It is difficult to predict when to commence potassium restriction, which is dependent on the patient's underlying renal disease and their medication and diet.

Serum biochemistry is the best guide; e.g. patients' taking diuretics other than those that 'spare potassium' will usually require restriction as their disease progresses, while those taking angiotensin converting enzyme (ACE) inhibitors, or with diabetes, could require restriction earlier. Polystyrene resins (calcium or sodium resonium) may also be required.

The introduction of phosphate-binding agents also depends on the serum biochemistry. If serum phosphate is <1.6 mmol/l, and serum calcium is not elevated, vitamin D_3 may be introduced. Phosphate-binders will be introduced if the 'calcium/phosphate product' is high (see Chapter 3).

Acid-base balance: Hydrogen ion generation is a normal result of metabolism. Between generation and excretion, hydrogen must be buffered to prevent a threat to the pH of blood.

The lungs excrete volatile acids produced as the result of intracellular metabolism, while the kidney excretes nonvolatile acids produced as the result of protein metabolism. When renal failure occurs, renal excretion is compromised and a metabolic acidosis results. While partial, or complete, compensatory mechanisms often keep the pH within normal limits for short periods of time, the person with chronic or end stage renal disease needs long term assistance to maintain normal acid-base status.

Prior to the commencement of dialysis this assistance is usually in the form of oral bicarbonate. Once dialysis has commenced, the most convenient way to supply a buffering substance is via the dialysate solution. Encouraging patients to adhere to protein restrictions will decrease the generation of nonvolatile acids, and hydrogen ion production will be reduced. In an attempt to overcome the malnutrition common among patients with end stage renal failure some countries are considering the use of guidelines that do not recommend restriction of dietary protein.

Cardiovascular

Cardiovascular disease is the leading cause of death in patients with CRF (Smith 1993). Apart from extracellular volume expansion, which increases cardiac preload, and anaemia, which exacerbates cardiac after load. The major contributors to cardiovascular disease are:

Hypertension: This may be due to the retention of salt and water (as with filtration failure) or to inappropriate activation of the renin-angiotensin-aldosterone system. An abbreviated explanation of the activation of this system is provided in

Chapter 4. For further details, the interested reader is referred to the recommended reading at the close of this Chapter.

Atherosclerosis: Hyperlipidaemia causes an accelerated atherosclerosis that contributes to the high incidence of cardiovascular disease in patients with CRF (Talbot and Curtis 1996, p 446).

Myocardial dysfunction: The combination of hypertension and atherosclerosis causes an increase in cardiac after load. The left ventricle hypertrophies in an attempt to deal with the problem, and, over time, as left ventricular muscle mass progressively enlarges, the contractility of the left ventricle falls. The coronary arteries have difficulty supplying blood to the increased muscle mass and ischaemia results, leaving patients vulnerable to arrhythmias, especially as serum electrolyte levels begin to fluctuate.

Hyperkalaemia: As already mentioned, the retention of potassium ions is dependent on factors other than the loss of significant renal function and differs between patients. Where potassium retention occurs, both pre- and current dialysis patients need to adhere to potassium restrictions (as discussed later in this chapter). As serum potassium rises, the gradient between intracellular and extracellular potassium decreases. This causes an increase in intracellular potassium and a decrease in the time required to reach the 'threshold' of the action potential; muscle becomes 'excitable' as the time for repolarisation is reduced, and muscle contraction occurs more easily. There are few symptoms of an increase in serum potassium until quite late, and patients may suffer severe arrhythmias (resulting in cardiac arrest) without knowing that their serum potassium was elevated.

Nursing care involves patient education relating to the maintenance of an acceptable blood pressure, adherence to fluid and dietary restrictions for potassium, and a reduction in serum triglyceride and cholesterol levels. Nurses should know, and tell their patients about, hidden sources of potassium, such as blood used in transfusions and medications, and should be aware of the emergency treatment of hyperkalaemia.

Musculoskeletal

The close relationship between calcium, phosphate, vitamin D_3, and the parathyroid gland is completely disrupted in CRF and ESRD. There are three primary reasons for this:

1. Decreased phosphate excretion by the kidney.

2.   Decreased gastrointestinal absorption of calcium, resulting from reduced hydroxylation (conversion to the active form) of vitamin D_3.

3.   Abnormalities in response to parathyroid hormone.

The importance of maintaining the correct balance between calcium, phosphate and vitamin D_3 will be fully examined in Chapter 3.

Pulmonary system

A reduced cough reflex, tenacious sputum and a reduction in pulmonary macrophage activity combine with the generalised immunosuppression that accompanies CRF to increase the incidence of pulmonary infection. These infections are usually bacterial, but viral and fungal infection is not uncommon (Crandall 1989, pp 71–72).

Nursing interventions include referral to a physician as soon as coughing is noticed or chest sounds indicate the presence of fluid, and close attention to physiotherapy to encourage the removal of secretions.

Haematological

White blood cells: Both specific and nonspecific arms of the immune response are depressed. Granulocytes are less mobile, and chemotaxis is reduced, resulting in suppression of phagocytic function and in a failure to attract 'B' and 'T' cells to the area of infection, and to keep them there. 'B' cell function fails, hence the increase in bacterial infection and 'T' cell failure results in an increase in viral infection (Crandall 1989, p 74). Decreased immune system activity results in a higher than normal incidence of malignancy.

Platelet function: Platelet numbers are usually within normal limits, but aggregation and adhesion are reduced, which results in prolonged bleeding times and bruising (Crandall 1989, p 72). This persists once dialysis has commenced and must be considered when cannulating the patient, although other factors can contribute to prolonged bleeding.

Erythrocytes: The reduction in red cell life by about one third, suppression of erythropoiesis, and loss of blood to laboratory testing and the dialyser if haemodialysis is undertaken, all contribute to the anaemia seen in CRF. Usually described as 'normochromic and normocytic', iron deficiency and megaloblastic anaemias also occur (Crandall 1989, p 73). Anaemia is less common now that the genetically engineered form of erythropoietin (Recombinant Human Erythropoietin [rHuEPO]) is available. rHuEPO acts in the same way as naturally produced erythropoietin. Both erythropoietin and rHuEPO promote proliferation and differentiation of red blood cell precursors in bone marrow cells. Erythropoietin is secreted in response to reduced oxygen content of red blood cells passing through peritubular capillaries (Wharon 1998, p 67).

Iron deficiency is often seen because iron stores may be depleted by the rapidly maturing red blood cells. Iron infusion may be required to enable appropriate use of available erythropoietin (Dennison 1999, p 409).

Nursing interventions include the early detection of infection, awareness of the prolongation of bleeding times, minimisation of blood loss to the laboratory, and the extracorporeal circuit if haemodialysis is the selected treatment option. Since the introduction of erythropoietin, the monitoring of ferritin levels, transferrin saturation and % hypochromic cells have become increasingly important and are addressed in Chapter 6.

The integument

Patients complain of itching, that is often due to the retention of urea and phosphate products. Scratching results, and causes bruising and ecchymosis due to capillary fragility. Oil gland activity is reduced resulting in dry skin that aggravates the itching. Skin often has a grey, bronze discolouration, or may appear yellow, despite the absence of hepatic disease. Anaemia can cause pallor of the skin and mucous membranes.

Uraemic frost is very rare now and refers to the appearance of a salt like substance on the skin of the face and chest. It is due to the excretion of urea crystals onto the skin and occurs in individuals with advanced end stage renal failure who require immediate dialysis.

The nails are often thin and brittle and frequently have dark tips with pale proximal edges that are scored by ridges.

Nursing interventions include avoiding the use of soap (use soap substitutes), selective use of antipruritic medications, assessment of the adequacy of dialysis if it has commenced, and of phosphate-binding agents if it has not. It is also worthwhile checking the patient's compliance with phosphate-binding agents because they are almost universally unpalatable, and many patients avoid taking them if at all possible (Crandall 1989, p 63).

Gastrointestinal

Changes to the entire gastrointestinal tract are associated with CRF, and nurses can play an important role in reducing the morbidity associated with these changes. For example, the anorexia that accompanies the approach of end stage disease may be minimised with frequent mouthwashes and small meals that are offered at a variety of intervals during the day.

Constipation that results from fluid and dietary restrictions, phosphate-binding agents and inactivity, must first be acknowledged as a complication of therapy, and then treated with agents such as fibre supplements and stool softeners.

Metabolic problems

End organ resistance to the action of insulin occurs, and results in an increase in the levels of circulating insulin. This results in an increase in glyceride production by the liver and a corresponding increase in the synthesis of triglycerides, and accelerates the rate of atheroma formation.

Patients are at risk of becoming malnourished as a result of protein restriction during CRF, especially as end stage approaches. Protein restriction is designed to reduce the generation of urea and hydrogen ions, both of which are removed by the kidney. Modification of the protein restriction may be required in severely malnourished patients as they approach end stage disease.

Nursing interventions include patient education about how to lower cholesterol and triglyceride levels, and encouraging patients to achieve a suitable protein intake using high biological protein products, discussed in the Chapter.

Neurological

Alterations to the neurological system can involve the central, peripheral and autonomic systems. In many patients, all three of these systems are involved.

Central nervous system: As early as 1839 it was recognised that 'normal mentation requires adequate renal function' (Brown and Brown 1995, p 244), and that the changes observed during renal failure ranged from subtle and nonspecific, when renal function was only moderately impaired, to gross and disabling, when the disease was far advanced. Signs and symptoms include a shortened memory span, memory loss, confusion and depression. Patients may be emotionally labile, irritable, difficult to engage in conversation and are often demanding (Crandall 1989, p 80). These changes, attributed to uraemia and characterised by alterations to 'cortical background rhythm', are often interpreted as a generalised slowing of cerebral activity (Crandall 1989, p 80). When untreated, this cerebral encephalopathy progresses to the coma and death that is the natural endpoint of end stage renal failure.

Peripheral nervous system: Peripheral neuropathy is most frequently confined to the lower extremities and, usually begins as a sensory loss, with paraesthesia that is 'accompanied by prickling, tingling or painful sensations' (Crandall 1989, p 81). As renal failure progresses, leg muscles weaken and muscle atrophy may develop. The 'restless leg syndrome' and the 'burning foot syndrome' are often described. In the former, the patient describes an irresistible desire to repeatedly move the feet, while the latter is associated with redness, swelling, and pain in the soles of the feet. These symptoms are usually symmetrical, are most often present in the distal portion of the limbs, and progress proximally. Foot drop and eventual loss of function in the lower limbs are the result of the axonal atrophy and demyelination of nerve fibres (Crandall 1989, p 81).

Autonomic nervous system: The depressed cough reflex, and an inability to compensate for either a reduction, or an elevation in, blood pressure are all thought to be due to the effects of uraemia on the autonomic nervous system. When pulmonary congestion is present it is difficult for the patient to cough and remove fluid exudate, which predisposes them to infection. The inability to increase cardiac rate and output impairs the response to hypotension. Similarly, although less frequently encountered, the sympathetic nervous system is unable to slow either cardiac rate or output to compensate for hypertension (Crandall 1989, p 82).

Reproductive

Alterations in both sexual and reproductive function are common in CRF and do not appear to improve once dialysis has commenced. Many factors are involved and include psychological disturbances, hormonal alterations, anaemia, and pharmacological agents, especially antihypertensive agents and steroids. Autonomic neuropathy and pelvic vascular insufficiency have also been implicated (Milde et al. 1996, p 307).

A reduction in testosterone secretion, combined with end organ resistance to follicle stimulating hormone, results in oligospermia and impotence in men. A similar organ resistance to follicle stimulating hormone, and decreased secretion of luteinising hormone, suppresses ovulation and results in decreased libido in women (Crandall 1989, p 87). Successful transplantation usually results in a return of normal sexual desire, function and fertility.

Nursing interventions include providing a comfortable, private area, where patients can discuss their concerns, and acceptance that such concerns are valid. If you do not feel able to discuss a patient's concerns about their sexuality, you should refer the patient to another person with whom they can discuss their concerns. Statements such as 'I don't have the information that you need, but I can tell you someone who does' saves the patient embarrassment. Also, 'did you know that many people with renal failure have problems like this?' can be helpful in letting patients know that the difficulties they are experiencing are part of their disease process rather than to a personal failing.

1.3 Slowing the progress to end stage disease

Factors that accelerate nephron loss

As stated earlier in the chapter, CRF is an irreversible disease, which, given sufficient time, will inevitably progress to end stage. However, early diagnosis and an appropriate therapeutic approach may prolong renal function and delay the need for dialysis for many years.

Finkel and DuBose (1997, p 151) recommend that the following questions need to be asked after an increase in serum creatinine is recognised:

1. Is the disease acute or chronic?

2. What disease process is involved?

3. Are the contributing factors reversible?

Diagnostic procedures should be undertaken to determine the underlying disease, and a renal biopsy may be required to determine the specific pathology and provide a guide to treatment and prognosis. In systemic diseases that involve the kidney, treatment of the primary disease may alleviate symptoms and preserve renal function. Diagnostic procedures and specific disease processes will be discussed later in this section.

Once CRF is diagnosed, intervention ranges from aggressive treatment of the primary disorder through to conservative management. There are specific factors that nurses should be aware of when educating patients about how to prolong of their renal function.

Dehydration: Reference has already been made to the different fluid requirements of patients with renal disease due to glomerular failure and those with disease due to tubular failure. If dehydration is allowed to occur the haemoconcentration that follows commences a cycle of worsening uraemia, increasing anorexia and vomiting and further dehydration. Patients may need intravenous fluid replacement if oral intake results in continued vomiting.

Hypertension: Elevated blood pressure can be the result of filtration failure, causing intravascular volume expansion, or renal artery stenosis, causing activation of the renin-angiotensin-aldosterone system, which results in vasoconstriction and the reabsorption of sodium and water if significant renal function remains. Either way, the increase in systemic pressure will cause a decrease in renal blood flow and a fall in glomerular filtration rate. Remember that, until blood pressure is extremely elevated, a patient will not experience hypertensive symptoms. Always emphasise the need to continue with prescribed medications unless they are ceased or altered by a physician.

Infection: An increase in catabolism with a corresponding elevation in serum urea usually follows infection that occurs within the kidney or elsewhere in the body. The increase in urea may be beyond the filtering capacity of the failing kidney and result in anorexia and dehydration, and increase the rate of nephron failure. Infection should be treated rapidly because these patients are already immunosuppressed with medication that has been modified to suit remaining renal function if the drug is renally excreted.

Obstruction: Obstruction to the outflow of urine eventually dilates the collecting system and aggravates the decline in function. Obstruction can be low in the urinary tract, as with prostatomegaly, or high, as with renal calculus or papillary duct obstruction. Patients with established renal failure can present with an 'acute-on-chronic' episode of renal failure. The mechanism behind this is similar to that for acute renal failure and follows the occurrence of an 'acute' assault on an already compromised kidney.

Medication: Nephrotoxic antibiotics are drugs that rely on glomerular filtration or tubular secretion for the removal of either the active drug or its metabolites. If the dose-interval, or dose, is not modified, there is a high risk of destroying remaining nephrons. Ascertain the appropriate information about dose adjustment in renal failure from a renal physician, a pharmacist or consult appropriate clinical practice guidelines. Dose adjustment is discussed in Chapter 5.

Diuretic therapy can aggravate renal failure by promoting dehydration (refer to the previous section), and can be especially problematic if cardiac failure is also present. If diuretic therapy is indicated, both cardiac and renal function should be carefully monitored. Potassium-sparing diuretics should be used with caution in patients with chronic renal failure.

Antihypertensive medication can reduce renal blood flow by causing vasodilation for e.g. drugs such as diazoxide, minoxidil. Others decrease glomerular capillary pressure by opposing constriction of the efferent arteriole, for e.g. ACE inhibitors such as captopril.

1.4 Nutrition

History

Prior to 1970 and the acceptance of dialysis as routine treatment for end stage renal failure, dietary management was the mainstay of therapy. Professors Sergio Giovanetti and Camello Giordano developed the original low protein diet and prescribed it for those patients approaching end stage disease who were not able to receive dialysis.

Dr. Geoffrey Berlyne modified the diet by replacing Italian foods with foods preferred by British patients. The modified diet consisted of 20 grams of high biological value (HBV) protein, which is protein that contains all the essential amino acids. Energy needs were met by supplying 50kCals/ kilogram of ideal body weight. The diet was prescribed for patients with a serum urea of slightly over 30mmol/litre and a glomerular filtration rate of 3mls/min, and patients often recovered sufficiently to be able to return to work. The diet was difficult to follow and required total commitment from the patient, but it was the only alternative to a uraemic death for many patients (Vennegoor and Coleman 1998, p 320).

As the availability of dialysis increased during the 1970's, protein restrictions were relaxed. However, there were numerous complications of dietary modification during this period that were due primarily to a limited understanding of the need to balance protein and energy requirements. When insufficient calories were consumed, energy requirements were met by using the protein that was meant for growth and tissue repair. The result was a calorie/protein malnutrition that increased morbidity and slowed the rehabilitation process. Although protein allowances are much higher today, many patients do not have enough protein in their diet, and exhibit signs and symptoms of protein malnourishment similar to patients in the early years.

Attitudes to protein restriction vary. Vennegoor and Coleman (1998, pp 321-324), wrote that the initial results of a long term research project commenced in 1985 indicate that patients with renal function below 20% of normal should reduce their protein intake, but that those with function between 20% and 40% of normal will have little benefit from protein restrictions. Preservation of renal function appears to correlate better with control of blood pressure and the absence of severe proteinuria. It also appears that a low protein diet may reduce the risk of renal disease in diabetic patients.

There is a growing body of opinion that suggests that once dialysis commences, protein intake of at least 1.2 gms/kg/ ideal body weight (IBW) should be encouraged, and that dialytic therapy should be adjusted to protein intake, *not* the other way around.

Sodium was initially restricted to 25 mmol/day, but was increased to 60 mmol/day, and potassium restrictions were increased from 50 mmol/day to 60 mmol/day with the modified diet (Vennegoor and Coleman 1998, pp 320-321).

Assessment

Malnutrition is common among renal patients (Rocco and Blumenkrantz 2001, p 374), and low serum albumin is the most reliable predictor of a compromised nutritional state (Burrows et al. 1993, p 671). Low serum albumin is second only to inadequate dialysis as 'the most potent laboratory predictor of mortality ... in the haemodialysis population' (Burrows et al. 1993, p 671). This is a reliable predictor of morbidity in the patient with chronic renal failure (Rocco and Daugirdas 2001, p 421).

Diet in chronic renal failure

The aims of protein restriction are to delay the need for dialysis and relieve the symptoms of uraemia. Each patient should have their diet tailored to their individual requirements. The diet should not become so tedious that the patient loses interest in food.

Protein is usually restricted to between 0.8 and 1.0 g/kgIBW when glomerular filtration rate is between 20 and 30mls/min and between 0.6 and 0.8 g/kgIBW when glomerular filtration rate is < 20mls/min. Protein restriction continues at this level until dialysis is commenced. At least 60% to 70% of dietary protein should be HBV protein (Vennegoor and Coleman 1998, p 325). There is usually no restriction with a GFR >30mls a minute.

Protein restrictions are eased once dialysis is commenced, usually to 1·2 g/kgIBW with haemodialysis, and 1.4 g/kgIBW during peritoneal dialysis. If you read widely you will see different figures quoted by different authors. Don't be confused by this, as experts often have different opinions. It is probably best to refer to a renal dietitian for specific advice.

Protein supplementation may be required by malnourished patiens. Supplementation is usually in the form of drinks such as Ensure, Fortisip or Resource plus. Parenteral supplementation may be required, especially if the patient is severely malnourished or if dialysis has commenced.

Energy: Between 35 kCals/kgIBW should be taken each day (CARI Guidelines, 2000, Dialysis adequacy, p 38). If too little is energy is consumed, protein catabolism resulting in a negative nitrogen balance, weight loss, and protein/calorie malnutrition will occur. If too many calories are consumed, a positive nitrogen balance will result in weight gain and attendant cardiovascular complications. Approximately 50% of energy requirements should consist of complex carbohydrates such as grains, cereals, rice and vegetables (Vennegoor and Coleman 1998, p 327).

Sodium: Restrictions are usually between 80 and 150 mmol/day unless the patient is a 'salt loser', in which case sodium replacement will be required. In practice, salt restriction can be achieved by not adding salt to food before or after cooking, and by avoiding canned vegetables and take-away foods. Patients should be warned not to use salt substitutes because they may contain potassium. They should be encouraged to use herbs and spices as flavour enhancers.

Potassium: Restriction is on an individual basis, as already discussed. Remember that there are nondietary causes of hyperkalaemia such as drugs, (e.g. potassium sparing diuretics, and cyclosporine), metabolic acidosis and cellular destruction (as with blood transfusion, surgery or injury).

Phosphate: Many foods, especially HBV proteins, contain large amounts of phosphate. Therefore, dietary restriction as a means of controlling serum phosphate is impractical. The administration of phosphate-binding medication is the only appropriate method of preventing hyperphosphataemia. When phosphate-binding medication is administered, dietary phosphate is bound to salts of magnesium, calcium or aluminium, and the resulting complex is excreted via the bowel. The administration of phosphate-binding medication should occur *with* food to ensure that it binds with dietary phosphate. As discussed earlier, many patients will avoid taking phosphate-binding medications because they are unpalatable. The importance of taking phosphate-binders with food should always be emphasised when teaching patients to participate in their own care.

Vitamin and minerals: Supplementation with water soluble vitamins, except B$_{12}$, usually begins once dialysis has commenced. Iron, zinc and calcium supplement are only required if body stores are low. Vitamin and mineral replacement prior to the start of dialysis occurs on an individual basis.

1.5 Indigenous issues

A world view

Indigenous people throughout the world are recognised as suffering renal impairment in numbers disproportionate to the rest of the population and becomes apparent once Aboriginal people begin to follow a 'western lifestyle'. Much of the renal failure that occurs amongst these people is due to diabetic renal disease that rapidly follows the introduction of highly refined diets that are common in much of western society.

In the United States of America, diabetic nephropathy is the major cause of end stage renal and is due primarily to the large numbers of 'Afro-Americans' who attend renal replacement programs failure (Finkel and DuBose 1997, p 151). It is the principal cause of end stage renal failure in New Zealand (ANZDATA 1999), accounting for approximately 44% of new patients, 88% of these had type 2 diabetes.

The UK Renal Registry produce an annual report. In December 2002 it reported that diabetic nephropathy is still more common in younger individuals and that the UK is not treating the increasing proportion of patients with diabetic nephropathy seen in the USA and much of Europe (UK Renal Registry Report, 2002).

References

In text references

ANZDATA Registry Report, 1999, 'Australia and New Zealand Dialysis and Transplant Registry, Adelaide, South Australia.

Brown, T., Brown, R., 1995, 'Neuropsychiatric consequences of renal failure', Psychosomatics, vol. 36, no.3, pp 244–253.

Briganti, E., McNeil, J., Atkins, R., 2000, 'Renal disease in Aboriginal Australians', *The Epidemiology of Diseases of the Kidney and Urinary Tract: an Australian perspective*, A Report to the Board of the Australian Kidney Foundation.

Burrows, J., Alto, A., Kaufman, A., 1993, 'Intradialytic parenteral nutrition: a practical approach', *ANNA Journal*, vol.20, no. 6, December, pp 671–677.

Caring for Australians with renal Impairment (CARI) Guidelines, 2000, A joint project between the Australian and New Zealand Society of Nephrology and the Australian Kidney Foundation, Excerpta Medica Communications, Sydney.

Crandall, B., 1989, 'Chronic renal failure', in *Nephrology Nursing: concepts and strategies*, Ulrich, B., (ed.), Appleton and Lange, California.

Dawborn, J.,1990, 'Dialysis', *The Medical Journal of Australia*, vol. 152, April, pp 367–372.

Dennison, H., 1999, 'Limitations of ferritin as a marker of anaemia in end stage renal disease', *ANNA Journal*, vol. 26, no. 4, August, pp 409–414.

Ewing, T. 1994, 'Aboriginal community makes a clean break with the past', *The Age newspaper*, Saturday 29th January, p 23.

Finkel, K., DuBose, T., 1997, 'Chronic renal failure', in *'Caring for the renal patient*, Levine, D., (ed.), 3rd ed., Saunders, Sydney.

Milde, F., Hart, L., Fearing, M., 1996, 'Sexuality and Fertility Concerns of Dialysis Patients', *ANNA Journal*, vol. 23. no. 3, pp 307–313, 315.

Rocco, M., Blumenkrantz, M., 2001 'Special problems in the dialysis patient: Nutrition', in *Handbook of Dialysis*, Daugirdas, J., Blake, P., Ing, T., (eds.), 3rd ed., Lippincott Williams and Wilkins, Philadelphia.

Smith, S., 1993, 'Uraemic pericarditis in chronic renal failure', ANNA Journal, vol. 20, no. 4, pp 432–43438, 508.

Talbot, L., Curtis, L., 1996, 'Cardiovascular assessment of the patient with renal problems', *ANNA Journal*, vol. 23, no. 4.

UK Renal Registry Report, 2002, Fifth Annual Report. UK Renal Registry, Bristol, UK.

Vennegoor, M., Coleman, J., 1998, 'Dietary management in chronic renal failure', in *Renal Nursing*, Smith, T., (eds.), 2nd ed., Bailliere Tindall, Sydney.

Wharton, S., 1998, 'Applied anatomy and physiology', in *Renal Nursing*, Smith, T., (ed.), 2nd ed., Bailliere Tindall, Sydney.

Recommended reading

Calkins, M., 1996, 'Pathophysiology of congestive heart failure in ESRD, *ANNA Journal*, vol.23, no. 5, pp 457–463.

Crandall, B., 1989, 'Chronic renal failure', in *Nephrology Nursing: concepts and strategies*, Ulrich, B., (ed.), Appleton and Lange, California.

Radke, K., 1994, 'The aging kidney: structure, function, and nursing practice implications', *ANNA Journal*, vol. 21, no. 4, pp 181–190.

Shoop, K. 1994, 'Pruritus in end stage renal disease', *ANNA Journal*, vol. 21, no. 2, pp 147–153.

Vander, J., 1995, *Renal Physiology*, 5th ed., McGraw Hill, Sydney.

Wade-Elliot, R., 1999, 'Caring for the Elderly with Renal Failure: Gastrointestinal Changes', *ANNA Journal*, vol. 26, no. 6, pp 563–569.

Acute renal failure

Introduction

Acute renal failure (ARF) develops in between 5% and 7% of hospitalised patients, but only a small number of these patients require renal replacement therapy. Of these, the mortality rate is approximately 50% and has not changed over the past several decades, despite the many technological advances in that time. If multiorgan failure is present, the mortality rate approaches 90%. The management of ARF, especially that requiring renal replacement therapy, presents a special challenge to renal nurses. Despite the current trend towards managing these patients in intensive care units, many present initially to the renal ward, or require post-acute management in renal areas. To provide appropriate care for these patients, renal nurses need to understand the differences between the pathophysiology of CRF and ARF, and appreciate the features that are shared by these two disease processes.

2.1 The development of acute renal failure

Definition

ARF is defined as any sudden fall in glomerular filtration rate (GFR) that is sufficient to cause uraemia. Oliguria occurs in many patients, however nonoliguric forms of ARF occur in a third to half of these patients (Neale 1986, p19). ARF secondary to severe burns and nephrotoxic damage is usually associated with normal urine output.

Causes of ARF

ARF is usually due to prerenal, intrinsic renal, or postrenal causes.

Prerenal failure: occurs when there is a fall in the blood supply to the kidneys. It be due to either hypovolaemia, or to a direct decrease in the renal blood supply (Saunders and Bircher 1998, p101). The early stages of ARF is characterised by lack of structural damage and the continuation of tubular function i.e. the ability to reabsorb water and electrolytes is retained (Dawborn 1986 p1309). This type of ARF is rapidly reversible with the restoration of blood pressure or correction of any obstruction of the blood flow to the kidney.

Causes of prerenal failure include:

- Extravascular volume loss
  - excessive diuresis
  -* third spacing
  - gastrointestinal tract (GIT) loss.

- Intravascular volume loss
  -hypoalbuminaemia
  -haemorrhage/burns
  -renal artery occlusion

- Decreased cardiac output
  -myocardial infarction
  -tamponade
  -cardiac failure

- Peripheral vasodilation
  -sepsis
  -antihypertensive agents

(Dawborn 1986 p 1310, Saunders and Bircher 1998 p 103).

* The Pathological accumulation of body fluid in a potential body space.

Most patients will demonstrate the classic signs of hypovolaemia but in those with septic shock the expected pallor, coolness and vasoconstriction can initially be replaced by vasodilation where the skin feels warm and the vessels appear full (Saunders and Bircher 1998, p100). The recognition of a prerenal cause for oliguria, and the rapid restoration of blood flow to the kidney, will result in the return of normal renal function within two to three days. If renal hypoperfusion continues, ischaemic damage results in a prolonged recovery phase.

Urinalysis will help to determine the difference between prerenal and intrinsic renal conditions. High, urine osmolality and low urinary sodium indicate that the tubules are still functioning and a quick recovery is likely. If ischaemia damage has already occurred to the tubules, the urine osmolality will be low and the urinary sodium will be high.

Because the progression to ischaemic damage is preventable in most cases, pro-active measures include: undertaking all complex surgery in hospitals with modern monitoring equipment and established management protocols; rapid transfer to such hospitals when risk factors are recognised; and the judicial use of diuretics and anti-hypertensive agents.

Intrinsic renal failure: occurs when there has been structural damage to the renal parenchyma. The difference between intrinsic renal failure and pre- and postrenal failure is that correcting the cause does not guarantee the return of full function. Recovery is often prolonged with residual loss of function. Intrinsic renal failure is classified as follows:

- Acute tubular necrosis (ATN)

    a) Postischaemic renal failure   - failure to reverse hypovolaemia
       (vasomotor nephropathy)

    b) nephrotoxic renal failure   - antibiotics/contrast media

- Glomerulonephritis

- Acute interstitial nephritis

- Vasculitis   - polyarteritis nodosa

- Intratubular obstruction   - myoglobin, Bence-Jones proteins

- Coagulopathies   - acute cortical necrosis
                                            - haemolytic uraemic syndrome

(Dawborn 1986, p 1310, Saunders and Bircher 1998, p 103).

Mechanisms of injury in intrinsic renal failure

The tubular injury that occurs in ATN is the one most frequently described and damage varies with the severity of the initial injury. Findings include the sequestration of glomerular filtrate in tubules where sloughed, necrotic tubular cells obstruct the lumen and the filtrate leaks back through damaged tubular cells into the interstitium (Myers 1996, p 444).

25

Changes occur to autoregulation. Despite an increase in the delivery of sodium to the macula densa, release of renin and subsequent generation of angiotensin 11 and endothelin, a local vasoconstrictor, result in constriction of the afferent arteriole, and a subsequent decrease in glomerular filtration pressure (Myers 1996, p 44f).

Activation of calcium channels results in an increase in intracellular calcium and the loss of the proximal tubular brush border. This results in decreased surface area and subsequent decrease in cellular transport. Brush border debris is able to be seen in the urine and may cause further obstruction to the tubule (Racusen 1997, p 4–5). Intercellular tight junctions and the loss of normal cytoskeleton lead to redistribution of sodium potassium ATPase away from the basolateral border where it is required for active transport.

Preservation of maximum renal function requires the recognition and aggressive treatment of glomerulonephritis and vasculitis, avoiding nephrotoxic drugs where possible, care with the use of combinations of drugs, especially in the elderly, and avoiding dehydration prior to procedures where fasting and/or bowel evacuation is required e.g. radiological examinations.

Postrenal failure: Bilateral obstruction to the collecting system above the bladder, and any obstruction below the bladder, results in an increase in pressure inside the kidney. As with prerenal failure, rapid correction of the cause will result in a return of full function. Long standing obstruction or incomplete removal of the obstruction can be associated with permanent loss of function.

Postrenal failure is classification as:

• Internal obstruction	- renal calculus (bilateral unless there is a single kidney), - urethral valves.
• External obstruction	- prostatomegaly, cervical cancer
• Disease within the wall of the collecting system	- bladder tumour

2.2 The management of established renal failure

Basic nursing care

Many patients, especially those not requiring renal replacement therapy, can be managed outside the critical care environment, preferably in a dedicated nephrology area. Nursing care includes an accurate fluid balance chart, daily weight, and daily review of fluid and nutritional status. Serum biochemistry should be examined at least daily in the initial stages, and regular assessment should be undertaken to exclude sepsis.

Note that undetected volume expansion can occur in patients with negative nitrogen balance because covert weight loss can be camouflaged by fluid gain. Hyponatraemia often indicates fluid excess, and salt intake should be curtailed, because sodium intake, especially that added during or after cooking, causes thirst and can lead to excess fluid intake.

Hyperkalaemia

As the GFR falls, serum potassium begins to rise. Patients with ARF will not tolerate the high serum potassium levels that are often seen in patients with CRF. Dietary potassium should be restricted, and oral or rectal polystyrene exchange resins, either calcium or sodium, are often required.

Signs of increased serum potassium are evident when levels rise above 5 mmol/litre (Saunders and Bircher 1998, p 109) and commence with peaking of the T wave. Myocardial excitability may be evident in the form of arrhythmias, and cardiac arrest becomes increasingly likely as the serum potassium increases.

Hypokalaemia can also occur but is much less likely in ARF. Patients with biochemical indicators of either hypokalaemia or hyperkalaemia should have continuous ECG monitoring.

Volume expansion

Fluid overload is most likely in patients with oliguria and tends to be confined to the extracellular compartment. This occurs because there is a corresponding inability to excrete sodium, and intracellular water is drawn into the extracellular compartment to re-establish normal serum osmolality. Most of this extracellular fluid accumulates in the intra-vascular space where the increase in circulating blood volume results in an elevated blood pressure in both central and peripheral blood vessels. As the hydrostatic pressure increases fluid is forced into the interstitial space where it contributes to peripheral oedema, pulmonary oedema and cardiac problems.

If renal failure is due to a cause where significant protein loss occurs, fluid may leak from the vascular space into the interstitial space. In this case the oedema occurs as a result of lowered oncotic pressure, rather than an increase in capillary hydrostatic pressure. Important nursing interventions include protection of the skin to maintain integrity. Oedematous tissue receives less oxygen and is at increased risk of breakdown and infection (Saunders and Bircher 1998, p 109).

Metabolic acidosis

The mechanisms that lead to metabolic acidosis are the same as those that occur in CRF. Treatment includes the use of oral sodium bicarbonate and the restriction of protein. If the acidosis is severe, buffers can be provided in the form of an intravenous sodium bicarbonate infusion, or dialysis. When mixed acid/base disturbances are present, e.g. with coexisting pulmonary disease, the patient is at increased risk of acidaemia because the normal pulmonary compensation mechanisms are compromised.

Renal replacement therapy

The development of the uraemic syndrome in ARF indicates the need for some form of renal replacement therapy. Signs that conservative management is no longer sufficient include persistent increase in serum levels for urea and creatinine, gastrointestinal (GIT) problems such as nausea and vomiting, wound infection, neurological symptoms such as changed mentation, irritability, and muscular twitching, and bleeding as a result of depleted clotting factors. As a general guide, renal replacement therapy is indicated when fluid overload is present, uraemic symptoms and hyperkalaemia are uncontrolled, or when the addition of fluids, such as the need for parenteral nutrition or blood transfusion, threatens volume status.

Peritoneal dialysis can be used as a renal replacement therapy in ARF providing that the patient is not oliguric, has a low catabolic rate, and was in reasonable health prior to the current illness. These requirements limit the usefulness of peritoneal dialysis as a treatment, but it is still used in some centres, especially to treat very young children, or when other forms of therapy are not available.

Intermittent haemodialysis, conducted for short periods on a daily basis, is suitable for patients with kidney failure alone, who are managed in the renal unit. It is also suitable for some patients in the intensive care unit (ICU), however these patients, especially those with multiorgan failure, are increasingly being managed by what are known as slow continuous renal replacement therapies (SCRRT). These therapies are examined in a later Chapter.

There are several SCRRTs. They are extracorporeal therapies that have the advantage of removing water and solute as it is gained i.e. continuously, and they do not expose the patient to the peak and trough effects seen with intermittent haemodialysis. Although peritoneal dialysis is also a slow continuous process, it is seldom used with ARF because it is often unsuited to the needs of the unstable ICU patient who is often hypercatabolic.

There are now numerous studies (Cheung 1990, Schulman et al. 1991, Hakim et al. 1994, Gasparovic et al. 1994) demonstrating the negative effect that cellulosic dialyser membranes have on several cascade systems in the body. The same studies demonstrate that the activation of these cascade systems retards recovery from ARF, and that the use of biocompatible membranes promotes tubular healing and recovery. Biocompatible synthetic membranes are now the preferred choice in patients undergoing extracorporeal renal replacement therapy for ARF.

Pharmacological treatment of acute renal failure

Diuretics: In post ischaemic ARF, diuretics such mannitol or frusemide can be given if oliguria persists, and after the circulating volume has been restored. Diuretics may also serve to protect tubular function by 'diverting energy from tubular transport to cellular metabolism, or by inhibiting tubuloglomerular feedback' (Dawborn 1986, p 1314). The use of diuretics in ACR remains controversial and has been disputed by some researchers.

Low dose dopamine: Dopamine stimulates alpha, beta and dopaminergic receptors depending on the serum concentration of the drug. Also known as 'renal dose dopamine', low dose dopamine is used to promote renal blood flow by selectively dilating renal and mesenteric vasculature. Its use is also controversial, primarily because of the possibility of cardiotoxicity. If a trial of low dose dopamine is considered to be appropriate, the results should be assessed within six hours, and the drug should be discontinued if urine output has not increased during this time (Vijayan and Miller 1998, p 527).

Antihypotensive agents: Vasoactive agents may be necessary to establish and maintain a blood pressure that is sufficient to perfuse the kidneys and to establish urine production. The appropriate blood pressure differs according to the patient's age and previous medical history (Dawborn 1986, p 1313).

Calcium channel blockers: Papadimitriou et al. (1998, p 653–654) wrote that calcium channel blockers such as verapamil play an important role in protecting the tubule from damage. The known and postulated mechanisms for tubular protection include:

- decreasing renal hypertrophy

- reducing metabolic activity in tubular cells

- ameliorating nephrocalcinosis

- reducing calcium entry into tubular cells

- decreasing free radical formation.

(Papadimitriou et al. 1998 p 653–654).

Drugs under investigation

Atrial natriuretic factor (ANF): ANF is a peptide hormone synthesised by cells in the cardiac atria. It is secreted in response to increased levels of serum sodium and promotes both natriuresis and diuresis. These processes occur when vasoconstriction of the efferent arteriole and vasodilation of the afferent arteriole are sufficient to increase glomerular filtration pressure and establish urine production.

Growth factors: Studies have shown that growth factors play an important role in the regeneration of both proximal tubular cells and cells of the medullary thick ascending limb of the loop of Henle. Their major role appears to be in the recovery of renal function following ischaemic damage (Vijayan and Miller 1998, p 527).

Endothelin antagonists: Animal studies, and a single study examining the role of endothelin antagonists in patients with chronic renal failure, (Gellai et al., 1995) indicate a possible prophylactic role for the use of this drug. Conclusive studies are yet to be published.

Nutrition

Patients with ARF secondary to damage caused by ischaemia or nephrotoxins usually retain GIT function and some urinary output. Recovery of renal function can be expected over a fairly short period, usually days to weeks. Patients with secondary ARF can usually be managed with enteral feeding and dietary restrictions. Protein may be restricted to between 20 and 30 gm/day (HBV) (Butler 1991, p 247) but only for a short period. The nutritional deficiencies that occur with severe protein restriction are associated with an increased rate of infection, delayed wound healing, and loss of muscle strength. Nutritional deficiencies contribute to the high mortality of patients with ARF and many of the dietary restrictions used in the past have been abandoned (Saunders and Bircher 1998).

Hypercatabolic renal failure, which is often the result of trauma, is characterised by oliguria and a nonfunctional GIT. These patients usually require parenteral nutrition and renal replacement therapy for the removal of nitrogenous waste that accumulates when nutritional requirements are met. In hypercatabolic states associated with renal failure, the fall in GFR is sudden and there is little time for adaptive mechanisms to occur and fluid and electrolyte abnormalities are often dramatic.

In ARF, protein degradation, gluconeogenesis, and amino acid release from cells are all increased, while protein synthesis and amino acid uptake by muscle tissue are decreased. High levels of insulin antagonistic hormones are present, resulting in carbohydrate intolerance and high levels of circulating insulin. Approximately 50% of patients with no previous diagnosis of diabetes require exogenous insulin Patients with pre-existing diabetes often require insulin dose to be reduced as a result of decreased insulin degradation by the kidney. Hyperlipidaemia, secondary to insulin resistance and impaired lipolytic activity is often present.

Critically ill patients have an increased demand for both calories and protein that results from inadequate use of available nutrients. Protein requirements are increased and may exceed 2 g/kg/day Protein intake *should not* be restricted to prevent or delay dialysis in the critically ill.

Providing adequate nutrition is one of the primary indications for dialysis. Extreme protein restriction (20 g/day), or the use of enteral solutions with low protein and amino acid content should only be used in patients who are not catabolic, and in whom renal function is expected to return in a few days.

Haemodialysis itself can contribute to protein catabolism and the loss of water soluble vitamins. Tissue catabolism is often the result of associated illness; therefore the decision to dialyse may depend on the amount of nutritional support that is required, not the severity of the renal lesion.

2.3 The changing clinical course

Progress from initial insult to recovery

People with ARF usually progress through four well-defined phases, if recovery is to occur. Traditionally these are described as the onset phase, the oliguric (or anuric) phase, the polyuric phase and the recovery phase. Nursing care will vary depending on the phase of the patient's recovery. Saunders and Bircher (1998) describe these phases as follows:

The onset phase: This phase lasts from the time of the initial insult to the kidneys until the occurrence of either oliguria or anuria. The duration varies depending on the cause of the renal failure. As discussed earlier, an examination of the urinary concentrating ability will provide a guide to the resumption of function in ARF due to prerenal causes. The presence of urinary sediment, and the type of sediment that is found, may provide a guide to the cause of renal failure that is due to intrinsic disorders.

The oliguric phase: This phase may last up to six weeks. As a general rule, the more protracted this phase is, the poorer the outcome is likely to be. Oliguria refers to a urinary output of < 400ml/day, and anuria refers to an output < 100ml/day. On an average western diet a person produces a metabolic solute load of approximately 600 mOsmol. The kidneys *must* produce at least 400mls of urine per day if the metabolic load is to be excreted. Thus the term 'oliguria' alerts the nurse to the fact that the patient cannot satisfactorily excrete their metabolites and that they will be retained within the body. The degree to which this occurs corresponds with residual glomerular and tubular function, and the level of dietary restriction that can be enforced to decrease the amount of solute that is generated. Remember that catabolic patients will generate a high level of waste product as a result of tissue breakdown, and that dietary restriction will be of limited value and possibly detrimental.

Just to confuse the picture, reduced urine output is not required for the diagnosis of ARF. Even though patients may have a normal, or even increased, urinary output, the ability of the kidney to concentrate urine can still be impaired, and solute excretion is impaired as a result. The normal kidney filters approximately 180 litres of water/day, but between 98% and 99% is reabsorbed. The benefit of this high filtration rate is that metabolic waste can be removed effectively. The downside is that many of the solutes that are needed are filtered along with waste products, and they must be reabsorbed (with most of the water), and there is little room for error. So, even though a patient has lost most of their renal function, they may still be able to filter a small amount of body water, and may appear to have an adequate urinary output. The trouble is, that very little of the daily generation of solute is present in this urine and serum levels will rise. Fluid restriction will not usually be required with nonoliguric ARF but replacement may be.

The diuretic phase: Usually commences over a relatively short period and lasts for several days. Some writers (Crandall 1989, p 49) subdivide the diuretic phase into two subphases:

1. The 'early' diuretic phase that commences when urine output exceeds 400ml/day and ceases when serum urea and creatinine stop rising.

2. The 'late' diuretic phase that commences when the urea and creatinine stop rising, and ceases when they return to near normal.

Crandall 1989 is an old reference, but has been included because her work is still relevant and is clear and easy to follow.

The basic rule of '500 ml plus the previous day's output' should be observed during this period because quite marked fluctuation in the urine output can occur. Rapid increases in urine output require altering the intake on a more frequent basis.

The recovery phase: After several days of diuresis, and a continued fall in serum urea and creatinine, the recovery phase commences. The length of time it takes relates to the length of the diuretic phase and individual metabolic states. Some authors extend the end of this phase up to when the patient can resume normal activities of daily living, which can be up to twelve months in some patients. Approximately 50% of patients who recover are left with residual renal impairment, and eventually decline towards chronic renal failure.

Causes of death: For those who do not recover, infection, often complicating progressive system failure, is the cause of death in over 50% of cases. The next two most common causes are those due to cardiac and pulmonary disorders, and a small number are caused by central nervous system disease, dialysis complications, 'technical mishap', digitalis intoxication and hyperkalaemia (Kjellstrand and Teehan 1996, p 828).

References

In text references

Butler, B., 1991, 'Nutritional management of catabolic acute renal failure requiring renal replacement therapy', *ANNA Journal*, vol. 18, no. 3, pp 247–259.

Cheung, A., 1990, 'Biocompatibility of hemodialysis membranes', *J Am Soc Nephrol* , vol.1, pp 150–161.

Crandall, B., 1989, 'Chronic renal failure', in *Nephrology Nursing: concepts and strategies*, Ulrich, B., (ed.), Appleton and Lange, California.

Dawborn, J., 1986, 'Acute renal failure', *Medicine International*, pp 1309–1316.

Gasparovic, V., Dakovic, K, Gasparovic, H., Merkler, M, Radonic, R., Ivanovic, D., Pisl, Z., Jelic, I., 1994, 'Do biocompatible membranes make a difference in the treatment of acute renal failure?', *Dialysis and Transplantation*, vol. 27, no. 10, October, pp 621–626, 674.

Gellai, M., Jungus, M., Fletcher, T., Ohlstein, E., Elliott, J., Brooks, D., 1995, Nonpeptide endothelin receptor antagonists, *Journal Pharmacological Experimental Therapy*, October, vol. 275, no. 1, pp 200–206.

Hakim, R., Tolkiff-Ruben, N., Himmelfarb, J., Wingard, R., Parker, R., 1994, 'A multicentre comparison of bio-incompatible and bio-compatible membranes in the treatment of acute renal failure', *J Am Soc Nephrol*, vol 5, pp 394–398.

Kjellstrand, C., Teehan, B., 1996, 'Acute Renal Failure', in *Replacement of Renal Function by Dialysis*, Jacobs, C., Kjellstrand, C., Koch, K., (eds.), 4th ed., Kluwer Academic Publishers.

Mehta, R., 1996, 'Modalities of dialysis for acute renal failure', *Seminars in Dialysis*, vol. 9, no. 6, November, pp 469–475.

Myers, B., 1996, 'Pathogenic processes in human acute renal failure', *Seminars in Dialysis*, vol. 9, no. 6, pp 444–453.

Neale, T., 1986, 'Management of Acute renal failure', *Practical Therapeutics*, pp 18–34.

Papadimitriou, M., Papagianni, A., Diamantopoulou, D., Mitsopolous, E., Belechri, A.' Koukoudis, P., Memmos, D., 1998, 'Acute renal failure-which treatment modality is the best?' *Renal Failure*, vol. 20, no. 5, pp 653–661.

Racusen, L., 1997, 'Pathology of acute renal failure: structure/function correlations' *Advances in renal replacement therapy*, vol. 4, no. 2, Suppl. 1, April, pp 3–16.

Rodriguez, D., Lewis, S., 1997, 'Nutritional management of patients with acute renal failure', *ANNA Journal*, vol. 24. no. 7, April, pp 232–241.

Saunders, P., Bircher, G., 1998, 'Acute renal failure', in *Renal Nursing*, in Smith, T., (ed.), 2nd ed., Bailliere Tindall, Sydney.

Schulman, G., Fogo, A., Badr, K., Hakim, R., 1991, 'Complement activation retards resolution of acute ischemic renal failure in the rat', *Kidney International*, vol. 40, pp 1069–1074.

Vijayan, A., Miller, S., 1998, 'Acute renal failure: prevention and nondialytic therapy', *Seminars in Nephrology*, vol. 18, no. 5, September, pp 523–532.

Recommended reading

Mehta, R., 1996, 'Modalities of dialysis for acute renal failure', *Seminars in Dialysis*, vol. 9, no. 6, November, pp 469–475.

Rodriguez, D., Lewis, S., 1997, 'Nutritional management of patients with acute renal failure', *ANNA Journal*, vol. 24. no. 7, April, pp 232–241.

Sutton, T., Molitoris, B., 1998, 'Mechanisms of cellular injury in ischemic acute renal failure, *Seminars in Nephrology*, vol. 18, no. 5, September, pp 490–497.

Vijayan, A., Miller, S., 1998, 'Acute renal failure: prevention and nondialytic therapy', *Seminars in Nephrology*, vol. 18, no. 5, September, pp 523–532.

Renal Osteodystrophy

Introduction

Bone disease was recognised as one of the major complications of renal failure shortly after the introduction of haemodialysis as a treatment for end stage renal disease. It is considered by some to be an unavoidable sequelae to treatment, and is apparent to some degree in all patients with end stage renal disease and many with chronic renal failure.

Osteodystrophy and its complications are an important cause of morbidity and occasionally mortality in patients with renal disease. The prevention of bone disease and the management of symptoms are among the most important goals of treatment and offer many challenges to nurses involved with the care of patients with renal disease.

3.1   The minerals and hormones involved

A fine balance

As mentioned in Chapter 1, the relationship between important vitamins, minerals and hormones becomes progressively disrupted as renal failure advances. The major players in relation to bone are calcium, phosphate, parathyroid hormone (PTH) and vitamin D_3.

Calcium: Calcium is absorbed from the GIT, stored in bone and excreted via the kidney. Approximately 99% of calcium is stored as the inorganic calcium/phosphate structure of bone. The remainder is found in plasma where approximately 40% is bound to protein and 50% is ionised. It is this ionised portion that participates in chemical reactions. Calcium is freely filtered at glomerular level and between 98% and 99% is reabsorbed in the renal tubule. When serum ionised calcium falls, the re*absorption* of calcium in the tubule increases, calcium *absorption* in the GIT is increased and re*sorption* from bone occurs (Smith 1991 p 130–144).

You will recall that protein malnutrition is not uncommon in renal patients. Malnutrition can lower the serum albumin level, decreasing the portion of calcium that is 'protein-bound' and can impact on the availability of medications that have a portion of the drug bound to protein.

Phosphate: HBV protein is the major source of phosphate, and is found in the extracellular fluid in both organic and inorganic forms. In its organic form it is protein-bound (phospholipid). Inorganically, it exists as either monohydrogen or dihydrogen phosphate. With a pH of 7.4 the ratio of monohydrogen to dihydrogen phosphate is 80% to 20% (Keyes 1990, p160). Phosphate is freely filtered at glomerular level and, while reabsorption from the tubule occurs as a regulatory mechanism as it does with calcium. Larger amounts of phosphate are required in the urinary filtrate if it is to function as a urinary buffer.

Vitamin D: Vitamin D is formed by the action of ultraviolet light on the skin, or ingested in the diet as cholecalciferol. It is hydroxylated to the 25 position in the liver, and to the active form on the 1,25 position by the action of the enzyme 1alpha hydroxylase, produced by the kidney. The active form of vitamin D is called 1,25 dihydroxy cholecalciferol, is usually abbreviated to 1,25 $(OH)_2D_3$.

1,25 $(OH)_2D_3$ is responsible for regulating the absorption of calcium and phosphate from the GIT. If serum levels are low, absorption increases, if they are high, absorption decreases. It also mediates the tubular reabsorption of calcium and the re-sorption of calcium from bone (Smith 1991 p 130–144). Low levels of 1,25 $(OH)_2$ D_3 can stimulate the release of parathyroid hormone (PTH) in the presence of normal serum calcium (Brunier 1994, p174).

Parathyroid hormone: The parathyroid glands secrete parathormone, more commonly known as parathyroid hormone or PTH. Secretion is increased by a low serum calcium level and decreased by an elevated level. Alterations in serum phosphate effect the release of PTH in a similar manner. PTH also mediates the release of calcium from bone in the presence of 1,25 $(OH)_2D_3$, decreases tubular reabsorption of phosphate and increases tubular reabsorption of calcium. The major effect of PTH is on bone while the major effect of 1,25 $(OH)_2D_3$ is on the GIT (Smith 1991 p 130–144).

When the balance is disturbed

As renal disease progresses and filtration starts to fall, serum phosphate levels increase. The retained phosphate complexes with calcium, causing ionised serum calcium levels to fall. The regulatory mechanisms are activated to increase serum calcium levels, but they encounter the following problems:

1. Calcium absorption from the GIT cannot be increased because renal hydroxylation of vitamin D to the 1,25 position is compromised because the enzyme responsible is not being produced.

2. Calcium reabsorption from the tubule cannot increase because of nephron loss. For the same reason, phosphate excretion cannot be increased.

The only available source of calcium is bone. Calcium resorption from bone results in a temporary increase in serum levels, but retained phosphate soon complexes with the newly available calcium, and the cycle starts again.

The aims of therapy are to supplement vitamin D in its active form, facilitating calcium absorption from the GIT. To achieve this aim calcium supplementation may be necessary. Phosphate-binding medication may be required to limit phosphate absorption. Since oral calcium can be used as a phosphate-binder, *or* a calcium supplement, it is important to determine the way calcium is given. Calcium given to bind phosphate should be given *with* food, whereas calcium designed as a mineral supplement should be given *between* meals.

3.2 Classification and management of bone disease

Osteitis fibrosa

Also known as hyperparathyroid bone disease, osteitis fibrosa is classified as a 'high turnover' bone disease that is the result of secondary hyperparathyroidism. The activity of both osteoblasts and osteoclasts increase, resulting in increased bone turnover (Brunier 1994, p174), however the activity of osteoclasts exceeds that of osteoblasts, resulting in progressive bone resorption. Uncontrolled disease results in the formation of eroded cyst like areas known as lacunae, and fibrosis of bone marrow.

The initial stimulation of the parathyroid glands causes relatively uniform hypertrophy that is usually considered a normal response. If the condition continues unchecked, one of the glands develops into an adenoma and commences autonomous and unregulated secretion of PTH, a condition known as tertiary hyperparathyroidism. Brunier (1994, p174) reports that children, young adults and women appear to have the greatest risk of developing high turnover bone disease, indicating that hormones other than PTH may play a role.

Signs and symptoms of osteitis fibrosa include low serum calcium and elevated serum phosphate, normal to slightly elevated alkaline phosphatase and elevated levels of PTH. Patients complain of muscle weakness, usually involving the shoulder muscles, and bone pain that is often worse at night and difficult to localise. Severe itching may be present and is due to the elevated levels of phosphate and subsequent deposition in the skin. If tertiary hyperparathyroidism occurs, serum calcium, phosphate, alkaline phosphatase and PTH levels all become markedly elevated.

Radiological findings include subperiosteal erosion, predominantly of the clavicles and the tips of the distal phalanges, and cortical defects of the skull known as pepper pot skull, and femur (Brown's tumour). Cancellous bone that lies beneath cortical bone can be subjected to sclerosis, especially of the vertebral bodies, the so called rugger jersey spine, where areas of bone resorption are in sharp contrast to areas of bone deposition, giving a striped appearance on X-ray.

Management involves the normalisation of serum phosphate and calcium, already discussed. Intravenous vitamin D_3 and low calcium dialysate combined with oral calcium are suggested alternatives (Moriniere et al. 1993, p 121). Other authors suggest using intermittent high doses of vitamin D_3 (Dahl and Foote1997). Long haemodialysis, daily haemodialysis, and aluminium- and calcium-free binding agents have been recommended to control serum phosphate levels (Norris 1998 p550–555). Parathyroidectomy is required for tertiary disease, and may be indicated for severe or refractory secondary disease.

Osteomalacia

Osteomalacia is one of two 'low turnover' diseases and is characterised by a decrease in osteoblast and osteoclast activity resulting in decreased bone turnover, and an increased osteoid, the organic matrix of bone that has not undergone calcification. The incidence of osteomalacia is declining in the renal population as a result of better control of vitamin D_3 and subsequent incorporation of calcium into bone (Catterson 1997).

Signs and symptoms of osteomalacia include low to normal serum calcium, elevated serum phosphate, and elevated PTH. Bones are soft and fracture easily. Fractures usually occur in the ribs and femoral neck. Bone pain and muscle pain are present as with high turnover disease.

Lack of the active form of vitamin D_3 results in failure to absorb sufficient calcium from the GIT, as a result there is not enough calcium available for normal bone mineralisation. Children are especially vulnerable to this type of bone disease where abnormal bone formation results in bowed legs, spinal and chest deformities and generalised body tenderness.

Adynamic bone disease

Adynamic osteodystrophy is the second of the two low turnover bone diseases. Osteodystrophy was first noted in the 1980's and has only recently been recognised as differing from osteomalacia. It is characterised by similar changes to the bone matrix but without the accompanying increase in osteoid. Adynamic bone disease is increasing in prevalence in patients undergoing dialysis, especially peritoneal dialysis (Catterson 1997). The condition is usually asymptomatic, and hypercalcaemia is the most frequent laboratory finding. It is thought to be due to suppression of the parathyroid gland even though serum levels are normal to slightly raised (Coburn et al. 1997, p181). The apparent anomaly can be explained by the fact that normal bone turnover in renal patients requires a PTH level of up to three times normal.

Treatment includes the use of low calcium dialysate, limiting the use of calcium as a phosphate-binding agent, and ceasing oral vitamin D_3 supplementation.

Aluminium bone disease

Sources of aluminium include the oral administration of aluminium-based phosphate-binders, intravenous administration of substances such as albumin and hyperalimentation fluid, exposure to untreated water, and the oral administration of food or medicines that increase aluminium absorption. For example, fruit juice and effervescent preparations.

Most of the problems associated with aluminium absorption have been resolved by using treated water for dialysate preparations and replacing aluminium salts with salts of either calcium or magnesium for phosphate-binding. However, aluminium bone disease, complicating primarily the low turnover diseases, is still occasionally seen.

Signs of aluminium toxicity include cerebral changes, microcytic anaemia and osteomalacia and should be suspected in any patient who exhibits changed mentation, microcytic anaemia or has osteomalacia that does not respond to the administration of vitamin D_3. Diagnosis is suspected when serum aluminium levels are elevated, and confirmed with bone biopsy after tetracycline tagging, which is also known as bone labelling. This procedure is also used to differentiate between the various types of bone disease. When aluminium toxicity is present it can be seen on the biopsy specimen.

Treatment involves the administration of the chelating agent desferrioxamine (DFO). Although aluminium is a small molecule, it is tightly bound to protein and therefore not available for removal during routine dialysis. DFO is usually administered during the latter half of dialysis and is small enough for removal via the dialyser membrane. It breaks the aluminium-protein bond and forms a complex with aluminium. This new DFO-aluminium complex is available for removal during the next dialysis. DFO also binds with iron, and iron deficiency is possible in patients being treated for aluminium toxicity.

Summary:

Remember that few, if any, renal patients suffer from one type of osteodystrophy exclusively. With the exception of aluminium bone disease, most show signs and symptoms of both high and low turnover disease; they have what is described as 'mixed bone disease'.

The price of normal serum calcium, phosphate and vitamin D_3 levels has been described as persistent hyperparathyroidism and eventual bone disease (Catterson 1997). The key to minimising the problem is early intervention, education about the use of phosphate binders and vitamin D_3, and parathyroidectomy where indicated. While this is easier said than done, renal nurses play a vital role in patient education, and monitoring serum biochemistry.

3.3 Complications

The dangers of poor control

The major signs of inadequate control of serum calcium and phosphate, and the symptoms associated with the various types of osteodystrophy have already been addressed, however there are some severe and potentially fatal complications that are worthy of separate discussion.

Metastatic calcification: The deposition of calcium and phosphate into peripheral blood vessels (vascular calcification), eyes (ocular calcification), and periarticular tissue (periarticular calcification) occurs in chronic renal failure, and often persists once dialysis has commenced. The deposits appear as nodules in the above tissues, and are due to sustained levels of the calcium/phosphate product (Catterson 1997). Central deposits in the viscera, especially the heart and lungs, occur less frequently, but are associated with higher morbidity and mortality than deposits in peripheral tissue (Lundin 1989, p 1135). The term 'tumoral calcinosis' is sometimes used to refer to the deposition of the calcium/phosphate product in tissues where it can be palpated as distinct nodules under the skin. Tumoral calcinosis is not a disease entity in itself, but an extension of the metastatic calcification that occurs when calcium/phosphate control is inadequate.

Calciphylaxis: This is a rare but serious complication of an elevated calcium/phosphate product, where there is progressive calcification of small and medium sized subcutaneous arteries resulting in ischaemia and necrosis of the skin. It is often precipitated by a specific event such as irritation or direct trauma, and progresses to nonhealing ischaemic ulcers that break down and become infected. Plaque like subcutaneous nodules, and any purplish discolouration of the skin, especially of the lower limbs, should be investigated. Treatment is by rigorous control of calcium and phosphate via the use of low calcium dialysate, cessation of calcium binders, urgent parathyroidectomy (where indicated) and the use of biphosphonates (Catterson 1997). Surgical debridement of wounds, with skin grafting if indicated, and specific antibiotic therapy should be included (Scurrah et al. 1997). Treatment with hyperbaric oxygen has been beneficial in some cases (Scurrah et al. 1997) but while patients with peripheral lesions tend to recover, central lesions are still associated with a high mortality (Catterson 1997).

Mucormycosis: Also known as Zygomycosis, this is a rare and potentially fatal fungal infection that is associated with immunosuppression (Deschamps-Latscha et al. 1999, p 272) and chronic debilitating illnesses (Anderson 1994, p 1686). The condition starts with fever and pain, and often commences in paranasal tissues where it is associated with nasal discharge. It spreads to the eyes and lower respiratory tract, and may infiltrate the brain and other organs (Anderson 1994, p 1686). The organism usually enters the body via inhalation, but may also follow direct inoculation after a puncture wound. There has been one reported case of the infection following renal biopsy (Dahl & Foote 1997 p 554). Treatment includes extensive debridement of craniofacial tissue and antifungal agents. In renal patients, the infection occurs in relation to a combination of chronic illness and immunosuppression and has been reported as a specific, but very rare, complication that accompanies the use of DFO (Vlasveld and van Asbeck 1991).

3.4 Associated disorders

Amyloidosis

Although not a bone disease as such, the retention of Beta 2 microglobulin, a substance normally eliminated by the kidney, and the formation and deposition of amyloid is included in this chapter for convenience as it is often associated with the bone disease experienced by people with renal disease.

Beta 2 microglobulin (B_2M) is a subunit of the Class 1 Human Leucocyte Antigen. In people with intact renal function, the daily production between 150–200 mg, is almost entirely removed by the kidney (Davison 1995, p93). With a molecular weight of 11 800 daltons, B_2M is too large for removal by standard cellulosic dialysers. As glomerular filtration rate falls serum levels of B_2M start to rise. The formation of amyloid occurs when the B_2M polymerises to form fibrils, but the precise mechanism is unclear.

It is uncommon for symptoms to occur before the fifth year of dialysis treatment and by fifteen years, over 50% of patients display some symptoms (Davison 1995, p94). Amyloid deposits occur in various locations, resulting in carpal tunnel syndrome, shoulder pain, effusive arthritis and bone cysts that can become quite large and cause pathological fractures. Deposits also occur in the skin, liver, spleen, rectal mucosa and blood vessels (Catterson 1997).

It was initially thought that amyloid formation was due to exposure to the haemodialysis membrane, but as B_2M deposits are now known to occur in predialysis patients, and patients who used peritoneal dialysis as their renal replacement therapy, it is now thought that the condition may be related to uraemia and not dialysis.

Definitive diagnosis is obtained from a biopsy, but ultrasonography and magnetic resonance imaging are also used. Surgical treatment, for example, for carpal tunnel syndrome, is effective in many cases, but the use of either haemofiltration, haemodiafiltration, or dialysers with a synthetic membrane, and the corresponding increase in sieving coefficient, are the only effective way of reducing plasma levels of B_2M. Transplantation usually results in the reversal of symptoms (Davison 1995, p 97).

Upper extremity problems

As with amyloidosis, a review of the upper extremity problems associated with dialysis are included in this chapter for convenience.

Wilson (1998, p149) writes that of the upper extremity problems that are associated with haemodialysis, hand dysfunction is amongst the most troublesome. The problems described by Wilson, an occupational therapist, include disturbances of joint structure and function, including osteodystrophy; tendon rupture and bursitis; nerve compression syndromes, including carpal tunnel syndrome and peripheral neuropathy resulting from ischaemia, and oedema with venous occlusion proximal to the site of vascular access construction.

Wilson suggests that nurses should be alert to signs that include swelling and weakness of the hand, numbness or tingling in the fingers, clumsiness with dropping objects or being unable to pick up small objects, finger stiffness and loss of finger movement. Nursing assessment includes measurement of hand oedema, determining grip and pinch strength, measurement of cutaneous sensitivity and hand dexterity.

References

In text references

Anderson, K., 1994, *Mosby's Dictionary,* Mosby, Sydney.

Brunier, G., 1994, 'Calcium/Phosphate imbalances, aluminum toxicity, and renal osteodystrophy', *ANNA Journal,* 1994, vol. 21, no. 4, June, pp171–178.

Catterson, R., 1997, Consultant Nephrologist, Royal North Shore Hospital, Sydney, Australia. Paper presented at Nurse Educators Study Day, sponsored Janssen-Cilag Pty. Ltd.

Coburn, J., Goodman, W., Salusky, I., 1997, 'Renal bone disease and aluminium toxicity in renal patients', in *Caring for the renal patient,* Levine, D., (ed.), 3rd ed., Saunders, Sydney.

Dahl, N., Foote, E., 1997, 'Pulse dose oral calcitriol therapy for renal osteodystrophy: literature review and practice recommendations', *ANNA Journal,* vol.24, no. 5, October, pp 550–555.

Davison, A., 1995, 'Amyloidosis in patients with end stage renal failure: uraemia associated or dialysis related?, in *Dialysis membranes: structure and predictions',* Bonomoni, V., Berland, Y., (eds.), Karger, Sydney.

Deschamps-Latscha, B., Witko-Sarsat, V., Jungers, P., 1999, 'Infection and immunity in end stage renal disease', in *Principles and Practice of Dialysis,* Henrich, W., (ed.), 2nd ed., Williams and Wilkins, Maryland.

Keyes, J., 1990, *Fluid, Electrolyte, and Acid base Regulation,* Jones and Bartlett, Boston.

Lundin, A., 1989 'Prolonged survival on haemodialysis', in *Replacement of Renal Function by Dialysis,* Maher, J., (ed.), 3rd ed., Kluwer, Boston.

Moriniere, Ph., El Esper, N., Viron, B., Bourgeon, J., Farquet, Ch., Gheerbrant, J., Chaput, M., Van Orshoven, A., Pamphile, R., Fournier, A., 1993, 'Improvement of severe secondary hyperparathyroidism in dialysis patients by intravenous vitamin D_3, oral $CaCO_3$, and low calcium dialysate', *Kidney International,* vol.42, S41, pp121–s124.

Norris, K., 1998, 'Toward a new treatment paradigm for hyperphosphatemia in chronic renal failure', *Dialysis and Transplantation,* vol. 27, no. 12, December, pp 767–772.

Scurrah, L., Miach, P., Dawborn, K., 1997, 'Calciphylaxis', Poster presentation for Research Week at the Austin & Repatriation Medical Centre, Melbourne, Victoria.

Smith, E., 1991, *Fluids and Electrolytes; A Conceptual Approach*, 2nd ed., Churchill Livingstone, New York.

Vlasveld, L., van Asbeck, B., 1991, 'Treatment with desferrioxamine: a real risk factor for mucormycosis', *Nephron*, vol. 57, pp 487–488.

Wilson, G.1998, 'Upper extremity complications in haemodialysis patients: recommendations and a review of the literature', *Dialysis and Transplantation*, vol. 27, no. 3, pp145–149, 153.

Recommended Reading

Brunier, G., 1994, 'Calcium/phosphate imbalances, aluminium toxicity, and renal osteodystrophy', *ANNA Journal*, vol. 21, no. 4, pp171–177.

Headley, C., 1998, 'Hungry bone syndrome following parathyroidectomy', *ANNA Journal*, vol. 25, no. 3, June pp 283–289.

Selected disease processes

Introduction

There are many diseases that can result in end stage renal failure. For the purposes of this chapter, the major syndromes causing renal failure will be discussed, as will some of the more frequently encountered diseases that are recorded as 'miscellaneous' in the ANZDATA registry. The bulk of the chapter will be devoted to the principal causes of end stage renal failure, as identified in Chapter 1 of this section. Not all the causes of end stage renal failure are addressed in this chapter, and the reader is encouraged to explore them as they encounter them in clinical practice.

4.1 Glomerular disease

Pathogenesis of glomerular disease

Possibly the easiest way to learn the pathophysiology of glomerular diseases is to think in terms of inflammation of the glomerular tuft, as evidenced by one or more of the following:

- Cellular proliferation where there is an increase in endothelial, epithelial and/or mesangial cells.

- Infiltration by polymorphonuclear or mononuclear leukocytes.

- The presence of complement and/or immunoglobulin, resulting in thickening of the basement membrane.

- Sclerosis, where the deposition of cellular debris causes hardening and the eventual destruction of the glomerular tuft.

(Meldrum 1998, p 133).

The majority of cases of glomerulonephritis are thought to be the result of immunological-mediated inflammation (Holdsworth & Atkins 1994, p 119). Mediators such as complement and coagulation promote the inflammatory response factors, while the immunological mediators are immunoglobulin, and, to a lesser extent, sensitised 'T' cells. The immunological response may be via either:

1. **Immune complex disease:** This accounts for the vast majority of cases, and occurs when circulating immune complexes become trapped within one or more of the three components of the glomerular filtration barrier. Antigens can be exogenous as with post streptococcal glomerulonephritis, correctly referred to as 'diffuse endocapillary proliferative glomerulonephritis,' or endogenous (but extra renal) as occurs with the autoimmune disease, systemic lupus erythematosus (SLE). Occasionally solid tissue and lymphoid tumours act as endogenous extra-renal antigens.

2. **Basement membrane disease:** where the glomerular basement membrane is mistakenly recognised as 'antigenic' and becomes the target of antibody production e.g. Goodpastures Syndrome. This syndrome is also an autoimmune disease, but the antibody-antigen complexes are formed in situ, as opposed to the entrapment seen in immune complex disease.

These two disease processes can be distinguished with immunofluorescence. Because immune complex disease results in the irregular deposition of immune complexes at random as they become trapped. Immunofluorescence reveals an irregular or lumpy pattern around the basement membrane. Basement membrane disease occurs because the entire basement membrane becomes antigenic and antibody attraction is uniform, resulting in a smooth and regular immunofluorescence around the entire basement membrane.

A third group of disorders often associated with glomerulonephritis was recently identified, and involves the presence of antineutrophil cytoplasmic antibodies (ANCA). The disorders are the forms of vasculitis associated with glomerulonephritis (Holdsworth and Atkins 1994, p 122), idiopathic crescentic glomerulonephritis and alveolar capillaritis (Wiseman 1993, p 18).

Many types of glomerulonephritis are of unknown aetiology, and various terms are used to describe them. The terms are often used in combination, when referring to lesions.

1. Diffuse lesions refer to damage that is apparent in the majority of glomeruli (over 80%).

2. Focal lesions refer to damage apparent in some (usually less than 80%) of the glomeruli.

3. Global lesions refer to lesions that affect the entire glomerulus.

4. Segmental lesions only affect a portion of each glomerulus.

5. Proliferative lesions where an increase in cellular nuclei can be seen (usually greater than 100), indicating cellular proliferation.

(Meldrum 1998, p133, Thomas 2000).

Thus, a glomerulonephritis classified as 'diffuse endocapillary proliferative glomerulonephritis' means that 80% of the glomeruli are involved, with changes observed in the endothelial cells, and with evidence of cellular proliferation is shown in figure 1.4.1.

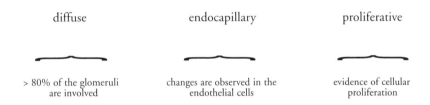

diffuse	endocapillary	proliferative
> 80% of the glomeruli are involved	changes are observed in the endothelial cells	evidence of cellular proliferation

Figure 1.4.1: Changes observed in glomerulonephritis (Terrill 1999).

Similarly, 'focal segmental glomerulonephritis' means that only a portion of each of the < 80% of glomeruli involved are affected. If you cannot remember the various classifications for glomerulonephritis, a difficult task for most of us, try to remember these definitions. They can help to resolve a multitude of problems!

Classification of glomerulonephritis

Remember that glomerulonephritis is the primary cause of end stage renal failure in Australia, and it is a frequent cause of acute renal failure. Gloerulonephritis is typically classed as either primary (where the disease process commences in the glomerulus) or secondary (where the glomerulonephritis results from systemic disease).

Primary glomerulonephritis: There are many ways of classifying this type of glomerulonephritis, but it is probably best to select one that uses the terms common among current nephrology texts, and used in this chapter. A complete review of each classification is beyond the scope of this text, and comprehensive reviews can be found in most nephrology texts.

Secondary glomerulonephritis: There are many systemic diseases that result in damage to the glomerulus. They include SLE, polyarteritis nodosa, Wegener's granulomatosis, progressive systemic sclerosis (Racussen 1998, p 603); anaphylactoid purpura and mixed essential cryoglobulinaemia (Cattran 1997, p 27). Most of these diseases are autoimmune, and are frequently seen in patients in nephrology wards and renal out patient clinics.

Syndromes associated with glomerulonephritis

An overview of clinical presentation of the syndromes associated with glomerulonephritis follows. Drug therapy will be mentioned later in this section. The use of renal biopsy to classify the type of disease process will be discussed in Chapter 6.

The Nephritic syndrome: This syndrome is associated with four primary features:

1. oliguria (due to glomerular damage and filtration failure)

2. haematuria (macroscopic or microscopic, and also due to glomerular damage)

3. oedema (particularly periorbital, and due to fluid retention)

4. hypertension (also due to fluid retention).

(Thompson and Charlesworth 1994, p 134).

The nephritic syndrome develops over a period of days to weeks and is often considered the most serious of the syndromes associated with glomerulonephritis (Cattran 1997, p 19).

The nephrotic syndrome: Proteinuria is the single cause of the nephrotic syndrome. To be classified as the nephrotic syndrome, urinary protein loss must exceed 3g/day (Thompson and Charlesworth 1994, p 132). The associated features of hypoproteinaemia, oedema, and lipidaemia are the result of protein loss. The nephrotic syndrome is not a disease in itself, but describes the manifestations that result from other renal diseases. Altered immunological responses are the result of immunoglobulin loss (particularly IgG), and place some patients at significant risk of infection.

Protein loss occurs when damage to the glomerular basement membrane causes an initial increase in permeability to small molecular weight proteins. As the disease progresses, permeability to larger proteins becomes a feature (Meldrum 1998, p138). While it is important that patients receive sufficient dietary protein to enable hepatic synthesis of albumen, it is not usual to increase protein intake above normal because it often increases urinary protein loss. Coggins (1997, p 17) suggested a protein intake of 0·8 g/kg/IBW and an additional 1 gram for each gram of proteinuria.

Goodpastures syndrome: This syndrome classically consists of interstitial lung disease with pulmonary haemorrhage, anaemia and glomerulonephritis. The discovery of antiglomerular basement membrane antibodies and antineutrophil cytoplasmic antibodies (ANCA), together with reliable detection methods, make it possible to detect and treat Goodpastures syndrome early. In the past, many people with Goodpastures syndrome suffered a fatal pulmonary haemorrhage, or developed renal failure that progressed to end stage.

Although rare, Goodpastures syndrome might occur even less frequently than was originally thought, because many patients with conditions that involved alveolar haemorrhage and glomerulonephritis were probably misdiagnosed. For a positive diagnosis the clinical presentation needs to be accompanied by antibasement membrane antibodies in blood, or in pulmonary or renal tissue (Wiseman 1993, p 17).

The differential diagnosis includes immune complex diseases such as Systemic Lupus Erythematosus (SLE), Henoch-Schonlein Purpura and Berger's disease, and the various forms of vasculitis such Wegener's Granulomatosis and Polyarteritis Nodosa.

Thin basement membrane disease: is also referred to as 'benign recurrent haematuria', 'benign familial haematuria' and 'recurrent haematuric syndrome'. It is characterised by thinning of the basement membrane and persistent microscopic haematuria. The disease is not commonly associated with renal impairment, and accounts for between 20 and 30% of people presenting with microscopic haematuria. Macroscopic haematuria and proteinuria are rare, but are occasionally observed (Thompson and Charlesworth 1994, p 139).

Evaluation and management

The following outlines the clinical evaluation and medical management of glomerulonephritis and provides a guide that can be applied to all glomerular disease processes. The nursing management is the same as that discussed in Chapter 2.

Table 1.4.1: Clinical evaluation and treatment of glomerulonephritis

General:	What is the age and gender of the patient? *
Aetiology:	Has there been a recent illness? **
Clinical:	Is the presentation classically nephritic or nephrotic (or is it a mixture of both)? ***
Laboratory:	What tests have been ordered and what do they show?

- What does the midstream urine reveal?

- Does the serum biochemistry or haematology show anything abnormal?

- Can serum antibodies be demonstrated? (As occurs with SLE).

- What is the blood glucose level? (Does the patient have diabetes?).

- Has urinary protein loss been estimated? If so, how much is due to glomerular damage (as with glomerular disease) and how much is tubular (as with interstitial disease).

- What does the renal biopsy reveal? Has the analysis included electron microscopy and immunofluorescence as well as light microscopy ****.

Treatment:	Implement appropriate *non drug* therapy (refer to Chapter 2)
	Are there any reversible factors? (Refer to Chapter 1)
	Implement appropriate drug therapy → steroids, nonsteroids, cytotoxic, anticoagulant, antiplatelet
	Is renal replacement therapy required? If so, what type?
Prognosis:	What is known about the prognosis and progression of the disease? Is there a need for advice about life style modification?
Follow up:	Any person who has had any renal disease should be followed up *for life*. This includes measurements as simple as a blood pressure check and a urinary 'dip stick' *whenever* the person attends a medical clinic (even if it is just for a 'flu shot' or advice about an ingrowing toenail) (Thomas 2000).

*   Some diseases occur primarily in certain age groups (e.g. minimal change glomerulonephritis).

**   Some occur primarily in a particular gender (e.g. SLE).

***   The pure nephritic syndrome is associated with post streptococcal glomerulonephritis while the pure nephrotic syndrome (especially in childhood) is associated with minimal change glomerulonephritis.

There are several glomerular lesions that are only identifiable after analysis of the biopsy specimen, and that are associated with specific disease process:

- Minimal change glomerulonephritis is associated with 'foot process fusion', where the podocytes are described as 'a smear along the basement membrane', which is most common in very young children.

- Membranous glomerulonephritis is associated with 'spiking' of the basement membrane, where the normally identifiable foot processes appear to be replaced by sharp spikes.

- Diffuse endocapillary glomerulonephritis (post streptococcal glomerulonephritis) is associated with 'humps' on the basement membrane that follow approximately two weeks after a streptococcal infection such as a 'strep throat' or impetigo).

- Mesangiocapillary glomerulonephritis is associated with what is described as 'tram tracking', where the basement membrane appears to be 'split'. This occurs as mesangial tissue pushes up between the basement membrane, splitting the tissue. This is a particularly aggressive form of the disease, usually with a 'mixed' nephritic/nephrotic presentation, and has a poor prognosis (Thomas 2000).

4.2 Interstitial and tubular disease

Interstitial nephritis

Acute interstitial nephritis: This term describes the pathology associated with an inflammatory response within the renal tubules and interstitium. It is a common condition, associated with a variety of infections and a number of drugs, and is a frequent cause of acute renal failure. Histological examination reveals interstitial oedema and infiltration by a mixture of lymphocytes, macrophages and infrequently, plasma cells. The glomeruli and blood vessels are essentially normal. The principal causes of interstitial nephritis are:

1. Drugs, especially methicillin. Others include penicillin, ampicillin, rifampicin, phenindione, sulphonamides, co-trimoxazole, thiazides and phenytoin.

2. Infection, either systemic or intrarenal. Organisms involved are bacteria, spirochetes, viruses, protozoa and rickettsia.

3. Immune related diseases such as Sjögren's syndrome.

4. Some cases of interstitial nephritis are idiopathic and are diagnosed by excluding all other causes.

The clinical presentation varies widely from an acute hypersensitivity reaction with renal failure, to an asymptomatic increase in creatinine and abnormal urinary sediment, with no evidence of a compromise in renal function. Diagnosis is made following renal biopsy, and any drugs that have been implicated as a cause of interstitial nephritis should be withdrawn. Most patients make a complete recovery but renal impairment may persist in a minority of cases. Steroids may shorten the course of the disease, but are not always used (Lynn and Robson 1994, p 215).

Chronic interstitial nephritis: There are multiple causes of chronic interstitial nephritis associated with interstitial fibrosis, the presence of chronic inflammatory cells and tubular atrophy. Disease progression varies with the causative agent, and follows the course of chronic renal failure described in Chapter 1. The most frequently encountered diseases known to cause chronic interstitial nephritis include:

1. Glomerulonephritis.

2. Drugs such as nonsteroidal anti-inflammatory agents and lithium.

3. Heavy metals such as mercury and lead.

4. Reflux nephropathy.

5. Malignancy such as myeloma and leukaemia.

6. Metabolic disorders such as gout, hyperoxaluria and hypercalcaemia

7. Infections such as leprosy, syphilis and tuberculosis

(Adapted from Lynn and Robson 1994, p 217).

As specified in the introduction to this chapter, those diseases listed by the

ANZDATA Registry (1999) as the principal causes of end stage renal failure will be the focus of discussion. For further information refer to specialised nephrology texts, or to the books noted as reference material at the end of the chapter.

Diabetic nephropathy

Diabetic nephropathy has been a steadily increasing cause of renal disease in Australia over the past decade. It is now the second largest cause of end stage renal failure, with 350 new patients, 22% of total new presentation, commencing treatment during 1998. Type 2 diabetics now out number type 1, with the number of non insulin requiring type 2 diabetics outnumbering those who require insulin.

The term 'diabetic nephropathy' is used to describe the renal lesions that occur in patients with diabetes mellitus. Proteinuria is usually apparent 10 years after diagnosis, and used to be considered the hallmark of diabetic renal disease. It is now recognised that protein loss actually commences much earlier and in a form not detected by Albustix (Jerums et al. 1994, p265). Early protein loss, or 'microalbuminuria' can be detected using Micral-test strips or twelve- or twenty-four hour urine collections. Persistent microalbuminuria is now considered the early phase of diabetic renal disease. There is evidence to suggest that excellent control of blood glucose levels and blood pressure reduce both the development of renal lesions, and slow their progression if they already present (Jerums et al. 1994, p 265).

Diabetic kidney lesions include:

1. Pyelonephritis, often the result of autonomic neuropathy that affects bladder function and accelerates the rate of disease progression.

2. Diffuse intercapillary glomerulosclerosis, causing damage to the basement membrane and mesangial proliferation.

3. Nodular glomerulosclerosis (Kimmelsteil Wilson nodules), which occurs as glomerular tissue is replaced by deposits of glycoprotein.

4. Arteriosclerosis, as hyaline deposits obliterate glomerular capillaries.

5. Papillary necrosis.

(Meldrum 1998, p 153).

Blood glucose control: As renal function declines, there is an increase in the end organ resistance to the effects of insulin. This does not result in an increased need for insulin or oral hypoglycaemic agents. Because the kidney is the final elimination pathway for insulin and oral hypoglycaemic agents, circulating drug levels actually rise because the half-life, $(t^1/2)$ is prolonged. Insulin doses may actually need to be reduced and patients on oral agents swapped to insulin to reduce the likelihood of hypoglycaemia.

Cystic Kidney Disease

Cystic disease makes up approximately 14% of all renal diseases (Douek and Bennett 1994, p 279). The major disease groups are:

1. Polycystic kidney disease (PKD)

    i)   Autosomal dominant PKD

    ii) Autosomal recessive PKD

2. Renal medullary cysts

    i)   Medullary cystic disease

    ii) Medullary sponge kidney

3. Acquired renal cystic disease

4. Cysts occurring in hereditary syndromes

    i)   von Hippel-Lindau disease

    ii) Tuberous sclerosis

5. Simple renal cysts

(Douek and Bennett 1994, p 279).

Polycystic kidney disease: The autosomal dominant form of this disease is often referred to as 'adult' polycystic disease because, although the cysts are present at birth, the disease usually becomes clinically apparent once adulthood is reached. The disease expression is variable, some patients develop end stage renal failure as young adults, but it mostly occurs in the mid to late 40's. Each child of a parent with polycystic kidney disease has a 50% chance of developing the disease, but the severity is not necessarily the same as that of the parent.

Three subtypes of the disease have been identified. Type 1 has the most aggressive course, and accounts for more than 90% of total presentations, with patients requiring dialysis early in the course of the disease. The gene responsible is located on the short arm of chromosome 16. The gene responsible for type 2 is located on the long arm of chromosome 4 and accounts for up to 10% of presentations. The third genotype, type 3, has yet to be assigned a genomic locus (McMullen 1997, p 46).

Renal function declines as cyst formation replaces normal renal tissue. Nocturia is common as tubular reabsorptive capacity decreases, bleeding into cysts causes haematuria that is often accompanied by loin or flank pain, and hypertension occurs as cysts expand. Cystic tissue often remains capable of producing erythropoietin, and many patients with polycystic disease condition will have acceptable haemoglobin levels. The tubular dysfunction that is an early presenting feature means that many patients continue to pass large amounts of urine, even after dialysis commences. Remember that oral fluid requirements are '500 ml plus the previous days output', and do not allow patients to become dehydrated. Adequate hydration is especially important prior to the development of end stage renal failure when dehydration can accelerate the progress of renal disease.

Cysts are common in areas other than the kidney, such as the central nervous system, ovaries, liver and heart and when bleeding occurs into the cysts the signs and symptoms correspond with disruption of the function of the organ concerned. The disease accounted for 115 (7%) of the total 1708 new patients commencing dialysis in Australia during 1999 (ANZDATA 2000).

Autosomal recessive polycystic kidney disease is a rare disease that usually presents in infancy. There is often associated hepatic fibrosis and pulmonary hypoplasia. If oligohydramnios is present secondary to limited urine output in utero, the infants usually succumb early due to renal failure or respiratory distress. Most infants who survive the first month of life usually do not develop chronic renal failure until late childhood or adolescence, where they may present with hepatic fibrosis or the bleeding complications that are associated with portal hypertension.

Because polycystic kidney disease affects the renal tubules, difficulties occur with the concentration and acidification of urine, and care needs to be taken when intercurrent illness or disease progression increases water loss and causes dehydration (Douek and Bennett 1994, p 285).

Renal medullary cysts: Medullary sponge kidney is a common disease that involves dilation of the collecting ducts in the medulla. It is a developmental disorder that is usually asymptomatic unless secondary complications, such as urinary tract infection or renal calculi, occur. Prognosis is excellent. Patients should be advised about the need to treat renal calculi and infection promptly to limit the possibility of long term renal disease.

Medullary cystic kidney disease does not have the same happy outcome. Most cases are diagnosed in childhood or adolescence, with multiple cysts and rapid progression to end stage renal failure. A similar condition is called 'juvenile nephrolithiasis' and presents in older children. It is an autosomal dominant condition, whereas medullary cystic kidney is autosomal recessive. Both diseases can occur sporadically (Douek and Bennett 1994, p 288).

Acquired renal cysts: Acquired cystic kidney disease occurs in dialysis-dependent patients who have not undergone bilateral nephrectomy. These cysts have the propensity to undergo malignant change, and should be suspected in any patients who have an unexplained increase in haemoglobin levels, as an increase in erythropoietin production occurs as renal tissue enlarges.

Reflux nephropathy

Reflux nephropathy occupies 6th place as a contributor to end stage renal failure programs in Australia (ANZDATA 1999). Reflux nephropathy is a congenital disorder where incompetence of the sphincter at the vesicoureteric junction allows the 'reflux' of urine upward towards the renal pelvis instead of downward towards the urinary bladder, as occurs during normal micturition (Meldrum 1998, p 129). If urinary tract infection is present because of the reduced length of the urethra and its proximity to the bowel), bacteria have the opportunity to access, and invade, renal tissue when this 'upward diversion' occurs. Urinary tract infection is more common in girls than boys.

Where the reflux is minimal and asymptomatic, improvement can occur to the point where renal function is never compromised. However, in severe, usually bilateral disease, repeated urinary tract infection results in scarring and contraction of areas of the kidney as the infected areas heal. Progression towards chronic renal failure is relentless as increasing amounts of renal tissue is destroyed. Presentation at chronic renal failure programs usually occurs as adulthood is approached. Early identification of severe reflux, and corrective surgery during childhood can dramatically alter the natural progression of the disease.

Hypertension

Hypertension is now the third highest contributor to end stage renal failure programs with 182 (12%) new presentations out of 1708 patients commencing treatment in 1999 (ANZDATA 2000). As mentioned in Chapter 1, hypertension can be the result of salt and water retention (as with filtration failure) or inappropriate activation of the renin-angiotensin-aldosterone system. When renal artery stenosis is present, the juxtaglomerular apparatus perceives the resulting decrease in blood flow to the kidney as hypovolaemia. The secretion of renin is followed by the conversion of angiotensin 1 to angiotensin 11, resulting in vasoconstriction and the secretion of aldosterone, resulting in an increase in the reabsorption of sodium and water from the distal convoluted tubule. The resulting (and relentless) attempt to restore 'blood volume' results in extracellular volume expansion, with hypertension and possible oedema. Figure 1.4.2 depicts the angiotensin cascade.

As community awareness of the importance of blood pressure control increases, it is hoped that hypertension will cease to be a major cause of renal impairment.

Renin (from juxtaglomerular apparatus) ↓	Angiotensin converting enzyme (from pulmonary capillaries) ↓	
Angiotensin → (from liver)	Angiotensin 1 →	Angiotensin 11 (vasoconstriction)
↑ Water reabsorption (from renal tubule) ←	↑ Sodium reabsorption (from renal tubule)	↑ Aldosterone secretion ←
Vasoconstriction plus volume expansion	→	HYPERTENSION

Figure 1.4.2: Angiotensin cascade

Analgesic nephropathy

The association between analgesic consumption and chronic renal failure first became apparent in the 1950's when it appeared that the regular consumption of preparations containing phenacetin was responsible for renal lesions associated with renal failure. Despite substantial opposition from the pharmaceutical companies involved, preparations containing phenacetin were withdrawn from sale in nonpharmaceutical outlets in most countries, and became available as prescription items only. While this curbed the development of the 'analgesic abuse syndrome', it did not eradicate it, and it is now generally accepted that any nonsteroidal anti-inflammatory drug that is taken in sufficient quantities, can cause renal failure (Buckalew 1994, p 192–193).

In the early 1980's analgesic nephropathy was responsible for 20% of new patients entering dialysis programs, second only to glomerulonephritis as the major cause. It was considered that most of these patients had sustained their considerable renal damage in the years prior to phenacetin being withdrawn from sale. The 1999 ANZDATA shows this number progressively decreasing and analgesic nephropathy now accounts for only 6% of new presentations.

The principal lesions found in analgesic nephropathy are renal papillary necrosis and tubulointerstitial nephritis. Renal manifestations include haematuria and colic which are due to the passage of sloughed papillae, repeated urinary tract infection, and an increased risk for the development of transitional cell carcinoma of the collecting system (Becker et al. 1992, p 282–283). Hypertension may be present, but hypotension and dehydration due to salt and water loss is more common (remember, this is a medullary lesion and renal concentrating ability will be compromised).

Nonrenal manifestations include the known side effects of nonsteroidal anti-inflammatory drugs (NSAID), such as gastrointestinal bleeding and ulceration. It is common for other addictions, such as cigarette smoking to be present. Accelerated atheromatous disease and premature aging occur, but the aetiology for this is not well understood (Becker et al. 1992, p 282–283).

Renal tubular disorders

All forms of renal disease affect the tubules to a greater or lesser extent, but some affect the renal tubules first and the glomerulus second, or not at all. The majority of renal tubular disorders are determined genetically, but some forms, especially those caused by drugs, are described with increasing frequency (Györy 1994, p 265). A brief summary of these diseases, as discussed by Györy is shown. Other authors are acknowledged as they are cited.

1. Specific isolated disorders of tubular transport

i) Carbohydrate

Glycosuria: Primarily an autosomal recessive condition characterised by glycosuria, and a normal to only slightly elevated blood glucose level. An autosomal dominant form is occasionally seen. No treatment is required.

ii) Amino acids

Hartnup's disease: Characterised by 'neutral amino aciduria, with a pellagra like skin rash, cerebellar ataxia, mental retardation, and the 'blue diaper' syndrome in infants' (p 266). The condition improves with age, and is treated is with nicotinamide and a high protein diet. Mono amine-oxidase (MAO) inhibitors should be avoided, as should exposure to sunlight while taking nicotinamide.

Cystinuria: This rare condition results in excess secretion of cystine, ornithine, arginine and lysine (COAL), and the formation of cystine crystals and renal calculi. It is more common in males, and is usually diagnosed between the first and fourth decade. The clinical course is that of renal stone disease, and general treatment is directed towards the preservation of renal function by preventing infection and secondary renal obstruction. Specific treatment involves the alkalinisation of urine and increasing urinary excretion between 2 and 4 litres/day, promoting dilution and a low specific gravity. Penicillamine might be required to decrease cystine excretion, and is replaced by tiopronin if side effects to penicillamine occur.

iii) Electrolytes

Renal tubular acidosis (RTA): There are three types of renal tubular acidosis. Proximal RTA, where the proximal tubule is unable to secrete sufficient hydrogen ion to reclaim all the bicarbonate that has been filtered, distal RTA, where the distal tubule is unable to secrete sufficient hydrogen ions to reduce the urinary pH to the accepted level of ~ 5.2, and hyperkalaemic, hypoammonuric RTA, where it is thought that the tubule is unable to respond to aldosterone, retarding tubular secretion of hydrogen. The features common to all three are a systemic metabolic acidosis, and persistently alkaline urine. Treatment is aimed at correcting the metabolic acidosis.

Bartter's syndrome: Characterised by hypokalaemia, systemic metabolic alkalosis, normotension and an increase in the secretion of both aldosterone and renin. Growth retardation may be seen in children. Signs and symptoms occur as a result of potassium depletion. Life long potassium supplementation is required. Aldosterone antagonists and drugs that interfere with renal prostaglandin synthesis are also be used.

Vitamin D-resistant rickets: This disorder is the result of a defect in phosphate reabsorption in the proximal tubule, and phosphate absorption in the jejunum, resulting in growth retardation. Treatment is with high dose vitamin D and phosphate supplementation.

iv) Water

Nephrogenic diabetes insipidus: In this condition, the distal tubule and collecting duct are unable to respond to either exogenous or endogenous antidiuretic hormone (ADH), resulting in polyuria, polydipsia, and elevated serum sodium levels. The condition 'may be hereditary, idiopathic, drug induced or due to a variety of renal and other disorder' (p 273). Treatment involves removing the causative agent if the condition is drug-induced, and adequate water intake, often up to four litres/day, for other causes. Sodium intake should be restricted.

Water retention: or nephrogenic diabetes insipidus, usually presents with a combination of hyponatraemia and central nervous system manifestations that occur as a result of the hyponatraemia. Since a basic defect in renal sensitivity to endogenous ADH is not known, most cases of water retention are due to drug therapy. Such drugs include vasopressin, oxytocin, cyclophosphamide, paracetamol, indomethacin, and the sulphonylureas.

2. Metabolic disorders with complex disorders of tubular function

The Fanconi syndromes: This is a group of disorders that may be either inherited or acquired, and that feature multiple abnormalities of proximal tubular function. In many instances, Franconi syndromes are due to the intracellular deposition, or accumulation, of abnormal amounts of metabolic substances. In the inherited form, clinical presentation is usually during childhood, and is characterised by 'renal tubular acidosis and hypokalaemia, muscle weakness, paralysis, nausea, vomiting, dehydration and failure to thrive'. In both adults and children, signs and symptoms of osteomalacia can be present. Prognosis is variable, and usually depends on the underlying condition.

Inherited disorders with symptomatology that includes the Fanconi syndromes are:

i) Cystinosis, also known as 'cystine storage disease', is an autosomal recessive disorder characterised by the intracellular accumulation of cystine crystals in multiple organs, including the kidney, cornea, brain, pancreas, conjunctiva, bone marrow, liver and spleen. Rapid progress to end stage renal failure occurs if the diagnosis occurs during childhood, or if the initial appearance of signs and symptoms can be traced back to childhood (Györy 1994, p 277). Disease progression can be slowed if effective treatment with cystamine, an analogue of cysteine, or with phosphocysteamine, is commenced during infancy. Once end stage renal disease has occurred, dialysis or transplantation is required for survival. The disorder does not re-occur in the transplanted kidney, however cystine accumulation in other organs continues, often with significant morbidity (Brodehl 1998). If diagnosis does not occur until adulthood, the prognosis is usually more favourable.

ii) Wilson's disease, also an autosomal recessive disorder, occurs due to the accumulation of copper within the renal cortex as well as other organs. Treatment is with the copper chelating agent penicillamine.

iii) Galactosaemia occurs when a deficiency of the enzyme galactose–1–phosphate uridyltransferaze' results in the accumulation of galactose–1–phosphate within the cells. Presentation includes the development of cataracts, hepatosplenomegaly and aminoaciduria. Young children may also present with failure to thrive and diarrhoea. Avoiding foods that contain galactose such as lactose, a simple sugar found in milk, usually successfully treats this autosomal recessive disorder.

iv) Hereditary fructose intolerance is a disorder that presents with proximal RTA and occasionally urolithiasis. It is due to a deficiency in aldolase activity in the renal cortex and the liver, resulting in a cellular accumulation of fructose–1–phosphate and phosphate depletion. Treatment consists of avoiding foods containing fructose.

v) Oxalosis, which may be primary (inherited) or secondary (acquired). The primary form is usually due to an autosomal recessive disorder, although some patients display a dominant form of the disease. Oxalosis is a disorder of oxalate-glyoxylate metabolism that results in increased levels of oxalate in the blood that usually causes urolithiasis and nephrocalcinosis. Calcium oxalate crystals are deposited in a variety of tissues, including the renal tubules, and diagnosis with progress towards end stage renal failure is usually made between the ages of two and ten years. Treatment is largely unsatisfactory, and dialysis is needed for survival once end stage has been reached. Transplantation is an option but the disease recurs in the transplanted kidney although several years free of dialysis can be expected, making this an acceptable treatment option for some nephrologists and their patients.

Acquired forms of the Fanconi syndrome can result from multiple myeloma, amyloidosis, Sjögren's syndrome the nephrotic syndrome, renal transplantation, and vitamin D deficiency (Györy 1994, p 276).

Drug-induced forms include the use of outdated tetracycline, 6-mercaptopurine, methyl-5-chrome, lead, cadmium, mercury, and gentamycin (Györy 1994, p 276).

4.3 Pregnancy and renal disease

Alterations to structure and function

Many normal changes occur in the kidneys of pregnant women.

1. The upper urinary tract dilates as a result of hormonal changes designed to promote muscle relaxation, and obstruction at the pelvic brim caused by the gravid uterus. This results in a degree of urinary stasis and increases the likelihood of urinary tract infection.

2. It is important to remember that the glomerular filtration rate almost doubles and creatinine levels fall. This means existing renal disease might not be recognised if the creatinine level is compared to usual values.

3. Peripheral vasodilatation results in a fall in blood pressure to about 10mmHg below the mother's normal level.

4. The kidneys increase in length by about 1 cm.

5. Sodium retention (between 500 and 900 mmol) occurs. Most of this is sequestered to the products of conception and contributes to the overall fluid gain of 6 to 8 litres.

6. Urinary anomalies, including glycosuria, lactosuria and the appearance of amino acids in the urine are common.

(Becker et al. 1992, 349).

7. Orthostatic proteinuria occurs due to forward rotation of the liver, which compresses the inferior vena cava, and to uterine pressure on the left renal vein, which increases filtration pressure.

Complications

1. Asymptomatic urinary tract infection is probably the most common complication, and occurs in up to 7% of pregnancies. The 30–35% risk of developing acute pyelonephritis dictates that all women with bacteriuria should be treated.

2. Hypertension can be divided into three categories:

    a) Essential hypertension, often not previously diagnosed.

    b) Secondary hypertension, as the result of renal or renovascular disease (adrenal and ovarian causes are also seen).

    c) Pre-eclampsia.

3. Acute renal failure, most commonly seen in the third trimester, is usually the result of pre-eclampsia, antepartum haemorrhage or acute pyelonephritis. Idiopathic postpartum renal failure is a rare cause and is one of the haemolytic uraemic syndrome spectrums of diseases associated with a particularly poor outcome. Another rare cause is the so-called fatty liver of pregnancy'.

4. Chronic renal failure used to be considered a contraindication to pregnancy, and while many women with renal failure experience a decrease in renal function as the result of pregnancy, many are managed successfully. The type of glomerulonephritis, the time of diagnosis in relation to the pregnancy, and

the presence of features such as hypertension impact on the outcome of the pregnancy and maternal morbidity (Gallery and Brown 1994, 404–407).

Dialysis and pregnancy: The two groups of women who receive dialysis are those who conceive while on dialysis because of pre-existing end stage disease, and those who require dialysis because of a decline in renal function as a result of the pregnancy.

References

In text references

ANZDATA Registry Report, 1999, 'Australia and New Zealand Dialysis and Transplant Registry, Adelaide, South Australia.

Becker, G., Whitworth, J., Kincaid-Smith, P., 1992, *Clinical Nephrology in Medical Practice,* Blackwell Scientific, Melbourne.

Brodehl, J., 1998, 'Cystinosis', in *Oxford Textbook of Clinical Nephrology*, Davidson, A., Stewart Cameron, J., Grunfeld, J., Kerr, D., Ritz E., Winearls, C., (eds.), Oxford Press, Oxford.

Buckalew, V., 1994, 'Analgesic abuse nephropathy', in *Primer on Kidney Disease*, Greensberg, A., (ed.), National Kidney Foundation, Academic Press, Sydney.

Cattran, D., 1997, 'Acute nephritic syndrome', in *Caring for the renal patient*, Levine, D (ed.), 3rd ed., Saunders, Sydney.

Coggins, C., 1997, 'Hematuria, proteinuria and nephrotic syndrome', in *Caring for the renal patient*, Levine, D (ed.), 3rd ed., Saunders, Sydney.

Douek, K., Bennett, W., 1994, 'Cystic renal diseases' in *Textbook of Renal Disease*, Whitworth, J., Lawrence, J., (eds.), 2nd ed., Churchill Livingstone, Melbourne.

Gallery, E. Brown, M., 1994, 'The kidney in pregnancy', in *Textbook of Renal Disease*, Whitworth, J., Lawrence, J., (eds.), 2nd ed., Churchill Livingstone, Melbourne.

Gyory, A., 1994, 'Renal tubular disorders', in *Textbook of Renal Disease*, Whitworth, J., Lawrence, J., (eds.), 2nd ed., Churchill Livingstone, Melbourne.

Holdsworth, S., Atkins, R., 1994, 'Pathogenesis of glomerulonephritis', in *Textbook of Renal Disease*, Whitworth, J., Lawrence, J., (eds.), 2nd ed., Churchill Livingstone, Melbourne.

Jerums, G., Cooper, M., Gilbert, R., O'Brien, R., Taft, J., 1994, 'Microalbuminuria in diabetes', *The Medical Journal of Australia*, vol.161, August, pp 265–268.

Lynn, K., Robson, R., 1994, 'Interstitial nephritis – acute and chronic', in *Textbook of Renal Disease*, Whitworth, J., Lawrence, J., (eds.), 2nd ed., Churchill Livingston, Melbourne.

McMullen, M., 1997, 'Autosomal dominant polycystic disease: pathophysiology and treatment', *ANNA Journal*, vol. 24, no. 1, February, pp 45–51.

Meldrum, E., 1998, 'Chronic renal failure' in *Renal Nursing*, Smith, T., (ed.), 2nd ed., Bailliere Tindall, Sydney.

Racusen, L., 1998, 'Autoimmune disease in the kidney', in *The Autoimmune Diseases,* Rose, N., Mackay, I., (eds.), 3rd ed. Academic Press, Sydney.

Thomas, G., 2000, Consultant nephrologist, 'lecture notes provided for 4th and 6th year medical students', Royal Melbourne Hospital, Victoria.

Thompson, N., Charlesworth, J., 1994, 'Classification, pathology and clinical features of glomerulonephritis', in *Textbook of Renal Disease*, Whitworth, J., Lawrence, J., (eds.), 2nd ed., Churchill Livingstone, Melbourne.

Wiseman, K., 1993, 'New insights on Goodpastures Syndrome', *ANNA Journal*, vol. 20, no. 1, pp 17–24.

Recommended reading

Headley, C., Wall, B., 1999, 'Acquired cystic kidney disease', *ANNA Journal,* vol. 26, no. 4, August, pp 381–387.

Hou, S., 1999, Pregnancy in chronic renal insufficiency and end stage renal disease, *NF* (Journal of the National Kidney Foundation), pp 1–24.

Kelly, J., 1996, 'Management of diabetes with renal involvement', *Current Therapeutics,* August, pp 45–50.

Racusen, L., 1998, 'Autoimmune disease in the kidney', in *The Autoimmune Diseases,* Rose, N., Mackay, I., (eds.), 3rd ed. Academic Press, Sydney.

Spilman, P., Whelton, A., 1992, 'Non steroidal anti-inflammatory drugs: effects on kidney function and implications for nursing care, *ANNA Journal*, vol. 19, no. 1, pp 19–25.

Wiseman, K., 1991, 'Nephrotic syndrome: pathophysiology and treatment', *ANNA Journal*, vol. 18, no. 5, pp 469–476,504.

Wiseman, K., 1993, 'New insights on Goodpastures Syndrome', *ANNA Journal*, vol. 20, no. 1, pp 17–24.

Pharmacology

Introduction

The elimination of many drugs is either partially or completely dependent on renal excretion. The therapeutic or toxic effect of drug therapy is related to the amount of free drug available. Therefore, drugs that rely on renal excretion for the elimination of either the whole drug, or its metabolites, require modification of either the dose, or the dose interval, if they are to be beneficial in the treatment of patients with compromised renal function. Although it is not suggested that renal nurses should memorise all of the drug modifications that are required, they should have a sound understanding of the reasons why drug modification might be necessary. They should also know how to access the necessary information to ensure that modification is undertaken as recommended.

5.1 Why are alterations to drug dosage necessary?

Pharmacokinetics

Pharmacokinetics is the study of the way drugs react when administered to the body (Anderson 1994, p1205). It includes the mechanisms of absorption and elimination, the commencement and duration of action, and the possible unwanted effects of administration.

Drugs, or their active metabolites, which rely on intact renal function for elimination, require adjustment when administered to people with renal failure (Swan and Bennett 1997, p 139). The dose adjustments are not based solely on the decrease in renal function. Other factors include:

1. The rate of absorption that will be affected by vomiting due to uraemia, sluggish gut mobility and delayed gastric emptying as occurs with diabetic autonomic neuropathy.

2. The degree of protein-binding that determines the amount of free drug available for therapeutic action.

3. The volume of distribution (V_d), which determines the compartmental distribution of a drug.

As defined by Golper et al. (1996, p 750) bioavailability refers to 'the fraction of an administered drug that reaches the systemic circulation'. Two processes determine drug availability:

1. The liberation of the drug from the form in which it is administered.

2. The systemic absorption of the drug.

Drug efficacy 'is determined by both the rate and quantity of drug input into the body' (Golper et al. 1996, p 751), which, in turn, determines the duration and the intensity of the effect of the drug on the body. Bioavailability is usually determined by estimating the 'peak' plasma level after a given dose (Golper et. al. 1996, p 751). Absorption reflects the characteristics of the membrane that the drug must cross prior to achieving its therapeutic effect.

Since the majority of drugs are administered orally, bioavailability reflects the state of the gastrointestinal system, which is affected by many factors including:

1. Drug dose.

2. Membrane permeability.

3. Absorption, surface area, and time of drug 'contact' with the cell wall.

4. Local pH.

5. Local irritant effect of drugs such as nonsteroidal anti-inflammatory drugs (NSAIDs).

6. Pancreatic exocrine dysfunction.

(Golper et al. 1996, p 751).

There is minimal interference when drugs are administered by alternate routes. By definition, the absolute bioavailability of a drug administered intravenously is 100% (Birkitt 1991, p 15). Local oedema is the major impediment to the absorption drugs administered intra muscularly (Golper et al. 1996, p 751).

Some drugs that undergo hepatic metabolism are subjected to substantial hepatic extraction after oral administration (Golper et. al. 1996, p 751). Known as 'first pass extraction', this only applies to drugs that have a 'high hepatic extraction' and becomes relevant when patients with renal failure develop liver impairment.

Volume of distribution

Following administration, drugs disperse throughout the body at a given rate. The volume of distribution (V_d) can be calculated by 'dividing the amount of the drug in the body by its plasma concentration' (Aronoff et. al. 1999, p126). This figure represents the amount of a drug that must be given to achieve a therapeutic plasma concentration, and does not correspond directly to the fluid volume of any body compartment. Drugs that are water soluble tend to be restricted to the extracellular compartment, while those that are highly protein-bound tend to remain in the plasma compartment where the majority of plasma proteins are found. Lipid soluble drugs are most likely to penetrate a number of organs and tissues, and will have the largest V_d.

Renal failure alters the V_d of drugs in a number of ways:

1. Fluid volume expansion can increase the V_d of drugs that are water soluble, resulting in low plasma levels. Similarly, dehydration may decrease V_d and result in high plasma levels.

2. Protein malnutrition results in a reduction in the number of binding sites available to protein-bound drugs. This is especially so for acidic drugs and increases the amount of free drug in the blood. The V_d, as well as the quantity of available free drug, and the degree of hepatic and renal excretion, are all influenced by the degree of protein-binding (Aronoff et. al. 1999, p127).

Since it is the unbound portion of the drug that is responsible for both the therapeutic effect and toxicity, drugs that are subjected to a high degree of protein-binding should have both total and unbound plasma concentrations measured when determining doses.

Metabolism

Metabolism refers to 'the biochemical conversion of a drug to another chemical form' (Golper et al. 1996, p 753). The liver is the primary source of drug metabolism, but many active (and often toxic) metabolites rely on intact renal function for excretion. While metabolites usually possess activity profiles that are different from the parent drug, some retain pharmacologically active properties, and toxic side effects may be increased when renal failure allows them to accumulate.

Clearance

Clearance refers to the volume of fluid (in this case plasma) completely cleared of a given substance per unit of time. When determining the clearance of a drug, all routes must be considered, and the effects are cumulative. As explained by Golper (1996, p 753) '[s]ystemic or total body clearance is the sum of regional clearances [and includes] hepatic, renal, respiratory, biliary and extra-corporeal [routes]'. Renal clearance is the result of excretion, including filtration, secretion, and reabsorption. Recall that drug elimination is usually expressed as 'half life ($t^1/_2$), i.e. the time it takes to decrease the amount of drug in the body by half. This figure reflects both clearance and V_d and is prolonged in situations where V_d is large, or where clearance is compromised. Most drugs rely on a combination of metabolism and renal excretion for elimination (Golper et al. 1996,pp 753-754), and consequently, many drugs given to patients with renal disease require modification of either the dose, or dose interval, or both.

Other considerations

Pharmacokinetics also alters with extremes of age. Children are not 'little adults' and dosage adjustments that would occur when renal function is normal also need to be considered when renal impairment is present. Renal function in the newborn is less than that for an adult on a weight-for-weight basis, but should approximate adult levels by one year (Harris and Spence 1998, p 478).

Similar difficulties can be encountered in the elderly. From the age of thirty, glomerular filtration rate declines by 10ml/minute/decade (more if hypertension and/or diabetes are present). This may not be accompanied by an increase in serum creatinine if muscle mass is lost. The aging kidney is also compromised in its ability to concentrate and acidify urine, and to retain sodium and potassium (Thompson 1995, p 543).

5.2 Drug administration in end stage renal failure

Assessment of renal function

End stage renal failure is usually considered to be present when the glomerular filtration rate has declined to 10mls/minute, although some patients may not commence dialysis until this rate approaches 5mls/minute. It can therefore be presumed that renal clearance of drugs is negligible and dose adjustments must be made for all drugs that rely on renal excretion for the removal of either the drug or its active or toxic metabolites. Remember that a few patients retain some degree of residual renal function, which needs to be considered when determining therapeutic drug doses for these patients.

According to Golper et al. (1996, p 754) safety is the primary reason for making dose adjustments. Convenience and cost are the other principal considerations. This is especially so for drugs that have a narrow therapeutic index, such as aminoglycoside antibiotics e.g. gentamycin and tobramycin, antiarrhythmics e.g. sotalol) and cardiac glycosides e.g. digoxin.

Calculating dosage adjustment

Loading dose: The goal of the initial dose is to rapidly achieve a therapeutic drug concentration. This may be achieved by delivering the same initial dose as is recommended for a patient with intact renal function (providing that the extracellular fluid volume is normal) (Aronoff et al. 1999, p128), or by administering multiple doses at short, regularly spaced intervals until accumulation and a steady state is reached (Golper et al. 1996, p 754).

Maintenance: Two approaches can be taken to deliver a maintenance dose designed to keep the drug level in a therapeutic range.

a) The normal dose can be given with an extended dose interval. This method is preferable for drugs with a wide therapeutic index and a prolonged t $^1\!/_2$ (Aronoff et al. 1999, p 128).

b) A normal loading dose followed by a reduced dose administered at the usual dosage interval. This is the preferred method for use with drugs that have a narrow therapeutic index.

The pharmacokinetics and the pharmacodynamics of individual drugs determine the choice of method, and occasionally both methods may be combined (Golper, et al. 1996, p 755).

Monitoring drug concentration levels: When the desired concentration of a drug, and the levels at which toxicity becomes apparent are known, the monitoring of concentration levels becomes a valuable tool in individualising therapy for a given patient (Golper, et al. 1996, p 754). Such monitoring enables the determination of both loading and maintenance dosage. The goal is to achieve a therapeutic concentration of drug as soon as possible, and to keep this concentration between the desired peak and trough levels. If serum concentration falls below the desired trough level, sub therapeutic levels will occur and treatment may be compromised. Alternatively, if concentration levels rise above the desired peak level, signs and symptoms of toxicity can develop.

5.3 Drug removal during dialysis

Factors affecting removal

The drug removal that occurs during conventional haemodialysis follows the same principles as those observed when removing accumulated electrolytes and metabolic waste products (see Haemodialysis, Chapter 1). The most effectively removed drugs are those with a size of less than 500 daltons, that are less than 90% protein-bound, and that have a V_d that is limited primarily to the extracellular space. More porous membranes will enable the removal of larger molecules. The molecular weight of a drug affects removal more with therapies that use dialysate, e.g. conventional haemodialysis, than it does with therapies that do not use dialysate e.g. slow continuous or intermittent therapies (Aronoff et al. 1999, p 130).

Recall that many patients with renal failure will have lower than normal serum protein levels as a result of compromised nutritional status. Low serum protein increases the amount of highly protein-bound drugs available. As nutrition improves, the amount of available free drug decreases with a corresponding decrease in the amount that is removed during dialysis. The message here is to remember to reassess dose requirements as the patient's clinical condition alters.

Aronoff et al. (1999, p 129) suggested the following calculation for determining the rate of drug removal during peritoneal dialysis and haemodialysis. When using this formula, remember the importance of protein-binding.

Haemodialysis: $\qquad$ Clearance $_{HD}$ = Clearance $_{urea}$ x $(60 \div$ MW $_{drug})$

Peritoneal dialysis: $\qquad$ Clearance $_{PD}$ = Clearance $_{urea}$ x $(\sqrt{60} \div \sqrt{MW}\,_{drug})$

Clearance $_{HD}$ refers to drug removal during haemodialysis.

Clearance $_{PD}$ refers to drug removal during peritoneal dialysis.

Clearance $_{urea}$ refers to urea removal by the dialyser.

MW $_{drug}$ refers to the molecular weight of the drug.

Peritoneal dialysis is much less effective than haemodialysis for drug removal, achieving clearance rates of around 20ml/minute. As a general rule, if a drug is not removed by haemodialysis it will not be removed by peritoneal dialysis (Aronoff et al. 1999, p129).

Supplementary dosage

Haemodialysis can be used as a sole therapy to effect the removal of a drug following accidental or deliberate overdose. In end stage renal failure drug removal usually presents as a further complicating factor to the determination of therapeutic drug doses. It is usual to administer drugs that are removed by dialysis following completion of the dialysis procedure. This is also the case for the administration of supplementary doses.

Many books addressing the care of patients with renal disease include sections that refer to the adjustment of drug doses that is required both before and after dialysis has commenced. For a listing of these drugs, please refer to the section by Aranoff et al, which is listed as recommended reading at the conclusion of the chapter.

Although peritoneal dialysis is not considered an efficient way to remove drugs, many drugs are absorbed well, when added to the peritoneal dialysis solution. This option will be further addressed in the section discussing peritoneal dialysis as a treatment option.

Pharmacological problems specific to renal failure

Golper et al. (1996, pp 755–756) describe the following problems as unique to the dialysis population.

Sensitivity: The relationship between drug effect and concentration at individual receptor sites (sensitivity) is altered by a number of factors. Examples of this are changes to the V_d that are seen in acidosis and changes to extracellular volume status, alterations to protein binding and increased blood/brain penetration with drugs such as salicylates and barbiturates. Hyperkalaemia enhances depolarisation, making muscle cells more reactive, while hypokalaemia has the opposite effect. Sudden electrolyte shifts predispose patients to arrhythmias and alter responses to drugs that have already been commenced.

Urinary tract infection: Despite apparently normal serum drug concentrations, decreased renal function may alter drug concentrations in the urine and/or renal parenchyma, making treatment of urinary tract infection difficult. Drugs such as aminoglycosides (which rely on glomerular filtration to enter the urine) and penicillins (which rely on tubular secretion) may never reach therapeutic levels without causing systemic toxicity. Patients with end stage renal failure due to reflux nephropathy and analgesic nephropathy are examples of patient populations with an increased likelihood of developing urinary tract infections.

Cystic kidney disease: The difficulties encountered when treating patients with cystic kidney disease are similar to those described in the previous paragraph, where the major problem is getting antibiotics to penetrate the cyst walls. Chloramphenicol, fluroquinolones, and trimethoprim-sulfamethoxazole are drugs that have been shown to be clinically effective.

Muscle paralysis: Accumulation of aminoglycoside antibiotics can potentiate the action of neuromuscular blocking drugs, and result in delayed spontaneous respiration following the administration of anaesthesia using these agents.

Metabolic load: Many drugs contain sodium and potassium and represent 'hidden' causes of elevated serum concentrations of these electrolytes. Always suspect medication when there is any unexplained change in the patient's clinical status e.g. vomiting can be the result of NSAIDs and their irritant effect on the gastric mucosa. If this is mistaken for worsening uraemia, the patient can commence the cycle of vomiting, dehydration and worsening uraemia that was discussed in Chapter 1 of this section.

5.4 Drugs used in the treatment of renal failure

Commonly used drug groups

The majority of drugs used frequently in renal failure have either already been discussed, or will be discussed in the relevant sections of subsequent chapters. The following listing is a summary only, and can be referred to during subsequent reading.

1. antacids and phosphate-binding agents—salts of either aluminium, calcium or magnesium

2. sodium bicarbonate

3. electrolytes—sodium or potassium

4. cation exchange resins—calcium or sodium polystyrene resins

5. water soluble vitamins (except vitamin B_{12}) and minerals

6. stool softeners and bulking agents

7. antianaemics—iron, rHuEPO, folic acid

8. antihypertensive agents

9. antimicrobial agents

10. cardiotonic agents

    a) inotropic drugs

    b) chronotropic drugs

11. chelating agents

12. diuretic agents (used primarily in ARF and before end stage is reached).

13. immunosuppressive agents (these will be discussed in the section addressing transplantation).

14. anticoagulant agents.

For patients with end stage renal failure, each drug or drug group carries its own specific risk factors and, like many drugs in use with patients with intact renal function, some interaction between drugs is not uncommon. Those more frequently encountered include:

- **Quinidine** will decrease renal clearance of **digoxin**, requiring a reduction in digoxin dose.

- **Metoclopramide** decreases **digoxin** absorption, requiring an increase in digoxin dose.

- **NSAID's** decrease the response to **loop diuretics**, requiring an increase in diuretic dose.

- **Antacids** decrease the absorption of **Betablockers**, therefore administer 1–2 hours prior to meals. Antacids also bind with iron supplements that are not administered in a 'slow release' form, therefore also administer several hours prior to meals.

- The hepatic clearance of **cyclosporine** is decreased by **phenytoin, phenobarbitol, rifampicin, erythromycin, ketaconazole and amphotericin B,** requiring a decrease in dosage, and careful monitoring of serum drug concentrations.

- **Allopurinol** decreases the metabolism of **azathioprine**, increasing serum levels and usually requiring a decrease in dose.

(Johnston 1994, p 319).

References

In text references

Anderson, K., 1994, *Mosby's Dictionary,* Mosby, Sydney.

Aronoff, G., Erbeck, K., Brier, M. 1999, 'Prescribing drugs for dialysis patients', in *Principles and Practice of Dialysis,* Henrich, W. (ed), 2nd ed., William and Wilkins, Maryland.

Birkett, D., 1991, 'Bioavailability and first pass clearance', *Australian Prescriber*, vol. 14, no. 1, pp14–16.

Golper, T., Marx, M., Schuler, C., Bennett, W., 1996 'Drug dosage in renal patients', in *Replacement of Renal Function by Dialysis,* Jacobs, C., Kjellstrand, C., Koch, K., Winchester J, (eds.), 4th ed, Kluwer Academic Publishers, Boston.

Harris, L., Spence, D., 1998, 'Drugs used in renal failure', in *Renal Nursing* (appendix), Smith, T., (ed.), 2nd ed., Bailliere Tindall, Sydney.

Johnston, J., 1994, 'Principles of drug therapy in renal failure', in *Primer on Kidney Disease*, Greensberg, A., (ed.), National Kidney Foundation, Academic Press, Sydney.

Swan, S., Bennett, W., 1997, 'Drug use in renal patients and the extracorporeal treatment of poisonings', in *Caring for the renal patient*, Levine, D., (ed.), 3rd ed., Saunders, Sydney.

Thompson, N., 1995, 'Drugs and the kidney in the elderly', *The Medical Journal of Australia*, vol. 162, May, pp543–547.

Recommended reading

Aronoff, G., Erbeck, K., Brier, M. 1999, 'Prescribing drugs for dialysis patients', in *Principles and Practice of Dialysis,* Henrich, W. (ed), 2nd ed., pp 131-140, William and Wilkins, Maryland.

CHAPTER SIX

Investigation of structure and function

Introduction

Numerous safe and accurate tests are available to evaluate the structure and function of the renal system. Technological advances improved imaging techniques, and computer processing enables rapid and accurate analysis of biochemical and serological data. Used in combination, these tests help diagnose disorders that previously required invasive techniques. Understanding these tests, recognising when they are indicated, and interpreting the results accurately, is essential for effective nursing management of renal disorders.

6.1 Urinary examination

Overview

Medicine has fortunately come a long way from the days when doctors occasionally tasted their patient's urine to assist with the diagnosis of disease. Nevertheless, urinalysis remains a vital part of the diagnostic armory available for investigating renal disease.

Urine should be collected with as little handling as possible, and in most cases, a midstream specimen is satisfactory. Suprapubic aspiration may be required in children, and either condom drainage or urinary catheter insertion may be needed in incontinent or unco-operative adults. It is usually best to examine a urine specimen when it is fresh because the cellular components disintegrate over time, and the chemical composition will alter. Bacteria multiply at room temperature, so urine that has been left unrefrigerated will probably have a bacterial count higher than when it was first voided (Greenberg 1994, p 23).

Physical and chemical properties

Normal urine is clear and pale yellow in appearance. The colour deepens as the urine becomes concentrated. Red or white blood cells and crystals can cause urine to appear turbid.

Specific gravity usually ranges between 1·001 and 1·035, and measurement using a hydrometer is generally considered to be the most accurate. Sufficient urine to suspend the hydrometer upright is required, but is not always available. The specific gravity of small amounts of urine can be determined using either a refractometer or a dipstick. Urine of a high specific gravity is concentrated, and urine of a low specific gravity is dilute. Tests measuring specific gravity can help to determine urinary concentrating ability, and often help to differentiate between prerenal ischaemia, where urinary concentrating ability is retained, and intrinsic renal failure, where concentrating ability has been lost due to tubular damage, see Chapter 2 of this section.

Urine dipsticks, plastic strips impregnated with chemical reagents, have replaced most of the older (and somewhat tedious) chemical testing methods. Some of these reagents are able to give a reliable reading in a variety of situations. Others can be affected by the presence of other substances in the urine, or be sensitive to time delays and give inaccurate readings.

Urinary pH indicates the degree to which hydrogen ion secretion, and bicarbonate ion reabsorption has occurred, and provides a rough guide only. When specific disorders of tubular transport are suspected, specially designed tests are required. Urinary pH will also be raised in the presence of urea-splitting organisms.

Both protein and red blood cells can appear in the urine of people with intact renal function, but more often than not, their presence indicates some degree of renal compromise. Urine that shows a positive reaction to blood should be further evaluated to determine the source. Crenated, also called 'dysmorphic', red blood cells indicate glomerular damage, while intact cells indicate bleeding in lower in the urinary system. Free haemoglobin indicates haemolysis, while myoglobin indicates muscle damage.

According to Greenberg (1994, p 25) the amount of protein is graded from 'trace to

++++' on dipsticks. The amount of protein loss can be roughly translated as follows:

i) trace = 5–20 mg/dL

ii) + = 30 mg/dL

iii) ++ = 100 mg/dL

iv) +++ = 300mg/dL

v) ++++ = > 2000mg/dL.

These figures are a guide only, and do not differentiate between the types of protein being excreted. All urine showing more than a trace of protein should be sent for further analysis, preferably using a specimen collected over a 24-hour period.

Remember that a protein loss of < 200mg/L (20 mg/dL) is not generally considered pathological, and that protein loss can be increased during febrile illnesses, after vigorous exercise, or following a period in the upright position (orthostatic proteinuria), and may not indicate renal disease. 'Fixed' proteinuria (proteinuria that is present all the time), that exceeds 200 mg/L, should always be investigated.

Glycosuria usually indicates hyperglycaemia, but it can also occur in renal disease when the tubular threshold for glucose absorption has been altered. It also occurs in patients with marked proteinuria (Whitworth and Lawrence 1994, p 64). In the early stages of renal disease when hyperfiltration and polyuria are present, urinalysis continues to reflect glycosuria, but as nephropathy progresses, the excretion of glucose slows as the glomerular filtration rate declines. In this situation the blood glucose estimations are the only reliable indicator of blood glucose levels.

The presence of ketones usually indicates that fat is being used as an energy source and are seen during starvation and fasting. Ketonuria` can precede ketoacidosis in type 1 diabetic patients who are dependent on insulin.

The presence of leucocytes in the urine usually indicates inflammation or infection, most frequently of the urinary tract.

Urinary casts are comprised of Tamm-Horsfall protein, a mucoprotein normally secreted by tubular cells, and a varied collection of cells. The most common being:

•   Hyaline casts, which consist of mucoprotein only.

- Granular casts are a mix of altered serum proteins and degenerated cells, and, while they can be shed after exercise, are often associated with renal damage.

- Waxy casts (also known as broad casts) form in tubules that have been widened as the result of renal damage, and indicate chronic renal failure.

- Red cell casts indicate glomerular damage, as opposed to intact red blood cells that indicate bleeding lower in the urinary system.

- White cell casts are associated with pyelonephritis, and are also seen with interstitial and tubulointerstitial disease.

- Tubular cell casts are associated with acute tubular necrosis, and indicate sloughing of tubular cells.

Urinary crystals are most frequently formed from calcium oxalate, magnesium ammonium phosphate, and cystine. Although many other crystals can appear in the urine, those listed here are frequently associated with renal pathology (Greenberg 1994, pp 23–33).

Tests of glomerular and tubular function

The standard test for glomerular function is the *creatinine clearance test*. The concept of clearance (C) can be understood in the following way.

1. The amount of any substance that appears in the urine (U) can be determined by multiplying its concentration by the volume of urine produced in a given time (V).

    This is expressed mathematically as U x V.

2. To then determine the amount of blood that would be contained in that amount of the substance, divide U x V by the plasma concentration of the substance (P).

    e.g. $C = U \times V \div P$

The final amount is then expressed with reference to a unit of time (e.g. 1.2 ml/second).

Glomerular filtration rate can be determined by performing the same calculation on what is called a *glomerular substance;* one that is freely filtered at glomerular level, and that is neither secreted into, nor reabsorbed from, the renal tubules. While creatinine does not meet all of these requirements, it comes close enough to enable it to be used to determine the glomerular filtration rate for most purposes. Creatinine is preferred to urea, as, with few exceptions, its production is relatively constant. Urea generation tends to vary over short periods of time in accordance with intake and a variety of catabolic challenges.

Tubular function is usually determined by testing the kidney's ability to concentrate and acidify urine. It is determined using a combination of the following methods:

1. Urinary concentration ability is measured by calculating the osmolality following either a period of water deprivation or the administration of antidiuretic hormone.

2. Reabsorptive capacity involves measuring urine sodium and potassium after two to three days of controlled low sodium dietary intake.

3. Acidification is determined by measuring urinary pH if metabolic acidosis is present, or following the administration of oral ammonium chloride that is designed to produce a short period of systemic acidosis (Whitworth and Lawrence 1994, p 69–71).

6.2 Haematological/serological examination

Serum biochemistry

Serum biochemistry has already been referred to in the initial chapters in this section and will not be reviewed again here. The reader is advised to become familiar with the normal values for urea, creatinine and electrolytes, and to note the alterations that occur when renal function is compromised. Do not forget to consider the previously mentioned (normal) variations that occur at both extremes of age.

Red blood cells and the importance of iron

As discussed in Chapter 1 of this section, the lack of erythropoietin (EPO) production (a function of normal kidneys) is compromised when renal failure occurs. As a result, red blood cell production is delayed, and oxygen delivery to body tissues is compromised. Each haemoglobin molecule contains four 'haeme' and one 'nonhaeme' molecule, and each haeme molecule can bind two iron ions.

Body iron content is approximately 50 mg/kg for men and 37 mg/kg for women. Either meat or vegetables, legumes and pulses, can supply dietary iron. Of these, iron derived from meat products is more readily absorbed than that obtained from other sources (Janssen—Cilag 1996, pp 6.5–6.6).

Following ingestion and absorption, iron is transported by the serum protein *Transferrin* to sites such as bone marrow or muscle where it is available for immediate use, or to storage sites such as the liver and the reticuloendothelial system. Iron is stored as either ferritin or haemosiderin. Ferritin is the most easily released when required. After its 120-day lifespan, which is often reduced to ~ 90 days in end stage renal failure, the red blood cell releases its iron content, which is returned to the circulation for redistribution for immediate use, or storage (Janssen-Cilag 1996, pp 6.5–6.6).

Once rHuEPO is given, red blood cell function can commence so rapidly that the available iron stores are rapidly used up. Alternatively, if iron stores are low when therapy is commenced, red cell production may not occur. In either case, the full effect of the EPO therapy will not follow its administration. It is therefore necessary to ensure that iron stores are adequate prior to commencing EPO therapy.

There are two types of iron deficiency.

1. **Absolute** iron deficiency, where iron stores are not sufficient to meet the requirements of the bone marrow.

2. **Functional** iron deficiency, where residual iron stores are adequate, but where they cannot be supplied quickly enough to meet the needs of the bone marrow.

(Janssen-Cilag 1996, pp 6.11–6.12).

Serum ferritin levels should be measured prior to commencing therapy, and should be above 100 micrograms/l if they are to meet the needs of the red blood cells. After commencing therapy, ferritin levels become less reliable as an indicator of iron levels. Thereafter, transferrin levels and the percentage of hypochromic red cells is a better indicator of the response to treatment. Transferrin levels show the amount of the protein available for transporting iron to the cells. The number of hypochromic cells, reflect the percentage of cells that reach the blood compartment with a low iron content.

To ensure that adequate iron stores are available to the red blood cells, serum ferritin levels should be > 100 mg/L; the percentage of transferrin saturation with iron (TSAT) should be >20%, and number of hypochromic red cells should be <10% (CARI Guidelines).

Other investigations undertaken to interpret anaemia are:

1. Full blood estimation (FBE). This is an automated five-cell count and is usually followed by a blood film and manual examination if one of the five cell counts is abnormal.

2. Reticulocyte count. A measurement of the number of immature red blood cells being produced.

3. Vitamin B_{12}. Vitamin B_{12} is required for the synthesis of nucleic acid, and therefore is important for cell division.

4. Folic acid. Also a 'B' group vitamin is required for cell division.

5. Bone marrow biopsy, if no cause for the anaemia can be found.

Miscellaneous

In diseases where the immune system is involved, serum complement levels can be measured to determine whether the classical or the alternative pathway is the means by which the cascade has been activated. The common pathway commences with activation of C3 and results in cell lysis. The classical pathway commences the process by activating C1 after contact with either, immunoglobulin (Ig) M, or IgG. The alternative pathway provides for direct (or alternative) activation of C3 after contact predominantly with the cell walls of microorganisms, or in the presence of Igs, other than IgG or IgM. Serum complement levels enable the immune stimulant involved to be determined.

Immune complexes. e.g. cryoglobulins, and autoantibodies are also occasionally measured, as are the hormones renin with phaeochromocytoma, accelerated and renovascular hypertension and dialysis-resistant hypertension, and aldosterone to diagnose primary or secondary hyperaldosteronism (Whitworth and Lawrence 1994, p 69–71).

6.3 Imaging techniques

Radiological imaging

Plain abdominal X-ray: This is a simple, noninvasive technique that provides information about the size and outline of the kidney, the presence of radio-opaque abnormalities such as calculi, and the presence of air that indicates the presence of a fistulae or infection with gas-producing organisms. X-rays can be combined with a tomogram, a film representing a cross section of tissue at a predetermined depth, or a zonogram, which is similar to a tomogram, but focuses on a small area of tissue. Developmental abnormalities can also be seen with a plain abdominal X-ray e.g. congenital absence of one kidney.

Intravenous urography: Also known as intravenous pyelography (IVP), this examination provides information relating to all structures containing urine. Following intravenous injection of a substance that is concentrated in the kidney and then excreted in the urine, radiographs of the renal system are taken at preset intervals. Studies are usually divided into the following stages:

1. The nephrogram stage that shows the contrast media concentrated within the renal tubules.

2. The pyelogram stage where the renal pelvis is examined to determine size, abnormalities of the calyces and papillae and the presence of space-occupying lesions. A constricting band is sometimes placed around the lower abdomen to constrict the ureters and delay emptying.

3. The cystogram, which is taken after micturition, and which reveals the presence of residual urine and vesicoureteric reflux, if it is taken after the contrast medium has cleared from the renal pelvis.

Delay in the appearance of contrast medium during the nephrogram stage usually indicates obstruction such as renal artery stenosis. Delay in the pyelogram stage usually indicates parenchymal damage. In this case, the contrast medium is concentrated in the area of damage (Becker et al. 1992, pp 14–17).

Voiding cystourethrogram: This is similar to the cystography phase of the intravenous urography. It is taken to detect urethral, as well as bladder abnormalities. It is usually reserved for lower urinary tract disorders.

Percutaneous antegrade urography: A fine gauge needle is passed into the renal pelvis under ultrasound guidance to guide the subsequent passage of a larger bore catheter or needle. Contrast media can then be injected directly into the renal pelvis. This is the procedure of choice when arterial obstruction is known or suspected, because the catheter can remain in-situ to provide urinary drainage (Becker et al. 1992, p 17).

Retrograde pyelography: A cystoscope is used to facilitate the passage of a catheter into either ureter. Contrast media is then introduced in a 'retrograde' manner, back towards the kidney (Becker et al. 1992, p 17). This technique enables visualisation of the ureter below the level of any obstruction.

Renal angiography: One of two techniques is usually employed:

1. Conventional angiography, where the renal artery or its sub branches is entered through a catheter placed into the aorta via the femoral artery. The catheter is advanced under televised control and direct visualisation of the renal vasculature is possible. Dilation of renal artery stenosis is undertaken using this procedure. Because of the risk of damage to the arterial puncture site, or haemorrhage, hospitalisation for twenty-four hours is usually required after the procedure.

2. Digital subtraction angiography (DSA), where a computerised subtraction process is used to 'subtract' an image recorded prior to the injection of contrast media, from that taken after the injection. The result is a record of the lesion only.

Renal venography: Similar to the renal angiography, but accesses the femoral vein to view the renal veins. It is used to diagnose renal vein thrombosis and is often accompanied by simultaneous injection of adrenaline into the renal arteries to decrease filling and enhance the retrograde filling with contrast media. Blood for renin assays can be taken at the same time (Becker et.al. 1992, p 19).

Computerised (axial) tomography: This is a relatively expensive procedure, and is usually employed only when diagnosis using other means was not successful. The procedure involves using a computer to reconstruct cross sectional images of 1cm slices of the chosen organ (Hattersely and Bell 1998, p 193). It is particularly useful with lesions involving the adrenal, perirenal, retroperitoneal and pelvic areas (Becker et al 1992, p 20), where malignant tumours or collections of fluid are otherwise difficult to visualise.

Ultrasonography

Ultrasonography does not carry the risks associated with radiation, especially for pregnant women and has replaced many X-ray procedures (Hattersely and Bell 1998, p 193). It is noninvasive and uses a transducer or 'sonar probe', to transmit high frequency sound waves through the kidney and extrarenal structures. The resulting echoes are amplified and converted into electrical images that are displayed on a screen, and reflect anatomical images.

Ultrasound examination is frequently used to determine the size and shape of the kidneys, where cystic or neoplastic lesions are suspected, and to guide the operator undertaking procedures such as renal biopsy. It is also used after renal transplantation where acute rejection, thrombosis of the renal artery or vein, or extravasation of urine from the ureteric anastomosis is suspected.

Radionuclide studies

When a radioactive substance is injected, the flow of isotopes through the kidney can be monitored enabling an image of renal perfusion, tissue integrity, and anatomy of the outflow tract to be obtained (Pollack 1994, p 46).

Depending on the information required, images are recorded at intervals ranging from seconds to several minutes. Radionuclide studies are most frequently used to provide information about:

1. Estimation of renal function, where glomerular filtration rate and renal blood flow are measured.

2. Measurement of 'divided' renal function, where the function of one kidney is compared with that of the other.

3. Detection of renal artery stenosis.

4. Where the use of contrast media is contraindicated.

5. Evaluation of function after renal transplantation.

6. Diagnosing intermittent obstruction.

7. Diagnosing inflammatory lesions.

(Pollack 1994, p 46).

Depending on the type of study to be performed, different radiopharmaceutical products are used.

6.4 Renal biopsy

The role of renal biopsy

Renal biopsy refers to the removal of tissue from the cortex of the kidney for pathological examination. The specimen is usually obtained by percutaneous puncture where a 'core' of tissue is obtained under local anaesthesia, or occasionally light sedation. Open biopsy where 'wedges' of tissue are taken, is possible, but is usually reserved for 'high risk' patients. Each core of tissue contains approximately twenty glomeruli. Since there are about one million glomeruli in each kidney, renal biopsy is usually only useful when renal disease is extensive and limited to the cortex.

The purpose of renal biopsy is to examine changes to the capillary endothelium, the basement membrane, mesangial cells and epithelial cells. It provides 'one of the few objective measurements of the type, nature, site, extent and … evolution of renal disease' (Striker et al. 1990, p 1). Biopsy assists in the management of renal disease by:

1. Providing information to assist in diagnosing glomerular disease.

2. Enabling the evaluation of disease progress and response to treatment.

3. Providing a guide to the prognosis.

4. Facilitating the diagnosis of coexisting systemic disease.

To accurately interpret the results of renal biopsy, a thorough knowledge of the structure and function of the kidney is required. This includes understanding the various changes that occur from infancy through to adolescence and adulthood.

Evaluation of biopsy findings

The cellular changes that occur with renal disease are examined after the biopsy using light microscopy, electron microscopy or immunofluorescence. The biopsy specimen should be handled with care to avoid damage that may either prevent accurate diagnosis of the disease process, or lead to confusion as to the extent of renal damage.

Once the biopsy specimen has been prepared for examination, information is obtained as follows:

1. Low power light microscopy enables the damage to be classified as diffuse, focal, global or segmental. The use of high power microscopy provides information about mesangial, epithelial or endothelial proliferation; basement membrane changes, e.g. thickening or 'splitting', and the presence of necrosis, hyalinosis and sclerosis.

2. Electron microscopy the damage to be located e.g. mesangial, subepithelial, subendothelial or intramembranous and the nature of any deposits to be determined, e.g. immunoglobulin or complement deposits.

3. Immunofluorescence differentiates between immune-complex disease and basement membrane disease, refer Chapter 4 of this section. It also provides more information about the precise location of these deposits.

The core of tissue taken during the biopsy is usually divided longitudinally. One half is processed for light microscopy and the remaining half is divided in half again. One half is for immunofluorescence is kept in a petri dish and covered with sterile gauze moistened with sterile, buffered saline and snap frozen for division and examination. The specimens for electron and light microscopy are fixed in a medium of choice. After being fixed, specimens are imbedded in a substance such as paraffin. Some will be stained. There is a battery of stains available to highlight specific lesions throughout the kidney. Specimens are then divided into thin slices and placed on slides for examination (Striker et al. 1990, p1–2).

Indications for biopsy

Life threatening haemorrhage is always possible with renal biopsy. It is usually reserved for situations where diagnosis cannot be confirmed, or where progress cannot be evaluated, by any other method. It is most commonly used in the following situations:

1. When proteinuria accompanies abnormal renal function, or when persistent proteinuria is present with normal kidney function. The latter can detect the presence of systemic disease in its early stages.

2. Haematuria where crenated (dysmorphic) red blood cells have been detected on microscopy.

3.   Nephrotic syndrome where the use of high dose steroids is considered of greater risk that the biopsy itself.

4.   Chronic renal failure with no apparent cause.

5.   Acute renal failure with no apparent cause.

6.   Where renal impairment is a known complication of a specific disease, e.g. diabetes, or where it occurs 'de novo'. Correct diagnosis is important because if the renal disease is presumed to be a complication of the primary disease, the opportunity to curtail the progress of a potentially treatable renal lesion can be missed.

7.   Following renal transplantation where it is important to differentiate between a decline in function due to nephrotoxicity (where immunotherapy may need to be decreased) and rejection (where immunotherapy may need to be increased).

(Taube 1986, p 1306).

Biopsy is not usually performed with lesions located in the medullary portion of the kidney. Renal biopsy is contraindicated in some situations. In these cases open biopsy is performed but is rare. Examples where open biopsy would be considered are:

1.   Where the kidney is not clearly visible on ultrasonography.

2.   Where there is only a small, single, or 'horseshoe' kidney.

3.   In the presence of bleeding disorders.

4.   When hypertension is present.

5.   Where a perinephric abscess is suspected.

6.   When pyelonephritis has been diagnosed.

7.   When a tumour is suspected.

8.   When the patient is unable to cooperate fully.

The biopsy procedure

Ultrasonography is used to locate the kidney and determine its depth below the skin. For a conventional biopsy, the patient is placed face down and the abdomen is supported with several rolled towels to reduce movement of the kidney with respiration. For a transplant biopsy, the patient is supine. The preferred biopsy site is the lateral border on the lower pole of the right kidney.

The patient is asked to hold their breath to prevent moving the kidney, and the needle is inserted. When resistance is felt, the renal capsule has been entered; this is confirmed by asking the patient to breathe—the biopsy needle will swing in rhythm with the patient's respirations. The needle is then marked at the skin surface to determine the kidney's depth below the skin and withdrawn. The biopsy needle is then inserted to the same depth and the specimen is taken. A pressure dressing is applied on completion of the biopsy and the patient is returned to the ward.

Nursing care: The patient should remain supine for approximately six hours after the procedure. Some bleeding is expected after the biopsy. The nurse needs to distinguish between frank blood that could indicate haemorrhage and post biopsy staining that diminishes over time. Serial urine specimens are collected for twenty-four hours to monitor blood loss. Blood pressure and pulse are recorded regularly to assist in the diagnosis of haemorrhage. If fluid restrictions are not required, drinking will increase urine output and reduce the risk of blood clots. It is usual to restrict activity for a fortnight after the biopsy.

Complications: These include haemorrhage, the formation of arteriovenous fistulae, perirenal haematoma and laceration of adjacent organs.

6.5 Summary

An approach to diagnosis

The following framework can be used to compile information to assist in determining the cause of renal impairment.

Investigation of Renal Failure

1. Clinical: History; take a detailed record of the presenting signs and symptoms, when they started and their frequency. Include psychosocial and quality of life questions. Include a physical examination based on standard nursing observations. Determine if there is obvious oedema, where it occurs, and whether it is pitting.

Assess skin turgor. Assess whether you can ballot the kidneys. If so, are they painful?

2. **Urinalysis:** Record all information available including reagent strip test results such as specific gravity and pH observation of the amount and colour, MSU results the presence of sediment, cytology and biochemistry to determine if the kidney is concentrating the urine and reabsorbing sodium.

3. **Serology:** Record the haemoglobin, haematocrit and other blood test parameters and consider what the heamatological biochemical analysis reveals.

4. **Renal function tests**: Consider the results of the renal function tests and what they reveal about the glomerular filtration rate and the renal status in general

5. **Radiology:**

6. **Ultrasound:** } Consider all information discussed under 6.3.

7. **Radionuclide:**

8. **Renal biopsy:**

Use the information to formulate a care plan for the patient that includes nursing care in hospital, self-care, education and counselling. Relatives and significant others should be involved after discussing their involvement with the patient.

References

In text references

Becker, G., Whitworth, J., Kincaid-Smith, P., 1992, *Clinical Nephrology in Medical Practice*, Blackwell, Melbourne.

CARI Guidelines, 2000, A joint project between the Australian and New Zealand Society of Nephrology and the Australian Kidney Foundation, Excerpta Medica Communications, Sydney.

Greenberg, A., 1994, (ed.), 'Urinalysis' in *Primer on Kidney Disease,* National Kidney Foundation, Academic Press, Sydney.

Hattersely, J., Bell, A., 1998, 'Investigations in renal disease' in *Renal Nursing*, Smith, T., (ed.), 2nd ed., Bailliere Tindall, Sydney.

Janssen-Cilag Pty. Ltd., 1996, Renal Disease Teaching Kit for Nurse Educators, Lane Cove, Sydney.

Pollack, H., 1994, 'Renal imaging techniques', in *Primer on Kidney Disease*, Greenberg, A., (ed.), National Kidney Foundation, Academic Press, Sydney.

Striker, L., Olson, J., Striker, G., 1990, *The Renal Biopsy,* 2nd ed., Saunders, Sydney.

Taube, D., 1986, 'Percutaneous renal biopsy', *Medicine International*, pp1306–1308.

Whitworth, J., Lawrence, J., 1994, 'Renal investigative techniques', in *Textbook of Renal Disease*, Whitworth, J., Lawrence, J., (eds.), 2nd ed., Churchill Livingstone, Melbourne.

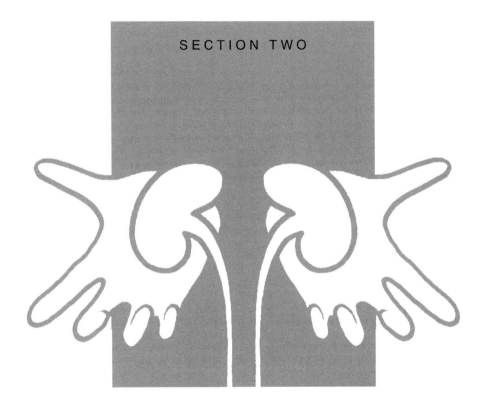

SECTION TWO

Overview of treatment

Introduction

Haemodialysis is undertaken by thousands of people world wide to replace renal function that has been lost due to acute or 'end stage' renal disease. In the acute setting, the goals of haemodialysis are to replace, or support, renal function until the kidneys recover. For people with end stage disease, replacement of renal function is ongoing, and ceases only when death, or successful renal transplantation, occurs.

This chapter is designed to acquaint the reader with aspects of the historical beginnings of haemodialysis, explain the principles underlying the procedure, and introduce relevant points about patient education. Understanding these basic principles, and their development over time, will assist the reader to safely undertake patient management and to help patients understand the reasons for alterations to their treatment.

1.1   A brief history of haemodialysis

Development

In 1861 Thomas Graham, a Professor of Chemistry at Anderson's University in Scotland, first used the term 'dialysis' to describe the separation of crystalloid and colloid substances via diffusion through a semi-permeable membrane. Although Professor Graham demonstrated that the process of 'dialysis' could be used to remove solute from fluids containing both crystalloid and colloid substances, he did not extend his experiments beyond the field of chemistry to medicine (Drukker, 1989, p 21).

John Abel, and his co-workers at the Johns Hopkins Medical School in Baltimore USA, took the next step. After anticoagulating the blood of a dog, it was passed through celluloid tubing within a glass container filled with either saline or a fluid resembling serum. They called this apparatus a 'dialyser' or 'artificial kidney'. Having demonstrated that nitrogenous substances could be removed using this process of dialysis, they were keen to try the treatment on humans, but were unable to do so (Drukker 1989, p 23).

Credit for the first human dialysis is attributed to a German physician, George Haas. Between 1924 and 1928 Haas performed a number of dialysis treatments on uraemic individuals. Although the treatments were well tolerated, they were too short to deliver significant therapeutic benefit. Although Haas performed the first human dialysis, a Dutch physician, Willem Kolff achieved therapeutic success in 1945.

The years following Haas' work saw the availability of purified heparin, and the development of seamless cellophane sausage tubing. This enabled dialysis using a well-tolerated anticoagulant and a dialyser membrane with relatively high efficiency. In 1945 a 67-year-old woman was bought to Kolff unconscious, with acute renal failure and severe uraemia, thought to be due to sulfonamide toxicity. Kolff subjected her to a single eleven-hour treatment after which she regained consciousness and eventually made a complete recovery (Drukker 1989, pp 29–33).

Following this demonstration of dialysis as an appropriate treatment for uraemia, improvements to the technique continued to be made and dialysis became an accepted form of treatment for acute renal failure of relatively short duration. Acute renal failure, with a prolonged anuric/oliguric phase, and chronic renal failure that required ongoing treatment, remained 'untreatable' until 1960. For haemodialysis to become a practical treatment, the availability of three major technological advances was required. These were:

- ready access to the circulation

- stable, semipermeable membranes

- reliable systems for the delivery of blood and dialysate.

(Wellard 1996 p 71).

Current application

Haemodialysis can be used to temporarily replace, or support, renal function in acute renal failure, or as a permanent form of renal replacement therapy when end stage disease has occurred. Because haemodialysis requires *direct* access to the blood compartment, as opposed to *indirect access* as occurs with peritoneal dialysis, reliable access to blood vessels is required. The *vascular* access may be temporary, when renal failure is acute and recovery of function is anticipated, or permanent, when a patient with end stage disease elects to accept haemodialysis treatment.

Currently, most patients with end stage renal disease dialyse for between four and five hours, three times per week. Patients with acute renal failure may dialyse between three and seven times per week, but fewer hours can be required (ANZDATA 1999).

These days, most of the population is aware of 'dialysis' as a treatment for renal disease, and ask about it when the signs and symptoms of renal failure start to compromise their quality of life. There is, however, seldom a corresponding knowledge of the complex nature of dialysis and the degree of commitment required to make it an acceptable form of treatment.

Haemodialysis has been described as a 'catabolic insult' (Dawborn 1990, p 369) with an increase in the generation of toxins and the activation of a variety of cascade systems. However, if renal failure is the primary problem and is considered amenable to treatment, a recommendation of dialysis or transplant is appropriate. Other forms of extracorporeal renal replacement therapies are available for both acute and chronic renal failure, and will be discussed in following chapters.

1.2 Overview of treatment

A brief review

Haemodialysis involves the use of a machine with a blood pump that moves blood around an extracorporeal circuit and through a dialyser before returning it to the patient. The blood pump operates in a peristaltic manner, occluding specific sections of the pump segment in a circular manner, propelling the blood ahead of it at a speed usually between 200 and 350ml/minute. The dialyser, or 'artificial kidney', is a part of the extracorporeal circuit and consists of two components, a blood compartment and a dialysate compartment. Both of these compartments are contained within a plastic casing called the 'dialyser housing'. Dialysers are manufactured in one of two designs: they may be cylindrical, called a 'hollow fiber' dialyser, or oblong and called a 'parallel plate' dialyser (Daugirdas et al. 2001 p46).

Although the shape is different, both dialysers function in a similar fashion. The blood passes through a compartment that is bounded by a semipermeable membrane made of multiple hollow fibres or multiple parallel membranes. Solute, metabolic waste and electrolytes, and water pass through pores in the membrane. The dialysate compartment is filled with a mixture of concentrated electrolyte (and sometimes non electrolyte) solution known as 'concentrate' and purified water. The mix of concentrate and water is known as 'dialysate', and it is the strength of the electrolytes in this mixture that helps determine the rate of solute movement through the semipermeable membrane.

During haemodialysis, blood is in continuous movement in one direction through the blood compartment of the dialyser and dialysate is in continual movement in the opposite direction. This is called 'counter current flow' and ensures maximum solute removal.

Water moves from the patient's blood in a different manner. In accordance with pressure generated within the dialyser, water will be either be 'pushed' or 'pulled' across the membrane and into the dialysate compartment. The used dialysate, now known as dialysate 'effluent', is discharged down the drain, and is continuously replaced by fresh dialysate.

The aims of treatment

Dialysis is defined in terms that refer to the separation of crystalloid and colloid substances via diffusion through a semipermeable membrane. The purpose of dialysis is to remove metabolic waste products and correct imbalances of body water and electrolytes. The correction is temporary, and often only partial, and the process of dialysis does not replace any of the regulatory functions of the kidneys.

Dialysis has two primary aims, the removal of solute and the removal of water. Solute removal is achieved primarily by diffusion. Convective solute transport does occur and, while it forms the basis of *other forms* of renal replacement therapy, its contribution to solute removal in *haemodialysis* is minimal. Water removal occurs primarily as a result of ultrafiltration with osmosis contributing in a minor way (Daugirdas and Van Stone 2001, pp 15–17).

1.3 Achieving the aims of treatment

The physiology of solute removal

Passive diffusion across the semipermeable membrane separating blood and dialysate enables solute removal during dialysis. This diffusion is 'restricted' and occurs in accordance with the pore size of the membrane, the size of the molecule, and the diffusion gradient established between blood and dialysate.

Solute size correlates quite closely with the molecular weight of a substance, and the term 'dalton' is used to identify molecular weight. Dialyser membranes are described as having a 'sieving coefficient', which refers to the largest molecule that can cross the membrane. Far fewer of these large molecules move across the membrane compared with much smaller molecules. For example, if one molecule weighing 5000 daltons, the sieving co-efficient of most cellulose-based dialysers, crosses the membrane at one point in time, 500 molecules weighing 10 daltons can cross in the same time.

To relate this to dialysis, 128 molecules weighing 39 daltons, which is the size of potassium, or 217 molecules weighing 23 daltons, the same size as sodium, can cross for each molecule weighing 5000 daltons (dalton size obtained from Chang 1988). Dialysers with larger sieving coefficients are available and will be discussed in the section examining the extra-corporeal circuit.

Although the sieving coefficient of most dialysers seems quite high (5000 daltons) only those solutes described as being in the 'small dalton range' will be removed effectively. Solutes of small molecular weight, or small dalton range, are generally described as weighing less than 500 daltons, but the numbers vary slightly in different texts.

Membrane resistance refers to the barrier to solute movement that is posed by the membrane itself. Characteristics such as membrane thickness pore size and the number of pores all affect clearance. For example, a thick membrane with fewer and smaller pores offers higher resistance to solute movement than a thin membrane with a large number of bigger pores.

You may read about the 'triple barrier' that haemodialysis poses to solute transfer. This refers to the combination of membrane resistance, and the areas of slower flow in the layer of blood and dialysate that lie immediately either side of the membrane (Daugirdas and Van Stone 2001, p 16). These areas of slower flow hamper the random movement of molecules that results in diffusion. In reality, dialyser design and the use of the maximum blood flow appropriate for each patient ensure that these factors are kept to a minimum. Careful priming of both the blood and dialysate compartments prior to dialysis is also required if the maximum surface area is to be available for solute transfer.

Where Qb refers to blood flow rate, Cb_{in} refers to the concentration of a given solute entering the dialyser and Cb_{out} refers to the concentration of a given solute leaving the dialyser. The formula Qb x $(Cb_{in}–Cb_{out})÷Cb_{in}$ enables the clearance for any given solute to be calculated.

Physiology of water removal

All dialyser membranes have an ultrafiltration coefficient, often termed 'K_{uf}'. 'K' expresses the 'clearance coefficient' and 'uf' means 'water'. In other words K_{uf} is the dialyser's ability to achieve water removal. The ability to remove water reflects the hydraulic permeability of the membrane (its 'leakiness') and its surface area (m^2). When expressing a dialyser's ability to achieve water loss, K_{uf} is expressed in ml/hour/millimetres of mercury 'TMP' (ml/hr/mm Hg TMP). TMP is the abbreviation for trans membrane pressure. During haemodialysis water moves from one side of the membrane to the other, in accordance with the hydrostatic pressure gradient that exists across the membrane.

The combined pressure reflects the pressure in the blood compartment minus the pressure in the dialysate compartment. The blood compartment pressure is recorded as 'venous pressure' (VP) and measures the pressure in the blood compartment at the outlet port of the dialyser. This pressure reflects both blood pump speed (Q_b) and the resistance offered by the patient's vascular access to the return of blood. During dialysis venous pressure is always positive. The dialysate compartment pressure (DP) is also measured at the outlet port and, with modern dialysis machines, can be either positive or negative, depending on the amount of water to be removed during treatment.

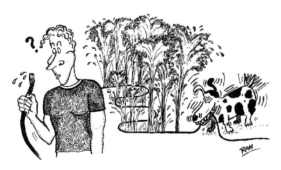

Figure 2.1.1: The contribution of venous positive pressure resistance to water removal
(Heintz 2000).

Figure 2.1.1 illustrates the contribution of venous positive pressure resistance to water removal.

Let's compare what happens to your garden hose. Think about the tap as the blood pump and the nozzle as the resistance that the patient's vascular access is offering to the return of blood. The hose itself becomes the membrane, and its 'K_{uf}' depends on the thickness of the rubber and number of holes that are in it. The holes can be intentional if it is a 'soaker' hose, or accidental if the dog has bitten it—it doesn't matter, the result is the same. The more you turn *on* the tap (your blood pump) *and/or* the more you *constrict* the nozzle (the patient's vascular access) the greater the pressure generated inside the hose (the 'venous pressure'). The higher the venous pressure becomes the further the water will squirt out of the holes and the more you will lose across the 'membrane'. If the pressure becomes excessive (or if you have a faulty hose) you may burst the hose itself. If this happens during dialysis the membrane has ruptured.

What about dialysate pressure? Let's stay with the garden hose analogy. If you want to move *more* water across the membrane than the pressure inside the hose can achieve alone, it's not safe to turn the tap on any further and the nozzle cannot be safely occluded any further, the dialysate pressure must be 'negative'. Forget hygiene for the moment, if you, and several friends, placed your mouths over the holes in the hose and sucked quite hard you would assist the movement of water from inside the hose as Figure 2.1.2 shows.

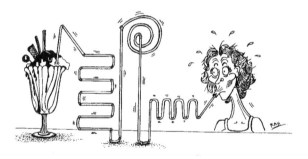

Figure 2.1.2: The contribution of negative dialysate pressure to water removal (Heintz 2000).

The combination of positive hydrostatic pressure (venous pressure) 'pushing' and the negative pressure that you create by 'pulling' achieves more water removal than venous pressure alone. The opposite is also true. Let's say you want less water removed than the venous pressure is achieving. This time you and your friends will need to oppose the water that the venous pressure is pushing across the membrane. You can achieve this by partially occluding the holes in the hose see Figure 2.1.3.

While this is not quite what happens during dialysis it is a good way to think of it. What actually happens during dialysis is, the pressure of dialysate leaving the dialyser is greater than the pressure of the dialysate entering the dialyser. This creates a positive dialysate compartment pressure that opposes the movement of

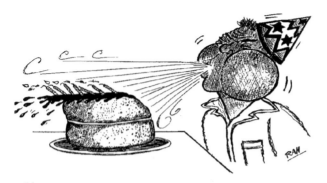

Figure 2.1.3: The contribution of positive dialysate pressure to water removal (Heintz 2000).

water from the blood compartment. Both positive and negative dialysate pressures are automatically or manually determined for each patient at the start of dialysis. **A**lthough the dialysate compartment pressure can be positive it must never exceed the patient's venous pressure.

It is rare for dialysate pressure to be displayed on modern haemodialysis machinery—but remember that the function exists. Although modern machinery reflects TMP, rather than dialysate pressure, and will alarm to alert you to problems, if you understand the principles of fluid removal you will be in a better position to effectively 'problem solve' in situations where alarm activation has occurred.

The combined pressure (TMP) needed to achieve each patient's required weight loss can be determined using the following equation:

$$TMP = \text{Fluid loss desired} \div (K_{uf} \times \text{hours for dialysis})$$

e.g. Where fluid loss is deemed to be 3000 mls, dialyser K_{uf} is 6.2mls and the time needed for dialysis is 5 hours, the TMP = 3000mls ÷ (6.2 x 5 hrs) = 97mmHg.

If the patient's venous pressure (VP) is 50mmHg a *negative* dialysate pressure of 47mmHg is required. If the patient's VP is 120 then a *positive* dialysate pressure of 23mmHg is required.

Some dialysis machines require the operator to manually program the TMP needed for fluid loss during dialysis while others only require the operator to determine the fluid loss required In this case the machine will automatically compute the required TMP to ensure successful fluid loss. Some older machines require a calculation of *negative* pressure, and for the figure to be programmed manually by the operator; if fluid loss exceeds that occurring as a result of venous pressure only, fluid *replacement,* either orally or intravenously is required.

When determining the amount of fluid to be removed during a given dialysis episode, factors such as 'prime,' the amount of 0.9% NaCl that is used to remove air from the dialyser and lines prior to commencing dialysis, and 'wash back', the amount of 0.9% NaCl that you will use to return the patient's blood at the end of dialysis, as well as fluid intake (and occasionally output) during dialysis need to be considered if the patient is to complete the dialysis session at their correct base weight.

One does not normally increase the Qb or induce alterations to the patient's venous pressure, to achieve fluid removal during dialysis. Alterations to fluid removal are a consequence of Qb and venous pressures. The only appropriate means of altering TMP to achieve the fluid loss required during dialysis is to alter the DP or fluid volume.

1.4 Isolated ultrafiltration

An alternative approach

During conventional dialysis, fluid and solute removal occur simultaneously. Hypotension is a frequent occurrence as a direct result of fluid removal and will be addressed in more detail in the section entitled related extracorporeal therapies. It is important for the common causes and appropriate nursing interventions to be understood early in the learning process. Put simply, when the removal of fluid from the vascular compartment exceeds the ability of the body to replace the volume with fluid from other body compartments, hypotension, sometimes profound, can occur.

Isolated ultrafiltration is the removal of body fluid only. No dialysate moves through the dialysate compartment, so there is no diffusive movement of solute. The procedure can be undertaken alone (in 'isolation') if only fluid is to be removed, or 'in sequence' if both solute and water are to be removed (sequential dialysis). During sequential dialysis the fluid removal process can be programmed to occur before, during, or after solute removal, and it may be employed to remove all, or part, of the interdialytic fluid gain.

The aim of sequential dialysis is to achieve asymptomatic fluid removal.

Separating the processes of water and solute removal can assist many patients and their carers avoid the problems associated with hypotension.

1.5 Patient Education

The importance of nursing involvement

For the majority of patients, nurses are the most frequently encountered health care professionals. Nurses are educators and their influence can occur as part of daily interaction with their patients or as part of specifically designed education sessions. In either case, nurses' attitude impact significantly on their patient's approach to illness, and influences their attitudes to, compliance with, food and fluid restrictions and to complex drug regimes.

Compliance with food and fluid restrictions are important if the overall goal of improving the quality of life of patients with end stage renal failure is to be achieved. Patients find fluid restriction especially difficult, and as a consequence can develop hypertension, cardiovascular disease, and pulmonary and peripheral oedema. Symptomatic fluid removal while undergoing dialysis is also required.

The inability to comprehend the need for fluid restrictions is the basis for many an argument between patients and their carers, and an empathetic attitude on the part of the nurse, combined with correct information, can go a substantial way towards problem solving.

References

In text references

ANZDATA Registry Report 1999, 'Australian and New Zealand Dialysis and Transplant Registry, Adelaide, South Australia.

Chang, R., 1988, 'Chemistry', 3rd ed., Random House, New York.

Daugirdas, J., Van Stone, J., 2001, 'Physiologic principles and Urea Kinetic Modeling' in *Handbook of Dialysis*, Daugirdas, J., Blake, P., Ing, T. (eds), 3rd ed., Lippincott Williams and Wilkins.

Dawborn, J., 1990, 'Dialysis', *The Medical Journal of Australia*, vol. 152, April, pp 367–372.

Drukker, W., 1989, 'Haemodialysis: a historical review', in *Replacement of Renal Function by Dialysis*, Maher, F., (ed.), 3rd ed., Kluwer Academic Publishers, Boston.

Heintz, R, 2000, Geelong Dialysis Unit, Victoria Cartoons Drawn on Request Specifically for this publication.

Wellard, S., 1996, 'Family connections? Exploring nursing roles with families in home based care', Unpublished Ph D Thesis, La Trobe University, Melbourne.

Recommended readings

Dawborn, J., 1990, 'Dialysis', *The Medical Journal of Australia*, vol. 152, April, pp 367-372.

Jenson, B., Dobbe, S., Squillace, D., McCarthy, J., 1994, 'Clinical Benefits of High and Variable Sodium Concentration in Hemodialysis Patients', *ANNA Journal,* vol. 21, no. 2, April, pp 115–116, 121.

Pierratos, A., Ouwendyk, M., Francoeur, R., Wallace, L., Sit, W., Vas, S., Uldall, R. (1995) 'Slow Nocturnal Haemodialysis', *Dialysis and Transplantation*, vol 4, no 10, October, pp 557–558,576.

Spital, A., (Series editor) 2001, 'Ethical issues in dialysis', *Seminars in Dialysis*, vol. 14, no. 1, p 22.

Friedman, E., 2001, 'Must we treat noncompliant ESRD patients?' *Seminars in Dialysis*, vol. 14, no. 1, pp 23–27.

Balint, J., 2001, 'There is a duty to treat noncompliant dialysis patients' *Seminars in Dialysis*, vol. 14, no. 1, pp 28–31.

Vascular access

Introduction

Haemodialysis requires direct access to the patient's blood compartment. The access can be permanent, as is seen in patients with end stage renal disease where maintenance dialysis is required to sustain life, or temporary, as occurs in acute renal failure when recovery of renal function is anticipated. In either case, the success of the dialysis procedure relies on creating and maintaining functional vascular access.

2.1 The development of vascular access for haemodialysis

Significant history of vascular access

Willem Kolff in the Netherlands performed the first reported successful haemodialysis where a patient survived and recovered in 1945. Vascular access was achieved by inserting wide bore glass cannulae into large vessels. Vessel availability was limited, consequently haemodialysis was only offered to patients with acute renal failure expected to resolve after a limited number of treatments (Drukker 1989, p 33).

In 1960 the development of the arteriovenous shunt enabled long-term access to the blood stream, and, for the first time, haemodialysis became available as a treatment for end stage renal disease. The first shunt was developed by Quinton, Dillard, and Scribner and consisted of two rigid Teflon 'vessel tips', one of which was implanted into a vein and the other into an artery. A short piece of silicon tubing (6–8 inches long) was then connected to each vessel tip, and a short, rigid Teflon connector joined the two. When dialysis was required, the connector was removed and the two pieces of silicon were connected to the extracorporeal circuit. When dialysis was completed, the silicon tubes were rejoined with a new, sterile connector. When not in use blood flowed continually through the shunt from artery to vein.

All forms of vascular access were associated with numerous complications, primarily related to clotting and infection, and it soon became apparent that other forms of access needed to be developed. A variety of shunts were developed during this early period in the history of dialysis but very few remain in use today.

Drs. James Cimino and Michael Brescia first reported the use of venipuncture for repeated haemodialysis in 1966. They used peripheral vein cannulation (as opposed to the earlier cannulation of large veins) and created a fistula between an artery and a vein. The selected vessels were usually in the forearm, and the high pressure of arterial blood prematurely entering the venous system dilated the vein. The vein eventually became permanently distended and thick walled enabling repeated cannulation with the wide bore needles necessary for successful haemodialysis.

Types of vascular access

Vascular access can be divided into four groups; internal, external, percutaneous and hybrid. A brief description of each group follows:

1. Internal devices

 i) native arteriovenous fistulae

 ii) graft arteriovenous fistulae.

Internal devices are preferred for access to the circulation because there are fewer complications associated with their use than with other forms of vascular access. A native fistula created by using the patient's own vessels, is the first choice, and the method of construction is the same as that developed by Cimino and Brescia. A 'graft' fistula is considered if the patient's vessels appear limited and unlikely to support the construction of a native fistula. The graft can be formed from the patient's own vessels, usually a saphenous vein graft, or from a variety of synthetic materials for example, polytetrafluoroethylene [PTFE].

The graft forms a subcutaneous 'bridge' between the patient's artery and vein, and again the forearm vessels are preferred. A 'straight' bridging graft is usually used to join the radial artery at the wrist to the basilic vein in the antecubital fossa. A 'loop' bridging graft usually joins the basilic vein (again in the antecubital fossa) to the brachial artery. Complications include clotting, infection, stenosis and aneurysms at sites where repeated cannulation weakens the vessels or the graft material.

2. External devices

The arteriovenous shunt is the only type of vascular access in this category. It is seldom used, but is included here to complete the categorization of vascular access. External devices were reviewed in the previous section and will not be discussed further.

3. Percutaneously inserted central venous catheters

i)   subclavian catheter

ii)   jugular venous catheter

iii)   femoral vein catheter.

The insertion, use and nursing care of these catheters are important for the survival of the catheter and the well being of the patient. These issues are addressed in detail in the following section.

4. Hybrid devices

i)   Bentley Button®

ii)   Hemasite®

Hybrid devices are a combination of an external portion, which is visible on the skin surface exiting between muscles on the upper arm or thigh, and an internal portion to which it is attached. One end of the internal portion is sutured to an artery and the other to a vein. The external portion contains a self-sealing port that offers 'no needle' dialysis (Aguilar, 1982).

These devices are expensive and are primarily of historical interest, however describing them is a good basis from which to introduce a new form of fully implantable vascular access known as the LifeSite®. This device consists of a subcutaneous valve usually located on the chest wall that is attached to the patient's vessel via a venous cannula. Vascular access is obtained by inserting a needle directly into the domed top of the valve.

2.2 Vascular access creation and revision

Internal devices

The construction of a reliable native or graft fistula depends on the availability of a surgeon experienced in creating vascular access for haemodialysis, usually a vascular surgeon. Vessels in the forearm of the non dominant arm are preferred. Once created, it is usually six to eight weeks before the device can be cannulated. The forearm is also the preferred site for graft fistulae, which can be cannulated usually between two and four weeks after they are constructed, depending on the material selected.

Both these access devices provide reliable blood flow and easy cannulation for many years. Complications may necessitate modification or replacement of the access. Skilled nursing management and thorough patient education are required to diminish the likelihood of such complications (Panno and Powell 1989).

General anaesthesia is sometimes required, but adequate analgesia is usually achieved with a regional nerve block. A mild sedative is often administered to alleviate anxiety.

Percutaneously inserted central venous catheters

Historically, the arteriovenous shunt was used to enable dialysis in patients who did not have a fistula, or for whom the fistula was unsuitable for cannulation. In recent years, new technology and materials with improved biocompatibility have made a centrally inserted vascular catheter the preferred means by which dialysis can be provided when peripheral vascular access is unavailable.

Centrally inserted catheters have a single, double or triple lumen and can be inserted into the subclavian, jugular vein or femoral vein. Catheters placed into the jugular or femoral veins are generally intended for short term use while those placed into the subclavian vein are used for either short or long term use.

(Athirakul and Schwab 1996).

2.3 Nursing management of vascular access

Peripheral vascular access

Patients with peripheral vascular access devices are at risk of thrombosis of the access, development of areas of stenosis, which make cannulation difficult, aneurysm formation and the risk of vessel rupture, local or systemic infection, haemorrhage and negative alterations to their self concept. The likelihood of developing these complications can be minimised by skilled nursing management prior to, and following surgery, and before, during and after cannulation.

Central vascular access

Preventing infection, haemorrhage and altered self-concept is important for patients with central venous access. In addition, the following precautions are required:

- The presence of comorbid conditions, such as a single lung could preclude the insertion of a subclavian catheter. If a catheter is required it should only be attempted on the opposite to the functioning lung.

- Femoral catheters are often preferred if a single procedure is anticipated, e.g. following exogenous poisoning.

- Chest X-ray, undertaken to confirm the safe positioning of the catheter should always be performed before dialysis is commenced because of the hazards associated with inserting a central vein catheter.

- The patient should always be visible during treatment, not sleeping under a blanket. If not, cardiac arrest can occur without being detected because arterial and venous pressure alarms do not always activate to alert carers to the fact that systemic circulation has ceased (Uldall 1988, p 190).

2.4 Cannulation of vascular access

Cannulation techniques

Most nurses new to dialysis find the prospect of cannulation the most stressful aspect of their job. So, if you are feeling concerned, you are not alone. All dialysis nurses have experienced what you are feeling at some stage of their careers.

The patient's vascular access is often described as their 'lifeline' and should always be treated with the utmost care. The patient and the nurse both play important roles in maintaining the lifeline and both need specific education. This section only addresses those aspects relating to staff. Patient education is addressed later in the chapter.

Most patients dialyse three times a week, inserting two fistula needles each time. While convention refers to an 'arterial' and a 'venous' needle, neither needle is inserted into an artery; both needles are inserted into the fistula, which is either an arterialised vein or a graft. The term 'venous' needle refers to the needle that is inserted into the proximal portion of the fistula and returns blood to the patient. The 'arterial' needle is inserted into the distal portion of the fistula and delivers blood to the dialyser. Many techniques are used to successfully cannulate vascular access: the following techniques accord with current practice in most contemporary dialysis units.

The venous needle is traditionally inserted with the bevel uppermost and aligned with the direction of blood flow (antegrade placement). The arterial needle is also inserted with the bevel uppermost and may point distally (retrograde placement) or proximally (antegrade placement). With few exceptions, the needle is introduced into the fistula at a 45° angle. Once the needle *tip* is *fully inserted* in the fistula, the 45° angle is reduced allowing complete introduction of the needle in a manner that accords with the alignment of the patient's fistula. Following insertion, the needle can be rotated 180° so that the bevel is facing downwards.

It is usual to vary needle puncture sites, and to cannulate along the entire length of the access. Local anaesthetic can be used to decrease sensation in the needle site prior to cannula placement (Brouwer 1995 pp 608–609). This method of cannulation is known as the 'rope ladder' technique. Two alternative methods of cannulation are also described.

1.   The 'button hole' method requires two pairs (usually) of cannulation sites to be selected. Following maturation of the fistula, needles are inserted into *exactly* the

same site for each dialysis, in the identical path of the previous cannulation. Proponents of this method claim that it results in less vascular trauma and prolongs the life of the vessel (Twardowski 1995 p 560).

2. 'Area' cannulation involves the selection of two or three sites where needles are inserted into the area surrounding the selected sites at each dialysis. This usually results in the formation of aneurysms that are separated by stenoses. This method is not generally recommended, but is be difficult to discourage because the dilated areas become 'easy' to needle, and the area is usually relatively pain free due to repeated cannulation and subsequent scar formation. Patients and staff should be cautioned against the use of this method unless there is no alternative.

When securing the needles with tape after cannulation, take care not to change the direction of the needle in the fistula or to tape so firmly that the bevel of the needle presses against the fistula wall. In patients with an aneurysm it may be necessary to support the needle with gauze or cotton wool placed underneath the wings of the needle. Use your fingertip to ensure the needle tip is not pressing against the wall of the fistula.

When removing the cannula at the completion of dialysis it is important to use strict aseptic techniques that do not traumatise the access, and to achieve haemostasis before the patient leaves the unit.

2.5 Complications

Summation

While the development of permanent vascular access has enabled haemodialysis for patients with end stage renal disease, the creation and use vascular access devices is complicated by a number of difficulties. Some patients have a vascular access that functions well for many years while others have complications from the outset and return frequently for modification or re-siting of the access.

Peripheral vascular access

Thrombosis, stenosis and infection are among the most common complications encountered. Thrombosis can occur during the immediate post operative period or after years of haemodialysis. Common causes are inadequate communication between the artery and the vein at the time of anastomosis, obstruction, stenosis, fibrosis and coagulopathy. Infection can be due to operative contamination, contamination of the needle during cannulation or skin infection that allows inoculation of the fistula with pathogenic organisms.

The high pressure of arterial blood entering the venous system prematurely via the fistula can cause congestive cardiac problems for some patients. Others develop venous engorgement or ischaemia in the hand of their access arm. Aneurysm formation is often seen in fistulae and occasionally causes the vessel to rupture.

Central vascular access

Pneumothorax, haemothorax, haemorrhage, cardiac arrhythmias and infection are among the most serious complications. Nerve injury, which is usually transient, can occur to the brachial plexus or the femoral nerve. Subclavian vein thrombosis was recently recognised as a complication of central vascular access and some practitioners do not consider subclavian vein catheterisation an appropriate method to achieve dialysis in patients without a functional vascular access.

Central subclavian vein occlusion, presenting as upper extremity oedema, occurs in patients who have permanent vascular access on the same side as prior subclavian vein catheterization. For this reason, most practitioners avoid subclavian vein catheterisation as a first line treatment. If it is required, the catheter is inserted on the opposite side to that in which the permanent access is constructed. It may be prudent to use progressive Doppler studies to assess blood flow through the subclavian vein. Anticoagulant therapy could prevent permanent occlusion if it is commenced before the clot becomes organised, and therefore not amenable to routine anticoagulant therapy.

2.6 Patient education

The role of the nurse

Patients undergoing maintenance haemodialysis vary in their ability to care for their vascular access. Many find the learning process difficult, especially when their cognitive ability is reduced due to the effects of uraemia.

Patients who are dialysing in their own homes need to learn cannulation skills similar to those learned by nurses. They also need to be able to problem solve, acquire an understanding of anticoagulation therapy, understand and apply infection control techniques and recognise risk factors that could threaten the viability of their fistula. Patients who are not responsible for their dialysis still need to be able to recognise risk factors, the same as the home dialysis patient, and should know when to contact the hospital in case of emergency.

References

In text references

Aguilar, M., 1982, 'Early Experience with the Hemasite Vascular Access Shunt'. *Nephrology Nurse,* May-June 1982, pp 36-39.

Brouwer, D., 1995, 'Cannulation Camp: basic needle cannulation training for dialysis staff', *Dialysis and Transplantation*, vol. 24, no 11, pp 606–612.

Drukker, W., 1989, 'Haemodialysis: a historical review', in *Replacement of Renal Function by Dialysis*, Maher, F., (ed.), 3rd ed., Kluwer Academic Publishers, Boston.

Panno, N., Powell, C., 1989, 'The Creation, Care and Complications of Subcutaneous Haemodialysis Access', *Dialysis and Transplantation*, vol. 18, no. 6, June 1989, pp 308–318.

Twardowski, Z., 1995. 'Constant Site (Buttonhole) Method of Needle Insertion for Hemodialysis', *Dialysis and Transplantation,* vol, 24, no. 10, pp559–560, 576.

Uldall, R., 1988, 'How should temporary vascular access for haemodialysis be achieved?' *Seminars in Dialysis*, vol. 1, no. 4, pp 189–190.

Recommended reading

Berkoben, M., Schwab, S., 1995, 'Maintenance of Permanent Hemodialysis Vascular Access Patency', *ANNA Journal*, vol. 22, no.1, February, pp17–24.

Brunier, G., 1996, 'Care of the Hemodialysis Patient with a New Vascular Access: Review of Assessment and Teaching', *ANNA Journal*, vol. 23, no. 6, December, pp547–556.

Ouendick, M., Helferty, M., 1996, 'Central Venous Catheter Management', *ANNA Journal*, vol. 23, no. 6, December, pp572–577.

Panno, N., Powell, C., 1989, 'The Creation, Care and Complications of Subcutaneous Haemodialysis Access', *Dialysis and Transplantation*, vol. 18, no. 6, June 1989, pp 308–318.

The extracorporeal circuit

Introduction

This chapter is designed to introduce the reader to components of the extracorporeal circuit used during haemodialysis. Dialyser designs are discussed together with their advantages and disadvantages, membrane types are reviewed, as are methods of sterilisation and the preparation that is required by the nurse prior to commencing treatment.

3.1 An historical review

… in the beginning

The use of semipermeable membranes to remove solute from blood dates from 1913 when Abel, Rowntree and Turner demonstrated that metabolites could be removed from the blood of animals by passing it through tubing bathed in saline. The membrane they used was quite fragile and consisted of colloidin hand cast from cellulose nitrate. George Haas modified the technique to enable dialysis to be used in humans. Although he is credited with performing the first human dialysis, lack of a suitable anticoagulant prevented his treatments lasting long enough to be of therapeutic benefit (see Chapter 1).

The discovery of heparin assisted in the development of haemodialysis as a therapeutic modality, but it was not until 1947 when Willem Kolff developed his 'rotating drum dialyser' that dialysis became accepted as a treatment for acute renal failure. Kolff's dialyser consisted of long strips of cellulose, in the form of seamless sausage casing, which was wound around a drum. The drum was made of metal or wooden slats and was rotated continuously through a container filled with dialysate (Drukker 1989 p 20–86). Although it enabled haemodialysis to be used therapeutically, it still presented many challenges.

a) The extracorporeal volume was large, often exceeding one liter. Initial priming of the lines and dialyser with blood, not saline was required, as is used for most dialysis treatments today.

b) Fluid removal was difficult because it was not possible to generate high positive pressures within the blood circuit. The addition of an osmotically active substance to the dialysate to enable fluid to be drawn across the membrane was needed.

c) Additional problems with fluid balance were caused by the lack of support of the outer surface of the membrane, allowing extra-corporeal volumes to fluctuate quite widely during treatment.

(Drukker 1989 p 20–86, Lysaght 1995 pp 1–9).

However, it was a start, and provided not only the framework for improvement, but it also prolonged many lives.

During the 1940's and 1950's regenerated cellulose, under a variety of trade names, remained the most widely used material in the manufacture of dialysers. Cellulose is a polysaccharide, which occurs widely in nature as the structural polymer of cotton, wood and many plants. To enable it to be used in treatments such as dialysis cellulose must first be purified and refashioned. This is achieved by dissolving the original polymer, reshaping the resultant substance, and reconstituting it either as a fibre, for hollow fibre designs, or a film, for flat plate designs. Alternatives, such as modified cellulose were introduced in the 1960's and synthetic membranes became commercially available during the 1970's (Lysaght 1995, pp 1–10).

Many different dialyser designs were tried during these early years. The 'hollow fibre' dialyser was the first, and was refined by Stewart to incorporate an outer perspex jacket. A 'flat plate' design, developed by Skeggs and Leonard, and a 'coil' dialyser, with many design modifications, followed.

The development of a permanent form of vascular access in the early 1960's (see Chapter 2) was accompanied by the implementation of dialysis as a treatment for end stage renal failure (ESRD). During this time the Kiil flat plate dialyser and the Kolff twin-coil dialyser were the two most popular designs. These early dialysers were not disposable. Disassembly, cleaning, reassembly and sterilisation were required between uses. This was not a favourite task of pioneer dialysis nurses.

Modern dialysers are either of the hollow fibre or flat plate design. There are other designs and the interested reader is referred to the recommended readings at the conclusion of this section.

3.2 Dialyser design

Hollow fibre dialysers

Hollow fibre dialysers are the most popular design in use in Australia at the time of writing. They consist of multiple hollow fibres; either cellulose or synthetic, with a surface area of between 1 and 2 meters square for an average adult. Much smaller surface area dialysers are available for use with children and neonates. These fibres, usually between 7000 and 15 000 in number for adults are called 'fibre bundles'. The fibre bundles are supported at each end of the dialyser in a polyurethane substance known as 'potting mix'. The potting mix/fibre bundle cohort is called the 'tube sheet'.

A plastic casing known as the dialyser housing surrounds the fibres and supporting structures. The blood inlet and outlet manifolds, known as 'headers', are cylindrical caps covering the tube sheets, and they can (usually) be screwed away from the body of the dialyser housing.

One of the main advantages of hollow fibre dialyser design is the *non compliant* nature of the membrane. This means that the fibres resist expansion in response to pressure changes, enabling them to retain a stable dimension and therefore a predictable K_{uf} over a range of blood flow rates. One of the major disadvantages is the possibility that the potting mix will retain the sterilising agent ethylene oxide (ETO). ETO is an extremely toxic substance that can cause anaphylactic reactions in previously sensitised people (Van Stone 1996, p 30).

Thorough rinsing prior to patient connection according to the manufacturer's guidelines for the recommended volume enables hollow fibre dialysers to be used safely. The need for thorough rinsing is less of a problem now that alternatives to gaseous/chemical sterilisation are available. Hollow fibre dialysers are also considered to increase the likelihood of clotting Increased doses of anticoagulant are often required compared to flat plate dialysers.

One potential problem with hollow fibre dialysers is the possibility of 'backfiltration'. Backfiltration can occur when the dialysate pressure at the outlet port exceeds the patient's venous pressure, which allows unsterile dialysate to enter the patient's blood. Although this possibility has always existed, it is only since the use of highly permeable dialyser membranes that clinical safety has been questioned (Gambro Basics, 1995, Section 4, p 19).

Parallel plate dialysers

Parallel plate dialysers, also known as flat plate dialysers, consist of sheets of membrane mounted on support screens and stacked in multiple layers. As is the case with the hollow fibre design, an outer plastic jacket surrounds both the blood and dialysate compartments. At the inlet points, manifolds distribute the blood and dialysate into the correct compartment.

Plate dialysers are said to have a 'compliant membrane', meaning that it will stretch more readily than hollow fibre membranes. This can be a disadvantage as higher blood flow rates can increase both the ultrafiltration capacity of the dialyser and its priming volume. In reality, stretch rarely causes a problem, because the manufacturer states the K_{uf} and the priming volume for a range of blood flow rates. It is of even less consequence when volumetric fluid loss is used. The compliant nature of the membrane can be an advantage in some situations. For example, when single needle dialysis is required there is no need to provide a compliance chamber for the extra-corporeal circuit because the blood compartment of the dialyser will expand without rupturing as the pressure in the circuit increases.

There is less risk of ETO infusion with parallel plate dialysers because no potting mix is used to provide membrane support. However, it is still necessary to rinse the dialyser with the recommended amount of fluid prior to connecting it to the patient.

3.3 Membranes

From past to present

As mentioned in Section 1, early membranes were made from cellulose, the structural polymers of cotton and many plants and trees. In its natural state cellulose is unsuited for contact with body fluids that are to be returned to the patient. Purifying the polymer and 'refabricating' it into the desired shape, either hollow fibre or flat plate confers partial biocompatibility. This is achieved by one of two processes:

a)   Solution spinning, where the polymer is dissolved in a chemical solvent and refabricated by extrusion through a mould.

b)   Melt spinning, where high temperatures are used to dissolve the material before following a similar process for shape design.

Both of these processes produce what is called 'regenerated cellulose' and the refabricated product is marketed under a variety of trade names (Radovich 1995, p11).

The chemical structure of cellulose membranes, even after regeneration and purification, retain elements that activate the immune system and elicit a variety of responses from the patient that are discussed in Section 5). The ions responsible are free hydroxyl (OH^-) groups that are a part of the cellulose molecule. In an effort to minimise these immunological responses a number of modifications to the membrane structure have been attempted.

These modifications have been achieved by either camouflaging the OH^- ion so that the body does not recognise it as foreign, or by binding the OH^- ion with another substance and then removing the resultant combination from the regenerated membrane. Where the free OH^- groups have been bound with acetate (the correct term is 'esterising'), the membrane is known as cellulose acetate. Where the OH^- groups are bound with a tertiary amine, the membrane is known as Haemophan (Lysaght 1995, pp 5–6). These modified membranes seem to be a convenient 'half way' step between the original regenerated cellulose and the newer synthetic membranes.

A truly biocompatible membrane probably does not exist, at least at the time of writing. Synthetic membranes, however, were a major advance towards achieving this goal. The AN 69 membrane, a copolymer of acrylonitrile and aryl sulphonate, was the first to be introduced and was followed by polysulphone and polyamide. They are mostly used for haemofiltration and were first used for haemodialysis in the 1980's. These three membranes are derived from petrochemicals and their adaptation for use in haemodialysis forms a small part of their application in numerous fields of engineering. The membrane structure leads to larger pore size with corresponding increases in ultrafiltration rates and diffusive solute transport (Lysaght 1995, pp 5–6).

3.4 Sterilisation methods

From old to new

The first sterilant used for early dialysis procedures was formalin, which remains in use in some renal units that reprocess (reuse) their dialysers and/or blood lines (see Section 6 of this chapter).

The most common method used to sterilise contemporary dialysers is exposure to the gas ethylene oxide (ETO). In many ways, this was a natural consequence of the development of dry and disposable dialysers, because it made preparation and shipment much easier. Today ETO is used in the preparation of many disposable medical supplies and has provided major health benefits because bacterial contamination has been markedly reduced. ETO is a highly reactive gas that is both flammable and explosive. It diffuses easily through porous membranes and is thought to achieve elimination of bacteria and other pathogens by disrupting nucleic acid synthesis and preventing cell replication. Its advantages as a sterilising agent include the fact that it has been used safely and effectively for many years, and it is simple to use and is reasonably cheap. The disadvantages include possible carcinogenic potential with long-term occupational exposure, its volatile nature and, for dialysis patients, the potential for hypersensitivity reactions (Daugirdas et al. 2001, pp 104–105, Gambro Basics, 1995, Section 4, p 19).

Steam sterilisation is becoming increasingly popular and is able to destroy many pathogens in a short time. Its use is limited by the ability of the device being sterilised to withstand high temperatures, moisture and pressure. Dialysis membranes are damaged by steam sterilisation and must be protected by pretreating them with glycerin. ETO and steam are unable to sterilise material without being directly contact with it. Therefore, all compartments of the dialyser must be left open and blood connection ports left unsealed during sterilisation. It is a highly biocompatible method of sterilisation and therefor causes no adverse reactions in the patient.

After steam sterilisation some dialysers are left filled with water as additional protection for the membrane. Before connecting the dialyser to the patient the extracorporeal volume should be discarded or recirculated for approximately 15 minutes with the dialysate flowing to enable the extra-corporeal fluid to reach isotonic levels. This process will prevent the patient from receiving an initial bolus of hypotonic saline when dialysis is commenced (Gambro Basics, 1995, Section 4, p 19).

A third method of sterilisation uses ionizing radiation. About one third of dialysers worldwide are sterilized by exposure to gamma rays (Cobalt 60) to split RNA and DNA strands, preventing microbial replication in a similar manner to ETO but without the potential side effects of ETO exposure. Gamma ray sterilisation does not require ports to remain unsealed as ETO and steam do, but the sterilisation process can damage the membrane so membrane protection with glycerine is required as with steam sterilisation.

Personal safety

A discussion of the issues involved in preventing cross infection between patients and/or staff members could appropriately be included in a variety of chapters. It is included here as most issues relate to either, the extracorporeal circuit, or its establishment.

When cannulating a patient, initiating the extracorporeal circuit, or intervening in an established circuit, staff should always wear gloves, protective clothing and protective eyewear. When gloves are potentially contaminated e.g. at the completion of cannulation, they should be changed before initiating blood flow through the circuit. Additional precautions, e.g. masks, are required if the patient has been infected with an organism that is transmitted during respiration, especially if coughing is one of the symptoms.

The prevalence of Hepatitis B and C among the dialysis population is high, although a steady decline in the incidence of both diseases has been evident over recent years. The decline probably reflects improved viral sceening of donated blood destined for transfusion and a decrease in the number of transfusions required by dialysis patients. However, occasional outbreaks of Hepatitis B continue to occur in dialysis units around the world, and the majority of hospitals offer vaccination against Hepatitis B to staff involved in the care of dialysis patients, and to patients undergoing regular dialysis (Lentino and Leehey 2001, pp 501–504). Staff should be especially vigilant in their infection control procedures when moving between patients. Although rare, there are several documented reports of Hepatitis B outbreaks among dialysis patients (Manette et al. 1989, pp 542–555).

3.5 Membrane reactions

A number of adverse reactions are possible as a result of the patient's blood contacting the extracorporeal circuit, specifically the dialyser membrane. These reactions, fortunately uncommon, range from those causing mild discomfort to those that are responsible for cardiovascular collapse and death. The reactions usually described are discussed in the following sections.

Complement reactions

When blood comes into contact with the membrane in dialysers using regenerated cellulose, the complement cascade is activated. This occurs when the free OH^-

groups on the cellulose membrane react chemically with complement factor three (C3), splitting it into C3a and C3b (Lysaght 1995, p 4). This results in sufficient systemic complement activation to produce a transient neutropenia, which is usually fully reversed by the conclusion of dialysis, as demonstrated by the white cell count. When the mobilised neutrophils move from the dialyser back into the circulation, they sequester in the first capillary bed they encounter; the pulmonary capillaries and the pulmonary surface area available for gaseous exchange is reduced. This appears to be a phenomena seen in *all* patients dialysed against regenerated cellulose membranes, however the majority remain asymptomatic.

Hypersensitivity

Hypersensitivity is variously described by a variety of authors as 'type A' and 'type B', 'type 1' and 'type 2' or 'mild' and 'severe', the best way to understand these reactions is to recognise that one is potentially life threatening and the other is not!

Mild hypersensitivity (the 'first use' syndrome):

In susceptible individuals mild hypersensitivity usually occurs *every time* a new dialyser is used. It is also known as the 'new dialyser' reaction. Some people use response from the patient to argue for dialyser reuse. Symptoms are usually mild, and occur during the first hour of dialysis. The patient complains of shortness of breath, low back or chest pain and nausea or vomiting. Some studies indicate an increased incidence of hypotension and non-specific fatigue following dialysis sessions. Symptoms usually subside during the dialysis session and there is seldom any need to discontinue treatment. It is not known whether mild hypersensitivity has a different pathogenesis from the severe form, or is simply milder.

Severe hypersensitivity

Although signs and symptoms are usually apparent during the first few minutes of dialysis, they can be delayed for up to thirty minutes. The patient complains of dyspnoea and a burning sensation, either at the access site, or throughout the entire body. Itching is common with urticaria, rhinorrhoea, and lacrimation, which can progress to angioedema, cardiovascular collapse and cardiac arrest. Causative agents include the use of EPO as a sterilising agent, and AN 69 dialyser membranes used in combination with ACE inhibitors (discussed later in this chapter). Contaminated dialysate solution and dialyser re-use have also been implicated (Bregman et al. 2001, pp 159–161). Reactions resulting from an allergic response *usually* occur during a patient's first dialysis, or during their first exposure to a cellulosic (usually regenerated cellulose) membrane.

Severe hypersensitivity also occurs in patients who have not reacted during previous dialysis if:

a)   The dialyser is inadequately rinsed.

b)   Recirculation prior to dialysis has been prolonged and the patient is connected without re-rinsing the lines.

c)   Recirculation is required *during dialysis* and blood that has been present in the lines is re-infused.

AN69 membranes

In 1990, a previously undescribed reaction was reported in patients using AN69 membranes who were taking angiotensin converting enzyme (ACE) inhibitors to treat hypertension. The proposed aetiology is as follows:

The coagulation pathway is activated when blood contacts the membrane. This initiates the generation of bradykinin from its precursors kallikrein and kininogen. Bradykinin is responsible for vasodilatation and its action is modified by the enzyme kininase. ACE inhibitors block Kininase and the subsequent increase in the hypotensive potential of bradykinin is thought to be responsible for the ensuing anaphylactoid reaction. Subsequent studies implicate AN 69 membranes in the pathogenesis of hypotension even without the concomitant use of ACE inhibitors (Churchill 1995, p 67).

The 'interleukin hypothesis'

When monocytes come into contact with the dialysis membrane (particularly regenerated cellulosic membranes) they become 'activated' and secrete the chemical mediator interleukin 1 (IL1). IL1 has a direct moderating role in the immune response. It activates T_4 cells, promotes fever, sleepiness, and increases the production of prostaglandins PGE_2, resulting in cerebral vasodilatation and headache, and PGI_2, resulting in generalised vasodilatation and hypotension. IL1 also promotes the degranulation of basophils, releasing histamine, and neutrophils, releasing lysozyme. These responses are thought to be responsible for many of the acute phase reactions of haemodialysis, as well as several of the longer term 'inflammatory' complications (Dinarello, Kock and Shaldon 1988, pp S 21–S26).

There are several ways nurses can reduce the likelihood of hypersensitivity reactions in their patients:

a) Always read *and follow* the manufacturer's instructions for rinsing the dialyser prior to connecting it to the patient.

b) Be alert to the patient with a history of allergic responses, such as asthma, dermatitis and 'hay fever'.

c) Rerinse ETO sterilised dialysers if longer than 20 minutes has elapsed between preparing them and connecting them to the patient, *especially* a patient undergoing an initial dialysis treatment.

3.6 Circuit reuse

The reuse of dialysers and blood lines

After the initial use of a dialyser, it can be rinsed with 0·9% NaCl to remove residual blood or chemically cleaned, usually with bleach, and then sterilised with a disinfectant, usually formalin to enable it to be reused. It is also possible to reuse the blood lines but this is practiced less frequently. Dialysers processed in this manner are reused on a varying number of occasions. The exact number depends on the policy of the unit, the membrane used and the efficacy of the rinsing procedure.

The advantages claimed for dialyser reuse are a decrease in the first use syndrome. Remember this usually only occurs the *first* time a new dialyser is used, but only if bleach is not used, cost savings, and a reduction in the amount of environmentally *un*friendly disposables.

Disadvantages include staff exposure to the cleaning and sterilisation chemicals, the possibility of dialyser contamination, cross infection, for this reason dialysers should only ever be reused on the same patient, and the increase in staff time needed to process the dialyser and to prepare it for patient connection. Some people also question the reuse of a product clearly labelled 'for single use only'. Any dialysis product prepared for reuse should be clearly labelled with the chemicals used.

Removal of these products before connecting the apparatus to the patient should be verified with an appropriate reagent and checked by two staff members to avoid errors.

Hollow fibre dialysers can lose a proportion of their surface area due to closure, or blockage, of fibres. Modern processing equipment can calculate the extent of fibre reduction enabling adjustment to dialysis time and/or TMP, should it be required.

Reuse is uncommon in Australia at the time of writing. It is common in the United States of America and to a lesser extent in Europe.

3.7 Bloodlines

Materials and function

The bloodlines deliver blood *from* the patient *to* the dialyser—the 'arterial' portion, and return dialysed blood *from* the dialyser *to* the patient—the 'venous portion'. Both arterial and venous sections are made from polyvinyl chloride (PVC) with a softer section designed specifically to fit between the blood pump housing and the rotor. Sampling ports are located on both the arterial and venous sections but are often absent on the arterial section between the patient and the blood pump. This absence is usually due to the negative pressure that exists in this portion of the circuit and the corresponding risk of drawing air into the blood lines and dialyser. A projection is available in the pre-pump portion of the arterial line to enable connection to an IV infusion (usually 0·9%NaCl); all connections, including those to the dialyser, should attach with Luer lock connections to reduce the possibility of accidental disconnection. Pressure monitoring devices are provided to enable monitoring of arterial and venous pressures during treatment and are always separated from the dialysis machine by a transducer protector (isolators). Some isolators cannot function properly if they become wet with either blood or saline during treatment and should be changed to ensure correct pressure measurement.

To ensure predictable blood flow rates, the rotor assembly should not under-occlude the blood pump segment, and the arterial portion of the blood lines should not be overly compliant. It is important to correctly rinse the bloodlines as well as the dialyser because plasticisers can leach from the lines and become lodged in the patient's tissues. ETO is the most common form of sterilisation for bloodlines and residual ETO needs to be removed as it does with dialysers. Gamma sterilisation has been used for blood lines but is not popular as the lines become discoloured and look unpleasant.

References

In text references

Bregman, H., Daugirdas, J., Ing, T., 1994, Complications during hemodialysis', in *Handbook of Dialysis*, Daugidas, J., Blake, P., Ing, T., (eds.), 3rd ed., Lippincott Williams and Wilkins, Philadelphia.

Churchill, D., 1995, 'Efficiency and biocompatibility of membranes', in *Dialysis Membranes: Structure and Predictions*, Binominal, V., Berland, Y. (eds.), Karger, Sydney.

Daugirdas, J., Ross, E., Nissenson, A., 2001, 'Acute haemodialysis prescription', in *Handbook of Dialysis*, Daugirdas, J., Blake, P., Ing, T., (eds.), 3rd ed., Lippincott Williams and Wilkins, Philadelphia.

Dinarello, C., Kock, K., Shaldon, S. 1988, 'Interleukin 1 and its relevance in patients treated with haemodialysis', *Kidney International*, S24, March, pp S21–S26.

Drukker, W., 1989, 'Haemodialysis: a historical review', in *Replacement of Renal Function by Dialysis*, Maher, F., (ed.), 3rd ed., Kluwer Academic Publishers, Boston.

Gambro Basics Part 4, 1995,'The Dialyser', Gambro Lundia AB, Lund. Sweden.

Lentino, J., Leehey, D., 2001, 'Special problems in the dialysis patient: infections', in *Handbook of Dialysis*, Daugidas, J., Blake, P., Ing, T., (eds.), 3rd ed., Lippincott Williams and Wilkins, Philadelphia.

Lysaght, M., 1995. 'Evolution of haemodialysis membranes' in *Dialysis Membranes: Structure and Predictions* Bonomoni, V., Berland, Y. (eds.), Karger, Sydney.

Manette, N., Penberthy, L., Alter, M., Armstrong, C., Miller, G., Hadler, S. 1989, 'Hemodialysis-Associated Hepatitis B: Report of an Outbreak'. *Dialysis and Transplantation*, vol. 18, no. 10, October, pp 542–555.

Public Health Laboratory Service Survey, 1976, 'Hepatitis B in retreat from dialysis units in the United Kingdom', *British Medical Journal*, vol.1 pp 1570–1581.

Radovich, J. 1995. 'Composition of polymer membranes for therapies of end stage renal disease' in *Dialysis Membranes: Structure and Predictions* Bonomoni, V., Berland, Y. (eds.), Karger, Sydney.

Daugirdas, J., Van Stone, J., Boag, J., 2001, 'Haemodialysis apparatus', in *Handbook of Dialysis*, Daugidas, J., Blake, P., Ing, T., (eds.), 3rd ed., Lippincott Williams and Wilkins, Philadelphia.

Recommended reading

Bonomoni, V., Berland, Y., 1995, *Dialysis Membranes: Structure and Predictions*. Karger, Sydney.

Henrich, W., 1999, (ed.), *Principles and Practice of Dialysis*, (2nd ed.), Williams and Wilkins, Maryland.

Schulman, G., Levin, N. 1994, 'Membranes for Hemodialysis', *Seminars in Dialysis*, vol. 7, no. 4, July-August, pp 251–256.

Stragier, A. 1992, 'Hazards With Disinfecting Agents in Renal Units', *ANNA Journal*, vol.19, no. 1, pp41–43, 87.

Anticoagulation

Introduction

This chapter encourages an exploration of the coagulation cascade, provides a review of traditional methods of anticoagulation during haemodialysis, and offers the opportunity to assess alternatives to the prevention of coagulation in the extra-corporeal circuit during dialysis.

4.1 The coagulation cascade

Activation of the coagulation cascade

Blood is pumped through vessels in the body under pressure. As a result, any disturbance to the integrity of the blood vessels results in the loss of blood. Maintenance of blood pressure is vital to the survival of the organism and the body has multiple ways of achieving adequate blood pressure. Haemostasis is the term used to describe the cessation of blood flow following injury. It involves three primary actions:

a) Vascular constriction—as a rule, the more trauma involved, the greater the degree of constriction.

b) Platelet plug formation—circulating platelets do not normally adhere to undamaged endothelial tissue. They only adhere when the subendothelial tissue is exposed by trauma.

c) Formation of blood clots—if the platelet plug is not sufficient to arrest bleeding the 'coagulation cascade' is activated and, results in the formation of a blood clot that adheres to the walls of the damaged vessel (Spence and Mason 1987, pp 516–518).

There are two mechanisms by which the coagulation cascade is activated:

a) The **intrinsic pathway**, which is initiated by contact with foreign surfaces or exposure to subendothelial tissue.

b) The **extrinsic pathway**, which requires the release of thromboplastin, a lipoprotein extruded from damaged tissue.

Activation during haemodialysis

The haemodialysis process offers multiple opportunities for activation of the coagulation cascade. Many patients experience minimal difficulty while others endure repeated clotting in the bloodlines, dialysers and access devices. Some of the most common causes are:

a) The extracorporeal circuit contains foreign material, has areas of lowered blood flow, is subjected to turbulence in a number of areas, undergoes interruption to blood flow and is subjected to heat loss.

b) The vascular access is subjected to repeated trauma during cannulation, experiences episodes of obstructed blood flow when a tourniquet is used to facilitate cannulation and during compression of the needle site following needle removal, and may be constructed using foreign material.

4.2 Anticoagulation

Anticoagulant drugs

Anticoagulant drugs interfere with the function of proteins required to activate the coagulation cascade and the ultimate formation of fibrin. Anticoagulant drugs are given for one or more of the following reasons:

a) To prevent thrombus formation.

b) To lyse an existing clot.

c) To prevent coagulation of extracorporeal circuits.

While preventing coagulation is the most frequent reason for using anticoagulants in patients undergoing haemodialysis, it should be remembered that many of these patients, especially the elderly, have comorbid conditions that require anticoagulant drugs for other reasons. Remember also, that the drugs used for these conditions can impact on anticoagulant requirements during haemodialysis. The most commonly used anticoagulants are:

a) Platelet inhibitors. Prevent the platelet aggregation and adhesion that activates both intrinsic and extrinsic pathways e.g. aspirin.

b) Thrombin inhibitors. Prevent the conversion of prothrombin to thrombin e.g. heparin.

c) Calcium binding agents. Complex with calcium and prevent it participating in the coagulation cascade e.g. tri-sodium citrate.

d) Vitamin K agonists. Disrupt the production of clotting factors whose synthesis depends on vitamin K e.g. warfarin.

e) Fibrinolytic agents. Drugs that break down the structure of stable clots e.g. urokinase.
    Please note: Genetically engineered fibrinolytic drugs also fall into this category e.g. the tissue plasminogen activators alteplase (Actilyse 10, 20, and 30), and reteplase (Rapilysin) are available for the lysis of stable clots, but they are rarely used in dialysis units.

Anticoagulation during haemodialysis

Recall that the development of the anticoagulant 'heparin' was a major step forward in the clinical application of dialysis for people with end stage renal disease, and it remains the mainstay of treatment in the majority of haemodialysis units.

Anticoagulant therapy can be administered as a 'regional' therapy that anti-coagulates the extracorporeal circuit only, or as a 'systemic' therapy that anti-coagulates the patient as well as the circuit. If the only the circuit is anticoagulated, the anticoagulant agent is administered before the dialyser and its action is reversed after the dialyser, in this way the patient is protected from the effects of the drug. The drug used for reversing the anticoagulant action of heparin is protamine sulphate. If tri-sodium citrate is the anticoagulant, it is reversed with a calcium infusion titrated to the patient's specific requirements (Hansen and Strutz 1999, p138–139).

There are disadvantages with both methods:

1. Regional anticoagulation with heparin and protamine sulphate can result in rebound anticoagulation if the heparin/protamine complex becomes unbound, anaphylaxis due to protamine sensitivity, and difficulties determining the appropriate protamine to heparin infusion.

2. Regional anticoagulation using citrate and calcium can result in systemic hypocalcaemia if sufficient calcium is not given, hypercalcaemia if too much is given, and alkalaemia resulting from citrate metabolism.

3. If the patient *and* circuit are anticoagulated, heparin is usually the drug of choice. A 'bolus' dose is administered via either the extracorporeal circuit (injected into the bloodlines) or the patient (injected into the patient during cannulation of the access device).

Anticoagulant therapy may be either continuous, where a small amount is administered through an infusion device, or intermittent, where the carer is required to administer specific amounts at prescribed intervals.

During the early years of haemodialysis 'heparin modeling' was common for all patients. This required access to bedside estimation of coagulation profiles, and a lengthy time commitment on the part of carers. This technique provided precise information about the required bolus dose of heparin, its hourly infusion rate, and the time when anticoagulants could be ceased in order to maintain satisfactory anticoagulation during treatment, but minimise the likelihood of bleeding post dialysis. This procedure is now uncommon in most units, as it has been recognised that the majority of patients respond to heparin in a predictable manner.

Patients who were at risk of bleeding e.g. those who had undergone recent surgery were usually submitted to a regimen known as 'tight heparinisation'. This involved prolonging the clotting time to no more than an *average* of 25% above the base line. While this is still practiced in many units, the preferred method of preventing clotting in the circuit is with repeated 'flushes' of normal saline, a technique commonly known as 'no heparin dialysis', or 'heparin-free dialysis' (Caruana and Keep 2001, 189–193).

Low molecular weight heparin

Apart from the difficulties associated with excessive anticoagulation, and providing adequate anticoagulation of the patient with coagulation disorders, possibly the major challenge to clinicians during recent years was the recognition of an immunologically-mediated syndrome associated with the use of heparin.

The Heparin Induced Thrombotic Thrombocytopenic Syndrome (HITTS) is an immunologically-mediated mechanism of platelet destruction, mediated by heparin-dependent antiplatelet antibodies. What this means is that the heparin molecule, by virtue of its size and derivation, is recognised as a foreign substance and the immune system becomes activated.

An immune response, mediated by immunoglobulin G commences; complement becomes fixed to platelet membranes activating the production of arachidonic acid and therefore thromboxane, platelet aggregation, adhesion and clot formation follows. The net result is a patient with a reduced platelet count and an increased likelihood of haemorrhage. The answer seems to be to use low molecular weight heparin. The heparin molecule varies in size between 5000 and 30 000 daltons (Street and McPherson 1996, p104). Molecules greater than 5000 daltons induce an immune response. The trick to preventing such a response lies in the ability to 'sieve' the crude heparin, and extract only those molecules that have a molecular weight between 4000 and 6000 daltons—a low molecular weight (Street and McPherson 1996, p104).

Anticoagulation is still effective because only a small portion of the heparin molecule is required to bind to antithrombin 111 in order to inactivate the coagulation pathway. This portion is present on both low molecular weight and conventional heparin. Because low molecular weight heparin has a longer $t^{1}/_{2}$ than unfractionated heparin, it can be given as a single predialysis dose. It causes less bleeding and improved lipid profiles, although the latter is still controversial (Ward and Aronoff 1999, p 75).

4.3 Complications associated with anticoagulant therapy

Bleeding tendencies

The uraemic syndrome is associated with abnormalities of platelet and red blood cell function, both of which lead to coagulation abnormalities and prolonged clotting times. When haemodialysis is commenced, the need for anticoagulation to prevent clotting in the extracorporeal circuit places the patient at additional risk of haemorrhage. Sites frequently associated with bleeding include:

a)   The gastrointestinal tract (GIT), where bleeding occurs in the upper and lower GIT.

b)   Intraocular areas, where vitreous haemorrhage can fill the vitreous chamber and disturb the transmission of light from pupil to retina.

c)   Intracranial structures, with bleeding into the various spaces surrounding the brain.

d)   Pericardial tissue, with bleeding into the pericardial space.

e)   The mediastinal space, with possible compression of the heart and lungs.

f)   Retroperitoneal areas.

(Swartz 1999, pp 162–168).

Vascular access clotting

The various contributions towards closure of the vascular access, either permanent or temporary, have been addressed in Chapter 2. An overview of the current methods of recovery, excluding access replacement/revision, that are available include:

a)   The instillation of fibrinolytic agents such as urokinase into the lumen/s of percutaneous devices.

b)   Mechanical declotting of peripheral devices with angioplasty balloon catheters.

c)   A combination of the two.

References

In text references

Hansen, S., Strutz, J., 1999, 'Anticoagulation and heparin administration' in *Hemodialysis for nurses and dialysis personnel,* Gutch, C., Stoner, M, Corea, A. (eds.), 6th ed., Mosby, St. Louis.

Hertel, J., Keep, D., Caruana, R., 2001, 'Anticoagulation', in *Handbook of Dialysis,*, Daugidas, J., Blake, P., Ing, T., (eds.), 3rd ed., Lippincott Williams and Wilkins, Philadelphia.

Spence, A., Mason, E., 1987, *Human Anatomy and Physiology*, 3rd ed.) Benjamin Cummings, Sydney.

Street, A., McPherson, J., 1996, 'The new heparins', *Australian Prescriber*, vol.19, no. 4, pp104–108.

Swartz, R., 1999, 'Anticoagulation in patients on haemodialysis', in *Principles and Practice of Dialysis*, Henrich, W. (ed), 2nd ed., Williams and Wilkins, Maryland.

Ward, R., Aronoff, G., 1999, 'Anti-coagulation strategies during hemodialysis procedures', in *Principles and Practice of Dialysis,* Henrich, W. (ed), 2nd ed., William and Wilkins, Maryland.

Recommended readings

Carbone, V., 1995, 'Heparin and dialyser membranes during hemodialysis: a literature review', *ANNA Journal*, vol. 22, no. 5, October, pp 452–455, 467.

Kinzner, C., 1998, 'Warfarin sodium (Coumadin) anticoagulant therapy for vascular access patency', *ANNA Journal*, vol. 25, no. 2, April, pp 195–203.

Northsea, C., 1994, 'Using urokinase to restore patency in double lumen catheters', ANNA Journal, vol. 21, no. 5, August, pp 261–264, 273.

Tranter, S., Donoghue, J., 2000, 'Brushings has made a sweeping change: use of the endoluminal FAS brush in haemodialysis central venous catheter management', *Australian Critical Care*, vol. 13, no. 1, March, pp 10–13.

Ward, D., Mehta, R. 1993, 'Extracorporeal management of acute renal failure patients at risk of bleeding', *Kidney International*, vol. 43, Suppl. 41, pp S 237–244.

CHAPTER FIVE

Dialysate preparation

Introduction

This chapter gives an overview of dialysate delivery systems, discusses the development of dialysis and examines the importance of concentrate preparation and water treatment in the provision of safe and effective dialysis.

5.1 History

Early experiences

The initial dialysate used for haemodialysis required precise amounts of electrolyte, usually in powder form, to be mixed by hand with large quantities of water. Enough solution for an entire treatment needed to be prepared. Small quantities were delivered to the dialyser during treatment and were circulated until they were saturated with uraemic toxins, then drained and replaced with fresh solution. Sodium chloride, potassium chloride and sodium bicarbonate were added first. Lactic acid and carbon dioxide gas were then bubbled through to lower the pH before calcium and magnesium could be added see Figure 2.5.1.

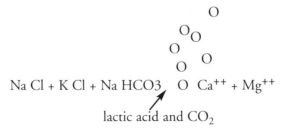

$$Na\ Cl + K\ Cl + Na\ HCO3 \quad O \quad Ca^{++} + Mg^{++}$$

lactic acid and CO_2

Figure 2.5.1: Provision of buffer via the addition of bicarbonate. This was an early method of preparing the dialysate using lactate and CO_2 to prevent bicarbonate precipitation
(Terrill 1999)

Because early dialysers did not have a closed dialysate compartment ultrafiltration could not be controlled, and it was not possible to program each patient's fluid loss requirements, as it is today. Glucose, an osmotically active agent, was added to the solution to encourage ultrafiltration.

The coil dialyser is an example of an early dialyser with an open dialysate compartment. It was immersed in a tank of dialysate that bathed the long membrane envelope. The addition of glucose to the dialysate encouraged the movement of water molecules from the blood compartment into the dialysate.

Central proportioning, where a number of patients were connected to a central unit through individual lines was the next development. A single large proportioning unit mixed the concentrate and water and delivered it to each patient station. One of the problems with this system was, that if contamination occurred in the proportioning unit, all patients connected to the central system, received an equal dose of the contaminant. Central proportioning units were soon replaced by individual proportioning units where each patient received dialysate through an individual unit.

The need to lower the pH of dialysate prior to the addition of calcium and magnesium had been overcome by using lactate instead of bicarbonate as a buffering agent.

Composition

Haemodialysis concentrate is an electrolyte solution with buffering agent added. Dialysate is a mixture of the concentrated solution and treated water mixed in a precise ratio, usually 34 parts of water to one part of concentrate. The dialysate is heated and deaerated remove any gases in solution from the mixture before it is delivered to the dialyser.

Dialysis machines are fitted with conductivity meters that measure the ability of ions in the dialysate to conduct an electrical current. This method determines the accuracy of the mix of concentrate and water. Dialysate must be isotonic with human plasma otherwise a hyper or hypo osmolar state can develop. In reality, the gradient between blood and dialysate is not steep. It is only sufficient to ensure the diffusion of electrolytes and metabolic waste products from blood to dialysate and occasionally, with electrolytes, from dialysate to blood. Steeper gradients exist for buffering substances where the molecules are required to move from the dialysate into the patient's blood in larger amounts.

Remember: because dialysate can cross the dialysis membrane and enter the patient's blood, it should be treated with the same caution as intravenous drugs.

5.2 Dialysate manipulation

Sodium

Serum sodium is the major determinant of extracellular osmolality as it is with dialysate. Early dialysis used very low sodium concentrations, < 120mmol/l, in the belief that preventing sodium accumulation during dialysis would control fluid gain and hypertension. There were no real problems with ultrafiltration, as we would expect today, because the dialysate compartment was not closed. Ultrafiltration was achieved by adding glucose, which more than made up for the osmotic reduction to the dialysate as a result of the low sodium. Difficulties did occur with low sodium preparations when dialysers with closed dialysate compartments were developed; glucose was no longer required to remove water and low serum sodium levels during treatment resulted in marked episodes of hypotension. A period of high sodium concentrations followed but problems occurred with thirst, excessive fluid gains and hypertension. The current trend is towards isonatraemic dialysate, allowing sodium to be removed along with water. A two litre fluid removal is usually sufficient to remove two to three days' worth of ingested sodium (Stewart 1989, p 200-201).

Potassium

Most chronic dialysis patients are dialysed against dialysate potassium between 1 and 2 mmol/l. This concentration seems to be sufficient to control potassium levels for a two to three day interdialytic period with an oral intake of 60 mmol/day (Stewart 1989, p 203–204).

Care should be taken with patients who are on digitalis preparations because hypokalaemia potentiates its action and higher dialysate concentrations may be required to prevent arrhythmias. Higher dialysate concentrations may also be required for patients with large or persistent gastrointestinal potassium losses. Be aware of patients who are catabolic, who have sustained tissue injury, or who have haemolysis for any reason. Low dialysate solutions may be required in this group of patients, because potassium is released from damaged cells and can cause a rapid increase in serum potassium levels.

Calcium

Normal serum calcium ranges between 2.1 and 2.6 mmol/l. Between 40% and 50% of this is protein-bound and the remainder is free to participate in chemical reactions. Stewart (1989, p 205) reported that, in renal failure the unbound portion could range between 57.6% and 64.3%. This means the dialysis patient can loose increased amounts of free calcium to the dialysate if their serum albumin is low and dialysate calcium is not increased.

Dialysate calcium tends to be highest when a patient first starts dialysis, often around 1·75 mmol/l, but decreases to between 1·3 and 1·6 mmol/l following weeks or months of treatment, when the serum calcium has stabilised. High levels can be used as an adjunct to treatment immediately following parathyroidectomy.

Although not common, hypercalcaemia can occur in patients taking Vitamin D supplements if serum calcium levels are not closely monitored. Symptoms include nausea, vomiting, confusion, constipation and soft tissue calcification.

Chloride and Magnesium

Both chloride and magnesium ions are important to maintain homeostasis but an alteration in the concentration is not usual during haemodialysis at this time. Some studies indicate that lower dialysate magnesium results in lower rates of osteodystrophy, improved nerve conduction, and a decrease in pruritis (Vaporean and Van Stone 1993, pp 46-51) but the literature is conflicting, and conclusive studies need to be completed. Low magnesium solutions can be used when oral magnesium is used to supplement phosphate binding (Palmer 1999, p33).

Chloride concentration tends to be predetermined by the need to maintain electrochemical neutrality. i.e. total anion content must equal total cation content (Ronco et al. 1996, p 266). Chloride salts, anions, are usually present with sodium, potassium and magnesium, cations, and sodium, the major cation, is present with both acetate, usually in very small portions in contemporary dialysis and bicarbonate, which replaces acetate as a buffer nowadays. Sodium concentration is, therefore, the major determinant of chloride levels.

Glucose

The historical use of glucose as an osmotic agent has already been addressed, as has its possible use as a caloric supplement. The addition of glucose to the dialysate in modern haemodialysis is considered to have a number of benefits. Some of these benefits are anecdotal and others have been the subjects of controlled evaluation.

Patients who have sepsis, diabetes or who are receiving betablocking agents should always be dialysed against a dialysate solution containing dextrose (Daugirdas et al. 2001, p 111). These patients are at risk of developing severe, symptomatic hypoglycaemia. The addition of glucose to the dialysate helps prevent this complication. Additional information about the use of glucose-containing dialysate is discussed in Chapter 7.

5.3 Buffering agents

Why bother with buffer?

Hydrogen ion generation is a normal result of metabolism. Between generation and excretion, hydrogen must be buffered to maintain normal blood pH. The lungs excrete volatile acids, which are produced as a result of intracellular metabolism. The kidney excretes non volatile acids produced as a result of protein metabolism. When renal failure occurs, renal excretion is compromised and a metabolic acidosis results. While compensatory mechanisms can often keep the pH within normal limits for short periods of time, the person with chronic or end stage renal disease needs long term assistance to maintain normal acid-base status. Therefore, oral bicarbonate is given before dialysis commences. Once dialysis is required, the most convenient way to supply a buffering substance is in the dialysate solution.

Acetate

Initial complexities with the addition of bicarbonate to dialysate resulted in the discovery of acetate, a buffering agent that was described as the second most important advance in dialysis history. By entering the Krebs cycle, acetate releases a bicarbonate ion for buffering, as part of its metabolism, see Figure 2.5.2.

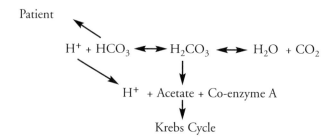

Figure 2.5.2: The metabolism of acetate as it enters the Krebs cycle (Terrill 1999).

While many people can metabolise acetate with no untoward effects, others develop signs and symptoms of acetate intolerance.

Bicarbonate

After the difficulties associated with the use of acetate as a buffering solution were recognised, attention was once again directed towards bicarbonate. The same problems arose, that is, the need to reduce the pH of the solution before the bicarbonate portion could be added. This problem was overcome, but other problems including the risk of bacterial contamination and expense were still present. The increased expense related to the limited amount of time that an opened bottle of solution could be kept without loss of carbon dioxide to the atmosphere and a corresponding reduction in the amount of available buffer. These problems have been overcome by using bicarbonate in dry powder form that is liquefied at the point of use. The use of bicarbonate as a buffer has completely superseded acetate in many countries because of the smoother correction it applies to acid-base imbalances.

Remember: This is not the case in all countries. Knowing the advantages and disadvantages of both agents is required for the safe dialysis of all patients.

Please note: Phosphate is not usually present in dialysate but it is now becoming apparent that patients undergoing slow nocturnal daily haemodialysis can actually require additional phosphate. Phosphate supplementation is needed because of the improved small molecule clearance that occurs. Some centres now add phosphate to the dialysate.

5.4 Water treatment

Why all the fuss?

Several years after the first successful treatments for end stage renal disease, many unexplained patient-related problems became apparent. It was soon recognised that many of these problems originated from using ordinary tap water to prepare the dialysate. Untreated water often contains many impurities, some of them added by councils to treat bacteria (chlorine) or to decrease sediment and provide clear water (aluminium). Others (copper and iron) can leach from pipes used to transport water, while others (nitrate) can leach into water storage depots from fertilisers.

While possibly not desirable, such exposure does not appear to cause difficulties for people with intact renal function. These people are usually only exposed to contaminants in water used for drinking and cooking of between one and two litres/day. Haemodialysis patients are exposed to between 120 and 150 litres of water per treatment (between 360 and 450 litres/week). Therefore exposure to very large amounts of contaminant is possible but they will only be absorbed if the molecules are small enough to cross the dialyser membrane. Common contaminants in drinking water that could cross the membrane include:

- Insoluble particles such as sand, silica and organic debris.
- Soluble organic compounds (disinfecting agents) such as chloramine.
- Soluble inorganic compounds such as copper, nitrate, and sulphate.
- Heavy metals and trace elements such as iron, zinc and aluminium.
- Bacteria and pyrogens.

A combination of some or all of the following are used to remove contaminants:

- Sediment filter.
- Water softener.
- Charcoal filter.
- Particle filters of various micron sizes.
- Ultra violet irradiation.
- Reverse osmosis.
- Deionisation.

References

In text references

Daugirdas, J., Ross, E., Nissenson, A., 2001, 'Acute hemodialysis prescription', *in Handbook of Dialysis,* Daugirdas, J., Blake, P., Ing, T., (eds.), 3rd ed., Lippincott Williams and Wilkins, Philadelphia.

Palmer, B., 1999, 'Dialysate composition in hemodialysis and peritoneal dialysis', in *Principles and Practice of Dialysis,* Henrich, W. (ed), 2nd ed., Williams and Wilkins, Maryland.

Ronco, C., Fabris, A., Feriano, M., 1996, 'Hemodialysis fluid composition', in *Replacement of Renal Function by Dialysis*, Jacobs, C., Kjellstrand, C., Koch, K., Winchester J, (eds.), 4th ed, Kluwer Academic Publishers, Boston.

Stewart, W., 1989, 'Composition of dialysate fluid', in *Replacement of Renal Function by Dialysis*, Maher, J., (ed.), 3rd ed., Kluwer Academic Publishers, Boston.

Vaporean, M., Van Stone, J. 1993, 'Dialysate magnesium', *Seminars in Dialysis,* vol. 6, no. 1., Jan–Feb, pp46–51.

Recommended reading

Almeida, A., Van Stone, J, 1989, 'Dialysate sodium', *Seminars in Dialysis*, vol. 2. no. 3, July–Sept., pp 176–179.

Hirsh, K., Amato, R, 1995, 'Setting up a water treatment system in an acute facility', *Nephrology News and Issues*, January, pp 44–47.

Hover, J., 1995, 'What to do when the water stops', *Nephrology News and Issues*, pp 42–43.

Ketchersid, T., Van Stone, J, 1991, 'Dialysate potassium', *Seminars in Dialysis*, vol. 4. no. 1, Jan.–March, pp 46–51.

Rosborough, D., Van Stone, J, 1993, 'Dialysate glucose', *Seminars in Dialysis*, vol. 6. no. 4, July–Aug., pp 260–263.

Ward, R., 1997, 'Water processing for hemodialysis (part 1): a historical perspective', *Seminars in Dialysis,* vol. 10, no. 1, Jan–Feb, pp 26–31.

CHAPTER SIX

The impact of chronic illness

Introduction

This chapter was written to introduce the reader to the differences between caring for patients with chronic illness and those suffering an acute illness. Aspects of spiritual care are addressed with the emphasis on the needs of people living with a disease that would be rapidly fatal without treatment. Nursing involvement, both personal and professional is discussed in relation to the discontinuation of treatment.

6.1 The effects of chronic illness

Acute versus chronic illness

The sick role, as defined by Parsons, the pioneer in much of this research, refers to a group of behaviors that an ill person is expected to adhere to (Callahan et al. 1966). These behaviors encourage dependence, and allow respite from former roles and social obligations. Paradoxically, there is also the expectation that the person will relinquish these behaviors and return to normal health as soon as possible. Such expectations infer that illness is acceptable as long as it does not last for long, and that the burdens of illness do not overly tax caregivers or those who are usually dependent on the person who is unwell.

This have been appropriate in earlier times when acute illness resulted in either rapid recovery or death and chronic illness was rare, but the results of recent improvements to medication and lifestyle mean that many previously untreatable diseases can now be cured or palliated. This means many people live with an incurable disease that often has periods of exacerbation that are unpredictable and leave many sufferers in continuing fear of relapse.

People with a chronic illness find their lives are altered in some way (Cameron and Greggor 1987, p 671). People with acute illnesses have a vested interest in compliance with societal expectations—their reward will be a return to wellness. No such reward exists with chronic illness. The best that can be expected is a possible reduction of symptoms with short periods of wellness, or that the natural progression of the disease will be slowed.

The Health Belief Model was developed in the USA in 1958 to explain preventative health behavior and is based on the premise 'that behaviour is determined by the subjective world of the perceiver' (Cameron and Greggor 1987, p673). The Health Belief Model has since been expanded in an attempt to explain compliance behavior in chronic illness (Mikhail 1981). The original model stated that people are more likely to comply with an enforced treatment regimen if they experience symptoms. The expanded model found that absence of symptoms decreases compliance if:

1. The person feels well or unchanged.

2. Medical interventions do not appear to alter progress.

3. Ongoing compliance is required.

4. No privileges are associated with compliance.

5. Compliance can involve intrusive behavior from health care personnel.

Cameron and Greggor (1987, p 671) wrote, 'a person with chronic disease assesses recommended treatments on how well they can be integrated into his life'. The individual's perception of their medical condition determines how well they will comply with treatment, and health care personnel who fail to recognise this, and incorporate the patient's viewpoint into educational programs can actually encourage non compliance.

Current health care delivery systems challenge us to think in terms of a 'partnership' between patients and health care professionals. While there will always be some patients who do not wish to participate in their care, those who do, should be encouraged to do so.

Psychological and social issues

Dialysis can be undertaken at home, in a community setting, or in an acute hospital facility. In order to encourage patients to accept responsibility for their care, most units aim to have all their patients dialysing at home, but this is not always possible. While some patients can manage their care effectively at home, the majority are cared for in satellite facilities and a small number will always dialyse in acute care settings.

Chronic illness creates many physical, social and psychological stressors on both patients and their families and it often very difficult to determine whether the therapy (the process of haemodialysis), or the condition requiring its use, is responsible (Eichel 1986).

Adaptability and uncertainty

Hilton (1992) defines uncertainty as 'a cognitive state created when an event cannot be adequately defined or categorised due to lack of information'. Most people experience a degree of uncertainty as part of their daily lives. However, uncertainty can become a significant stressor when it occupies a large part of life. Many chronic illnesses are characterised by the unpredictable exacerbation of symptoms. The uncertainty engendered by the emergence of these exacerbations becomes a major factor influencing the patient's expectations about the final outcome of their condition. It also has important ramifications for how the patient and their significant others adjust to the disease (Terrill and Morris 1997).

As a result of the ongoing uncertainty, stress is often present for most of the person's waking hours. It becomes threatening because it limits the individual's sense of control over their illness and, as feelings of helplessness develop, fear and anxiety become an ongoing part of the person's life.

The nurse's role in alleviating uncertainty

The uncertainties associated with critical and chronic illness cause stressors that are evident through emotions as well as through particular behaviors. The process of adjusting to an illness is heavily influenced by these uncertainties, and nurses have an important role in assessing and alleviating uncertainty.

Initial assessment involves being aware that not all the person's uncertainty relates to a lack of knowledge about the future. It also involves feelings of not being safe or cared for, being in doubt, lacking trust, and fear of pain and death. Distortion of the facts, or simple misunderstanding, can compound a problem and a clear explanation can relieve some fears (Terrill and Morris 1997).

It is helpful to distinguish between those processes that can be altered, and those that cannot. Differentiating between behaviours and attitudes that can be altered and those that cannot allows the person to begin to accept at least some aspects of their illness and make informed choices about their compliance. Patients also need help to interpret events, and to identify cause and effect in order to identify the consequences of their choices. Discussing the issues can help a patient differentiate between the areas where they need assistance to make decisions and the areas where they can act independently. Independent action can reduce feelings of helplessness (Terrill and Morris 1997).

It is equally important to identify those patients who do not wish to have input into understanding and managing their illness. Some people are happy to know that they are ill, but do not want the details. If information is forced on such a patient, their level of anxiety could be increased unnecessarily.

Coping strategies

Levy (1976) developed a model of coping by observing patients on chronic haemodialysis. The model described three stages. In the first stage, the honeymoon period, the patient is hopeful and confident after the initiation of treatment. There is often a great sense of relief when dialysis is established and the patient realises that the treatment is not as bad as they had imagined. This realisation is often accompanied by an alleviation of some of the adverse physiological consequences of chronic renal failure. There is also a degree of anxiety and concern as the realities of dependence on a machine, coupled with the need to return to normal social activity, are recognised.

Recognition heralds the commencement of the second stage that usually occurs between three and twelve months. The patient experiences the first conflict between remaining in the sick role and returning to normal duties. The treatment has not cured the underlying condition, and the relentless nature of dialysis is faced. The patient can be sad, withdrawn, discouraged and feel 'out of control'.

The final stage is that of adaptation. The patient begins to accept that there are limitations to treatment and there is evidence of the return of hope. Because illness is a subjective experience, patients with similar conditions can have vastly different methods of coping. Coping strategies are usually working when distress is kept within manageable limits, hope is generated, and self-worth is maintained or restored.

Summary

The most important point for health professionals is to recognise when a person's usual coping strategies are no longer effective. Nurses can help patients to discover new coping strategies, design ways of controlling new stressors and use resources they have not used before. In this way the patient benefits and nurses are rewarded by satisfaction in the care they give and are less likely to experience 'burn out' when caring for the chronically ill.

6.2 Spirituality

Spiritual needs of the sick

All people are spiritual, and all people have spiritual needs. Although we tend to link spirituality with theology and matters of religion … spirituality has a broader scope. In this sense, our spirituality is the complex set of emotions, thoughts, and relationships that is derived from the ability to comprehend, reflect, and, in some ways, control our existence.

(Sommer 1989, p 225).

Most of us relate spirituality with organised religion, but as Sommer suggests, spirituality is much more than religion. As humans, we have a sense of destiny. We know what it is to be strong, to strive for, and achieve, goals. We have a sense of self-worth and most of us have been taught to value others as well as ourselves. In countries such as Australia, most people do not experience the constant struggle to survive that is present in some other countries.

In many cases, just as we are feeling invincible, we are faced with our own mortality. As a race, humans are gregarious; we seek out others of our kind for love, approval, support and care, especially in times of crisis. As nurses, we often find ourselves as providers of many of these needs. Undergraduate nurse education programs seldom address these issues and it can be exhausting, confronting and confusing when a patient requires spiritual assistance and we are not equipped to provide it. Sommer (1989, p231) suggests:

> ... to understand how another person is limited, we must understand our own limitations. To enter another person's pain, we must identify that pain in ourselves. To help another face death, we must be able to imagine our own death.

Some authors (Piles 1990, Soeken and Carson 1986) have suggested that a limitation in the nurses own spiritual resources could be the reason for the discomfort that they experience when a patient is having an emotional crisis.

Nurses as spiritual providers

Patients and staff in many dialysis units often enter into relationships that are not unlike those of a family unit. Birthdays are celebrated and weddings and engagements are times for celebration. Like most 'families' squabbles and disharmony occasionally occurs. This closeness, together with the amount of time spent in treatment, means that patients often approach their nurses with their spiritual needs.

6.3   Death in the dialysis unit

Unexpected death and its consequences

Death is a reality in all dialysis units and impacts heavily on both carers and fellow patients. The quasi-family relationships that develop often cause intense grief for staff. Those who feel the strongest need to say goodbye, often attend funeral services for the deceased person. While patients know that their disease is life threatening, and that without treatment they will die, usually in a very short time, they can deny the reality for extended periods of time if they, and their fellow patients, remain well.

The death of any person with whom a relationship has developed, always affects those who go on living (Hudson 1988, p 15)). Therefore, the care that nurses provide for themselves, as well as for their colleagues requires that 'attitudes about death should not be put aside, but exposed, articulated and recognized' (Hudson 1988, p 15).

The strong sense of bonding that often occurs between patients who share a common but controlled threat can cause some patients to experience extreme guilt at their survival, when a fellow patient succumbs. Vamos (1997) likens these phenomena to the post combat syndromes that occur after shared trauma in theaters of war or situations of natural disaster.

The use of advanced directives

A study conducted by Terrill (1996), explored the use of advanced directives in dialysis units and the role of the nurse in promoting their use. It is interesting to note that, while the nurses participating in the study endorsed the use of advanced directives, and their role in promoting them, patients did not appear keen to use them. The reasons for this may include the belief that no active treatment means no treatment at all '… [and] that many patients fear that all nursing care will immediately be withdrawn should unexpected intercurrent illness occur' (Terrill 1996, p14). Preliminary findings in a research project currently being undertaken (Terrill and Sullivan) indicate that even the most seriously ill patients are not provided with information about their prognosis or given the opportunity to explore treatment options, even prior to a terminal event.

Withdrawal from treatment

All dialysis units are familiar with this complex and distressing need to withdraw treatment. The following discussion does not include mentally incompetent patients for whom a medical officer has discontinued treatment after examining all the facts, deciding that recovery is unlikely, and that the burden of continued treatment outweighs any possible benefits.

Respect for a patient's request to discontinue treatment is grounded in the ethical principle of autonomy. After making such a request, patients are asked to undergo psychiatric examination to determine the absence, or otherwise, of depressive illness that, if corrected, could alter the patient's decision.

Family members are frequently consulted, as are social workers and clergy who are known to the patient. Once a decision has been made, the patient is usually asked if they wish to die at home or in hospital, and every effort is made to comply with their wishes. It should be made clear that the decision to discontinue treatment is not irrevocable and a change of mind is 'OK,' and that no recriminations will be bought to bear if the patient wishes to recommence dialysis.

Most patients want to know what their dying will be like and they should be assured that the team who has cared for them for so long would not abandon them at their death. Isolated ultrafiltration might be offered to relieve any respiratory distress and the patient should be told that this would in no way affect the dying process.

References

In text references

Callahan, E., Carrol, S., Revier, Sr. P., Gilhooly, E., Dunn, D., 1996, 'The sick role in chronic illness: some reactions' *Journal of Chronic Illness,* vol.19, pp 883–897.

Cameron, K., Greggor, F. 1987, 'Chronic illness and compliance', *Journal of Advanced Nursing,* vol. 12, pp 671–676.

Eichel, C., 1986, 'Stress and Coping in patients on CAPD Compared to Haemodialysis', *ANNA Journal,* vol. 16, no. 1, pp9–13.

Evans, R., Manninen, D., Garrison, L., Hart, G., Gutman, R., Hull, A. Lowrie, E., 1985, 'The quality of life of patients with end stage renal disease', *New England Journal of Medicine,* vol. 312, no. 9, pp 553–559.

Hilton. B. 'Perceptions of uncertainty' *Critical Care Nurse* Vol.12, No. 2, pp 70–73).

Hudson, R., 1988, 'Whole or parts—a theological perspective on 'person'', *The Australian Journal of Advanced Nursing,* vol. 6, no. 1, Sept, pp 12–20.

Levy, N., 1976, 'Coping with Maintenance haemodialysis-psychological considerations in the care of patients', in *Clinical Aspects of Uraemia and Dialysis,* Massry, S., Sellers, A., (eds.), Springfield, Illinois.

Piles, C., 1990, 'Providing spiritual care', *Nurse Educator,* vol. 15, No. 1., pp 36–41.

Soeken, K., Carson, V., 1986, Study measures nurses attitudes about providing spiritual care', *Health Progress,* vol. 67, no. 3, pp 52–55.

Sommer, D., 1989, 'The spiritual needs of dying children', *Issues in Comprehensive Pediatric Nursing,* vol. 12, pp 225–233.

Terrill, B, 1996, *'Dialysing acutely ill patients: the lived experience of renal nurses',* Unpublished Masters thesis, Deakin University, Geelong.

Terrill, B., Morris, M., 1997, Renal Clinical Teacher and Course Co-ordinator, *'The human Machine Interface',* a learning package developed for the Austin and Repatriation Medical Centre.

Recommended reading

Colvin, E., Hammes, B., 1991, 'If only I knew: A Patient Education Program on Advanced Directives', *ANNA Journal,* vol. 18, no. 6, pp557–560.

Cramond, W., Fraenkel, M., Barratt, L. 1990, 'On letting go: the patient, haemodialysis and opting out', *Australian and New Zealand Journal of Psychiatry,* vol. 24, pp 268–275.

Henderson, M., 1995., 'Facilitating a good death in patients with end stage renal disease', *ANNA*

Journal, vol.22, no. 3, pp 294–300.

Laidlaw, J., Beeken, J., Whitney, F., Reyes, A., 1999, 'Contracting with outpatient hemodialysis patients to improve adherence to treatment' *ANNA Journal,* vol. 26, no. 1, pp 37–40.

Nordberg. M., 1990, 'When patients die: handling grief in the dialysis unit', *Dialysis and Transplantation,* vol. 18, no. 4, April, pp 164–168, 215.

Reed, P., 1991, 'Preferences for spiritually related nursing interventions among terminally ill and non-terminally ill hospitalized adults and well adults', *Applied Nursing Research,* vol.4, no. 3., August, pp 122–128.

Ross, L., 1994, 'Spiritual aspects of nursing', *Journal of Advanced Nursing,* vol.19, pp 439-447.

Rotarius, T., Liberman, A., 1999, 'Managing non-compliant patients with behavioral contracts', *Dialysis and transplantation,* February, pp 87–88, 89.

Vamos, M., 1997, 'Survivor guilt and chronic illness', *Australian and New Zealand Journal of Psychiatry,* vol.31, pp 592–596.

Wellard, S., 1998, 'Constructions of chronic illness', *International Journal of Nursing Studies,* vol. 35, pp 49–55.

CHAPTER SEVEN

Dialysing the acutely ill patient

Introduction

Haemodialysis of the acutely ill patient presents the nurse with a different set of challenges from those encountered during the dialysis of stable, end stage renal failure patients. People who require dialysis during an episode of acute illness are frequently haemodynamically unstable, experience sudden alterations in serum biochemistry and acid-base status, and may have multiple organ failure.

Frequent assessment of fluid and electrolyte status is indicated, and alterations that occur can require modification of the dialysis orders several times during a single treatment. It follows that the nurse caring for acutely ill patients requires a heightened awareness of the alterations in fluid and electrolyte balance that can occur once haemodialysis is commenced and of the appropriate nursing interventions to implement.

7.1 Indications for treatment

Initial reminders

As explained in Chapter 2, General nephrology, only a very small proportion of patients in acute renal failure require renal replacement therapy. The choice of treatment modality depends on physician preference, available equipment, nursing skill mix, and a variety of other considerations including the area in which the patient is receiving care and comorbid risk factors. This chapter focuses on the use of *haemodialysis* only.

Patients with end stage renal failure can become suddenly unwell and require treatment in an acute setting. The only real difference between acute illness in patients with end stage renal failure and other renal patients with acute illness, is that the 'gentle' dialysis procedure used when patients first commence maintenance dialysis is often omitted. All other features of an acute dialysis prescription apply. For the purposes of this chapter, the maintenance dialysis patient with an acute illness is discussed at the same time as the acutely ill patient with compromised renal function. Be aware that references to any return of renal function *do not* apply in the acutely ill person with end stage renal failure.

The aim of treatment

The aim of haemodialysis in acute illness accompanied by renal failure is to support, or replace, renal function until recovery. Because dialysis in acute illness is considered to be a temporary measure, it is often undertaken with a different prescription from that used in maintenance dialysis. Daily dialysis may be required for hypercatabolic patients, or for patients whose parenteral nutrition or intravenous medication requirements dictate the need for fluid removal. Daily treatment may also be required for patients with scalds, burns or crush injuries where tissue damage causes a massive efflux of potassium from within cells.

According to Hutchison (1994, p161) the absolute indications for dialysis are:

1. The development of uraemic symptoms.

2. Signs and symptoms of uraemic pericarditis.

   The relative indicators include:

1. *Volume expansion.

2. *Hyperkalaemia.

3. *Metabolic acidosis.

4. 'Other' electrolyte abnormalities.

* If conservative management is unsuccessful or contraindicated.

Whilst most nephrologists broadly accept these indicators, a number of controversies remain. These include the likely prognosis for the patient and therefore the appropriateness of dialysis, the type of dialyser and membrane, treatment modality and treatment intensiveness (Conger 1998, p534).

7.2 The haemodialysis prescription

Initial considerations

If patient survival was the only consideration, it would be relatively easy to determine the level of uraemic toxicity at which dialysis should be started. This is rarely the case however, and much debate centers on determining if patient survival is the only consideration. It is not as easy to determine the *optimum* time to commence treatment to maintain quality of life and prevent comorbidity (Kjellstrand and Teehan 1996, p839).

Infection and gastrointestinal bleeding are the two major contributors to mortality in patients with acute renal failure and in whom dialytic support is required. The most appropriate time to commence dialysis to avoid these complications is not clear. Currently treatment is started well before the accumulated azotaemic solutes reach levels likely to produce uraemic symptoms. In many cases treatment is required to maintain fluid balance, especially in oliguric patients receiving large amounts of intravenous fluids. In these patients, fluid overload 'may precede significant azotemia by several days' (Kjellstrand and Teehan 1996, p839).

If the commencement of dialysis has been delayed and uraemic solute accumulation is advanced, the occurrence of neurological, musculoskeletal and cardiovascular complications can be minimised by using short, gentle and frequent treatments. These complications are discussed fully in the next chapter.

The dialysis prescription will be altered for each episode of dialysis, especially for patients who are septic and catabolic. Changes may also be required *during* the dialysis session. Limiting the reduction of accumulated urea to <30% each dialysis minimises the likelihood of disequilibration where rapid changes in serum biochemistry results in movement of fluid into cells and cerebral cellular oedema.

Important considerations

The dialysis 'dose': According to Daugirdas et al. (2001 p 102) the most important determinants of the amount of dialysis to be delivered are the length of the treatment and the blood flow rate. When solute accumulation is extreme, and the chances of either disequilibrium resulting from rapid decreases in serum urea, and cardiac arrhythmias due to sudden alterations in serum potassium are high, treatment times should be reduced to between two and three hours. Blood flow rates between 150 and 200 ml/min are usual. Individual dialysis units have preferred protocols for the commencement of dialysis for acute and end stage patients.

If anticoagulation is not required during the treatment, the high blood flow rates that are often recommended with no heparin dialysis can result in higher solute clearances of urea. than those suggested in the preceding paragraph. One way to avoid high urea clearance is to connect the dialysate lines so that a cocurrent flow is established between blood and dialysate. This will decrease diffusive clearance as serum concentrations of blood and dialysate reach equilibrium towards mid point along the dialyser membrane (author's personal experience). The reduction in clearance applies to all solutes, and adjustments to dialysate electrolyte concentrations, especially potassium may be needed.

The dialyser and membrane: Most practitioners now accept that the use of biocompatible, synthetic membranes offers the acutely ill patient the best chance of survival once acute renal failure requiring renal replacement therapy develops. The common reasons for using such membranes include:

1.   The increased infection rates associated with the use of unsubstituted cellulosic membranes (Hakim 1992 p 367).

2.   The activation of the complement cascade and the generation of bradykinin that is also associated with the use of unsubstituted cellulosic membranes (Schulman and Levin 1994 p 251–253).

3.   The lack of adsorptive qualities common to cellulosic membranes (Schulman and Levin 1994 p 253).

Dialysate composition:

1.   **Sodium:** Kjellstrand and Teehan (1996, p 844) suggest that the sodium composition of the dialysate used with end stage renal failure patients might not be appropriate for patients with acute renal failure, but much controversy surrounds the use of both higher than 'normal' and lower than 'normal' solutions. The use of sodium profiling is discussed in the next section, and the reader is encouraged to obtain the referenced to broaden their knowledge in this area. Current studies into variable sodium concentrations are limited primarily to end stage renal failure and may not apply to patients with acute renal failure.

For practical purposes, the dialysate sodium concentration is usually the same as that used for stable, chronic patients, with the exception of patients with hyper or hyponatraemia. Of special note, is a condition known as central pontine myelinolysis that occurs predominantly in women after rapid correction of hyponatraemia (usually <125 mmol/l). In such situations it is recommended that dialysate sodium be adjusted to correct serum levels by no more that 10 mmol/l per treatment (Hansen 1992, p 5).

3. **Potassium:** Careful consideration of the dialysate potassium concentration is required, especially in patients who have significant pH alterations, and those who have ischaemic heart disease and patients receiving multiple inotropes or preparations containing digitalis. The standard K1 or K2 bath definitely does *not* apply in these situations

   Correction of acidosis leads to a decrease in serum potassium, and the correction of alkalosis increases it. Hypokalaemia potentiates the action of digitalis, and the rapid correction of acidaemia can cause cardiac arrhythmias. Similarly, hypokalaemia can cause an increase in skeletal muscle resistance and in the coronary vascular bed (Kjellstrand and Teehan 1996, p846).

3. **Calcium:** The major consideration with patients receiving dialysis for acute renal failure is the lowered serum calcium that follows the correction of acidosis. Approximately 50% of calcium is protein-bound and protein is an important blood buffer that resists alterations in pH. When pH falls, binding the excess hydrogen ions to protein resists the resulting increase in hydrogen ions and displaces calcium from its usual binding sites. As serum pH is corrected, hydrogen ions are released from their binding sites on the protein molecule. As calcium ions bind to their 'normal' sites on the protein molecule again the amount of *ionised* calcium falls. Although total serum calcium is not altered, neurological changes associated with a fall in ionised calcium, tetany—tingling numbness cramps, carpopedal and laryngospasm, can result.

4. **Dextrose:** It is common to use dialysate containing dextrose in patients with sepsis, those receiving beta blocking agents and those who have diabetes mellitus (Daugirdas et. al. 2001, p 111). The consequences of using dialysate that does *not* contain dextrose include the development of a negative nitrogen balance that occurs as glucose passes across the dialyser membrane, and symptomatic fluid removal as extracellular osmolality falls in relation to the intracellular fluid. There is also an increase in the removal of total body potassium because the lack of dialysate glucose can decrease the 'intradialytic translocation of potassium into cells' (Ward et al. 1987, in Daugirdas et al. 2001, pp109–110).

5. **Dialysate buffer:** All acutely ill patients should receive bicarbonate as a buffering solution.

It is not usual to alter dialysate magnesium or chloride levels. While phosphate is not added to the dialysate for patients with end stage renal failure due to their almost universal hyperphosphataemia, patients with acute illness receiving dialysis can develop hypophosphataemia. If hypophosphataemia occurs, it is usually corrected with intravenous phosphate rather than by modifying the dialysate solution.

Vascular Access

Unless the patient has either chronic renal, or end stage renal failure with an established vascular access, the only appropriate means of obtaining access to the circulation is through a centrally inserted venous catheter. Nursing management of these catheters can be found in Chapter 2 of this section.

Anticoagulation

The extracorporeal circuit is as prone to clotting in acutely ill patients as it is with end stage renal failure patients, and heparin remains the most frequently selected anticoagulant. However, for patients with coagulopathies e.g. disseminated intravascular coagulation, who are at risk of bleeding, anticoagulant-free dialysis is indicated.

The method recommended for heparin-free dialysis (Kjellstrand and Teehan 1996, p842) is as follows:

1. After the dialyser and lines have been rinsed with the recommended amount of normal saline, recirculate the extracorporeal volume after adding between 2000 and 5000 units of heparin.

2. Prior to commencing therapy flush the heparinised saline from the extracorporeal circuit.

3. Use blood flow rates between 250 and 300 ml/min. Remember the increased solute removal can cause disequilibration.

4. Flush the extracorporeal circuit with 50 to 100 mls of normal saline every 15 to 20 minutes, remembering to add the total amount of fluid to be used to the fluid removal calculations. Kjellstrand and Teehan (1996) report a 95% success rate using this method to prevent clotting in the extracorporeal circuit.

Post dialysis assessment

Patient assessment after acute haemodialysis is similar to assessing the dialysis of a stable, maintenance end stage renal failure patient, except that more detail is required. Comparison of the pre, post, and intradialytic blood pressure helps guide the fluid removal technique and blood pressure support for the next treatment. Special attention should be paid to the efficacy of anticoagulation, after dialysis or intradialytic bleeding problems, especially in a patient who has recently had surgery, rapid changes to the acid-base status and any signs of disequilibrium.

It takes between one and two hours for electrolytes to be redistributed between the intra and extracellular fluid compartments. This means that serum biochemistry results from immediate post dialysis blood samples do not reflect the biochemistry some hours later. As electrolytes move slowly from within the cells, extracellular levels increase. It is therefore, important to recognise that analysing blood samples taken one to two hours after the completion of therapy best assesses the effect of treatment on the patient's blood chemistry.

This is also true for end stage renal failure patients, but as they are considered to be 'stable' it cannot usually be justified to keep them waiting for some hours after dialysis finishes to enable the correct estimation of serum biochemistry. The same *is not* true for the acutely ill patient who is already in hospital, has an established intravenous route for the collecting blood samples, and in whom the next treatment may well be guided by the results of the preceding treatment.

7.3 The use of profiling techniques

Beginning comments

If you wish to start an argument in the dialysis unit, introduce the subject of dialysis profiling. It is probable that few nephrologists or nephrology nurses share the same opinion. The term 'profiling' refers to the use of specific techniques to preprogram fluid and solute removal in a graduated manner over a given time period.

Profiling techniques explore the idea that a 'set' value for fluid removal and/or solute removal is not necessarily beneficial for all patient groups, or for each hour of their individual dialyses. Rather, profiling suggests that for any given amount of dialysis time, the volume of fluid and/or solute removed should be individualised for each patient.

Dialysis patients probably recognised this many years ago. They knew that a Vegemite sandwich or biscuit with morning tea stopped them experiencing hypotension or cramps during dialysis. Why? —Because the increase in extracellular fluid sodium and therefore osmolality enabled their bodies to 'pull' fluid from the intracellular space into the extracellular fluid from where it could be removed during ultrafiltration. Current technology allows therapy to be individualised using profiling options available as a part of the usual dialysis program data on many modern haemodialysis machines.

Sodium profiles

When haemodialysis was in its infancy, dialysate sodium was deliberately kept at a low level compared to the accepted values for normal serum sodium. This was intended to reduce the patient's desire to drink associated with an increase in serum osmolality, due primarily to an increase in serum sodium. Low sodium dialysate kept the interdialytic fluid gain, and more importantly the blood pressure, to within acceptable levels. It was not uncommon for dialysate sodium levels to be as low as 130 mmol/l during these early years (Ronco et al. 1996, p258).

Low dialysate sodium levels were often associated with hypotension and neurological symptoms because the reduction in extracellular osmolality compared to intracellular osmolality opposed vascular refilling. This encouraged fluid to enter cells where it caused cellular swelling associated neurological symptoms when cerebral cells were involved, and hypotension, as fluid moved from the interstitial space into the intracellular space in an attempt to equalise osmolality between these two major body water compartments.

As early as the late 1970's, researchers demonstrated that the use of high dialysate sodium, again with respect to normal serum values, was associated with fewer major intradialytic complications of disequilibrium and hypotension. Unwanted interdialytic fluid gain could be prevented if the dialysate sodium was reduced to lower than physiological levels (130 mmol/l) for the last hour of a four-hour treatment (Kjellstrand and Teehan 1996, p 844–845).

These findings led to the manual use of 'variable' sodium concentrations during the dialysis procedure. The operator was required to change the strength of the dialysate sodium each hour of treatment or per treatment aliquot (period of time), which proved to be cumbersome and labour intensive. The market demand for further research into this variation of conventional sodium delivery dialysate soon led to the development of haemodialysis machines able to deliver sodium dialysate concentrations that could be preset by the operator at the commencement of each treatment.

High sodium dialysate, concentrations between 145 and 150 mmol/l of sodium are delivered for the first two to three hours of treatment. The amount of dialysate sodium is then gradually decreased to between 135 and 138 mmol/l by the end of the treatment. The decrease can be achieved by either linear or incremental adjustment, and is usually determined in accordance with the operator's assessment of the patient's response to fluid removal. A major component of using high sodium dialysate is the predialysis assessment that includes a review of the patient's cardiovascular status.

Ultrafiltration profiles

As with sodium profiling, there is controversy about water, or ultrafiltration, profiling. Whether the idea of water profiling precedes or follows sodium profiling is irrelevant The technique remains an option that can decrease the symptoms so often associated with fluid removal. If sodium profiling results in increased extracellular sodium, it follows that the increase in serum osmolality encourages vascular refilling, enabling an increase in fluid removal demand to be reasonably well tolerated.

Let's explore this concept further. If, during sodium profiling, the extracellular sodium value is greatest at the commencement of dialysis, the largest amount of fluid should be able to be removed at this time. Why? —Because the high extracellular sodium concentration should support fluid movement from the intracellular compartment to the extracellular compartment, i.e. the high extracellular sodium concentration encouraged by the high sodium dialysate promotes fluid movement from inside the cells to the vascular compartment where it can be accessed and removed.

Many proponents of sodium and water profiling consider that the amount of water removed during dialysis should be complemented by the sodium concentration of the dialysate. Please note, there are multiple variations available between 'linear' and 'variable' sodium and ultrafiltration concentrations. Many haemodialysis manufacturers recommend correlating the fluid removal profiles and the dialysate sodium concentrations.

Bicarbonate profiles

Bicarbonate profiling is an option provided by only a few haemodialysis machine manufacturers. It is offered as a means of enhancing phosphate removal. The suggested mechanism is as follows:

Serum bicarbonate levels are kept at the lower end of the normally accepted physiological range when commencing dialysis and for a variable period of time thereafter. The operator determines the length of time after reviewing the patient's serum calcium, phosphate, and pH. The maintenance of a slightly acidic environment in the vascular space prevents the dissociation of phosphate and hydrogen as would occur if bicarbonate was added. Thus phosphate remains in the vascular compartment where it is used to buffer the hydrogen ions that maintain the serum pH at the lower end of the normal range. Towards the end of the dialysis treatment the bicarbonate levels in the dialysate are increased to free hydrogen from its bond with phosphate and allow phosphate to be removed during the latter part of dialysis.

Bicarbonate profiling is an adjunct to the correct use of phosphate-binding medication and appropriate phosphate dietary restriction. It does not replace either of these management strategies in good patient management.

Summary

The various profiling techniques are tools that can be used to individualise fluid removal and normalise electrolyte status in selected patients. By promoting a more physiological movement of fluid and solute, haemodialysis that incorporates these techniques often results in greater stability of blood pressure during treatment and reduces the neurological and cardiovascular symptoms associated with disequilibrium.

Profiling is a *tool* to assist in patient management. It does not replace the recommended predialysis thorough patient assessment that should precede any haemodialysis treatment.

References

In text references

Conger, J., 1998,'Dialysis and related therapies', *Seminars in Nephrology*, vol.18, no. 5, pp 533–540.

Daugirdas, J., Ross, E., Nissenson, A., 2001, 'The acute haemodialysis prescription', in *Handbook of Dialysis*, Daugirdas, J., Blake, P., Ing,T. (eds.), 3rd ed., Lippincott Williams and Wilkins, Philadelphia.

Hakim, R., 1992, 'Use of biocompatible membranes improves outcome and recovery from acute renal failure', (abstract), *Journal of the American Society of Nephrology*, vol. 3, no. 3 p 367.

Hansen, S., 1992, 'Patient assessment in acute haemodialysis', J CANNT, vol. 2, no. 1, pp 17–9.

Hutchison, F., 1994, 'Management of acute renal failure', in *Primer on Kidney Disease*, Greenberg, A., (ed.), Academic Press, Sydney.

Kjellstrand, C., Teehan, B., 1996, 'Acute Renal Failure', in *Replacement of Renal Function by Dialysis*, Jacobs, C., Kjellstrand, C., Koch, K., (eds.), 4th ed., Kluwer Academic Publishers, Boston.

Ronco, C., Fabris, A., Feriani, M., 1996, 'Haemodialysis fluid composition', in *Replacement of Renal Function by Dialysis*, Jacobs, C., Kjellstrand, C., Koch, K., (eds.), 4th ed., Kluwer Academic Publishers, Boston.

Schulman, G., Levin, N. 1994, 'Membranes for hemodialysers', *Seminars in Dialysis*, vol. 7, no., 4, July-August, pp 251–256.

Recommended readings

Ebel, H., Saure, B., Laage, C., Dittmar, A., Keuchel, M., Stellwaag, M., Lange, H., 1990, 'Influence of computer-modulated profile haemodialysis on cardiac arrhythmias' Nephrology, Dialysis and Transplantation, Suppl. 1, pp 165–166.

Meers, C., Toffelmire, E., McMurray, M., Hopman, W., 1999, 'Reducing complications during haemodialysis using gradient ultrafiltration and gradient sodium dialysate', *ANNA Journal*, vol. 26, no. 5, pp 496–501,505.

Sadowski, R., Jabs, K., Alfred, E., 1993, 'Sodium modelling ameliorates intradialytic and interdialytic symptoms in young haemodialysis patients', *Journal of the American Society of Nephrologists*, vol. 4, no.5, pp1192–1198.

CHAPTER EIGHT

Acute complications of haemodialysis

Introduction

Despite the numerous technological advances that have occurred since the acceptance of haemodialysis as an appropriate treatment for acute and chronic renal failure, the procedure is not risk free. Elderly patients with significant comorbid disease are increasingly being accepted into end stage renal disease programs. Nurses are frequently required to dialyse medically unstable patients, often with multiple organ failure, in intensive care environments. Knowledge of the risks inherent in extracorporeal therapy, as well as the risks associated with haemodialysis as a treatment modality, will enable the dialysis of these patients to be accomplished with minimal risk.

8.1 Hypotension

Occurrence

Hypotension requiring intervention by either medical or nursing staff is reported to occur in up to 30% of all dialysis treatments (Bregman et al. 2001, p 148; Kaufman et al. 1993, p 109). This does not mean that all patients become hypotensive at every third treatment. Some patients seldom have any symptomatic fall in blood pressure while others have problems during most treatments. However, hypotension is the most frequent adverse event during treatment and a major cause of morbidity and occasionally mortality.

Apart from the discomfort of muscle cramps, nausea, vomiting, and diaphoresis, hypotension is associated with vascular access clotting, cardiac arrhythmias, myocardial infarction, cerebral ischaemia and infarction, and convulsions (Sherman 1988, p136). Sherman (1988 p 136), suggests that an understanding of the physiological basis of hypotension is best facilitated by reviewing the factors that determine blood pressure, which he summarises this as follows:

> *Mean arterial blood pressure is determined solely by peripheral vascular resistance (PVR) and cardiac output. Cardiac output is a function of heart rate and stroke volume, with stroke volume, in turn, depending upon intrinsic myocardial contractility and plasma volume. Ultrafiltration of blood during haemodialysis will lead to a reduction in plasma volume and will result in hypotension unless compensatory changes occur in PVR, heart rate, or myocardial contractility.*

The ability to activate responses that enable blood pressure to be maintained is compromised in many patients with renal disease, even moderate ultrafiltration rates result in hypotension in some patients.

Pathophysiology of hypotension

Ultrafiltration: As fluid is removed during ultrafiltration in conventional haemodialysis, the oncotic pressure in the vascular space rises and encourages fluid to move out of the interstitial space in order to equalise the oncotic pressure between these two extracellular spaces. As a result the combined oncotic pressure of the extracellular fluid is higher than the pressure of the intracellular fluid. This in turn promotes the movement of water out of the cells. This process is known as vascular refilling and is encouraged by techniques such as sodium profiling.

Hypotension often results if ultrafiltration is excessive, especially when it is accompanied by inadequate vascular refilling, compromised cardiac function or impaired autonomic responses. Further, hypotension can be compounded when urea is removed rapidly from the vascular space, as occurs during high efficiency dialysis, and results in higher concentrations of urea in the cells. This encourages extracellular water to move into the cells and depletes the extracellular fluid volume (Kaufman et al. 1993, p 110).

Autonomic nervous system dysfunction: Autonomic neuropathy is a frequent finding among patients with end stage renal failure and potentiates dialysis-related hypotension (Sherman 1988, p 137). It is characterised by abnormal functioning of the afferent portion of the baroreceptor reflex arc and the parasympathetic efferent response (Leunissen et al. 2000, pp 72–73) and is thought to be responsible for failure of the normal cardiac and vascular responses to reduced circulating blood volume. As circulating blood volume falls, especially when vascular refilling is inadequate, cardiac output and peripheral vascular resistance fail to increase enough to support normal blood pressure and hypotension results.

Dialysate buffer: The use of acetate as a buffering agent during haemodialysis is a well-established cause of hypotension (Bregman et al. 2001, p 153; Mujais et al. 1996, p 692; Sherman 1988, p137). Acetate is a known cardiac depressant and vasodilator and therefore its role in hypotension is greater in patients with existing impaired cardiac function. Acetate is metabolised primarily in the liver and its hypotensive effect is greater in patients with small muscle mass or liver disease.

Although acetate is no longer used as a buffering agent in Australia, it is still used in some other countries. As discussed earlier, there are implications for patients who have never been exposed to acetate who wish to travel to countries where acetate is still used. These patients need to be advised accordingly. Acetate-based dialysate is also recommended for use when natural disasters require international intervention because acetate can be transported and managed in the field easily, and for use of mechanical-based machines, rather than electronic machines (Solez et al. p1450).

Dialysate sodium and serum osmolality: The maintenance of 'high' serum osmolality with respect to intracellular osmolality, and its effect on blood pressure during dialysis was discussed in the preceding chapter.

Dialysate temperature: For reasons that are not well understood, end stage renal failure is associated with a lower core body temperature (Bregman et al. 2001, p 151). The haemodialysis procedure itself is frequently associated with a transitory increase in temperature that is, in turn, associated with central vasodilatation and a fall in blood pressure. The possible cause is explained as follows:

1. The combined effects of blood membrane interaction, the transport of inflammatory mediators from dialysate to blood, and the loss of amino acids and glucose to dialysate, all support increased catabolism that is associated with haemodialysis and which cause core body temperature to rise.

2. The increase in heat is normally dissipated through the peripheral circulation as blood is exposed to atmospheric temperature.

3. This normal response to heat generation is hampered, because peripheral vasoconstriction, which often follows ultrafiltration, prevents the patient from responding normally (Woods 1998, pp 5–6).

The use of 'cool' dialysate (36°) can be helpful for patients whose blood pressure falls during treatment where no obvious cause is apparent.

Postprandial hypotension: The ingestion of food results in the secretion of fluid into the stomach and intestine to facilitate digestion. A typical meal can result in 'the secretion of up to 700mls of gastric juice' (Spence and Mason, 1987, p 638). The effect of this fluid shift can last several hours and can represent fluid loss from the extracellular compartment that was planned as part of the patient's ultrafiltration requirement. Patients who develop hypotension after eating should be advised not to eat during dialysis.

Antihypertensive medication: Some patients become hypotensive as a result of taking their antihypertensive medication on the morning of, and occasionally on the evening prior to, treatment. Such patients may benefit by modifying the dose or occasionally omitting the predialysis dose.

Management of hypotension

It is likely that anyone who commences work in an acute haemodialysis unit will witness a major hypotensive episode within a very short time. Immediate treatment includes laying the patient as flat as possible (remember that some patients will have respiratory disorders that make lying flat difficult), and elevate their feet if possible. Ultrafiltration should be lowered or stopped completely, and 0·9% NaCl infused in increments usually not exceeding 200mls. Frequent monitoring of the blood pressure and pulse are required and the saline infusion titrated against the results. Some patients require intranasal oxygen.

When hypotension is anticipated, especially in patients with large volumes of interstitial fluid, the infusion of hyperoncotic albumin, containing 20g of albumin per 100 ml bottle, (Albumex 20), can assist vascular refilling and prevent hypotension. The use of sodium and water profiling and isolated ultrafiltration may also be of benefit, especially with patients who are prone to hypotension.

It is important to accurately assess fluid loss before dialysis. There is no point aggressively removing large amounts of fluid, only to have the patient become hypotensive and need an equally large infusion to be adequately resuscitated.

Hypotension is an emergency and should always be treated as such. For some patients there is a very small margin between hypotension and cardiac arrest. Other patients can move from apparently normal conversation to loss of consciousness in seconds. Always check for the presence of circulation and respiration in these patients and assume cardiac or respiratory arrest if one or both are absent.

Always follow a hypotensive episode with a review of the ultrafiltration assessment and the parameters that have were programmed into the dialysis machine. If is no trace of an error in these places review the patient's base weight, cardiac status, and the appropriateness of the fluid volume that you were attempting to remove as well as the possibilities discussed in the preceding paragraphs. Always discuss your findings with the medical staff, because the correct estimation of weight range can be difficult at the best of times.

8.2 Dialysis disequilibrium

Definition

Bregman et al. (2001, p 158) define the disequilibrium syndrome as 'a set of systemic and neurologic symptoms associated with characteristic electroencephalographic (EEG) findings that occur either during or following dialysis.' Numerous descriptions of the disequilibrium syndrome can be found, but all refer to the development of a clinical syndrome related to intracellular swelling.

Development and clinical manifestations

While the precise pathogenesis of the disequilibrium syndrome is still obscure. It is accepted that the intracellular swelling is most probably the result of water entering the cerebrospinal cells, which can be preventing a concentration gradient between the intra and extracellular spaces developing. (Bregman et al. 2001, p 158; Mujas et al. 1996, p 706; Hansen 1992, p 5; Wakim 1969, p 406). This occurs most frequently with patients who are extremely uraemic, and in whom the rapid biochemical correction of the uraemic state is attempted.

The most frequently accepted cause of water entering the cerebrospinal cells, is the ease with which urea appears to be removed from the extracellular compartment compared with its removal from the intracellular compartment. As a result, the extracellular osmolality decreases and the osmolality in the cells increases. Extravascular water crosses the cell membrane and enters the intracellular fluid in an attempt to equalise osmolality across both compartments. This is known as the 'reverse urea effect'. The demonstration of higher cerebrospinal urea levels post dialysis compared to plasma levels, lends support to the theory that urea passes more slowly from brain tissue than it does from plasma (Mujais 1996, p 706).

The most recent focus for the development of the disequilibrium syndrome is the generation of osmotically active substances inside the cells. It has been suggested that the accumulation of organic acids during dialysis could be the cause of the lowered intracellular pH, and subsequent intracellular swelling (Biasioli 2000, p 576).

Whatever the cause, the symptoms of mild disequilibrium are common, and include headache, nausea and lethargy that often trouble patients at the completion of therapy (Kaufman et al. 1993, p 113). The major symptoms of disequilibrium include confusion progressing through delirium to seizures and coma, and death. The symptoms can be accompanied by nausea and vomiting because of unphysiological fluid shifts, and cardiac arrhythmias from rapid alterations in pH and electrolyte levels. The disequilibrium syndrome can occur up to 24-hours after dialysis and the signs and symptoms often persist for two to three days (Biasioli 2000, p 576).

Management

Increased awareness of the difficulties associated with dialysis and high serum urea levels in both acute and chronic settings have resulted in a very low incidence of dialysis disequilibrium in its life-threatening form. However, the syndrome is still seen when aggressive dialysis of the extremely uraemic patient is attempted. By far the best form of management is prevention. If at all possible, dialysis should be commenced *early*, before urea levels become excessive. It should be undertaken *frequently*, daily if necessary, and it should be *gentle*, and reduce urea by no more than 30% of the predialysis value (Bregman et al. 2001, p 158). Initial treatment times should be between two and two and a half-hours.

Mujais et al. (1996, p 707) suggested that consideration be given to using the following as methods that could reduce the likelihood of disequilibrium:

1. Prophylactic osmotic agents such as glucose, fructose or mannitol administered either the intravenously or in the dialysate.

2. Reducing dialysis 'efficacy' by using slower blood and dialysate flow rates and dialysers with a low urea clearance.

The continuation of dialysis should be questioned if discrete signs of disequilibrium are suspected and treatment should be discontinued if overt signs appear. Seizures are managed with medication such as diazepam, and nursing care is the same as that for any patient requiring airway management and protection from harm.

A word of caution—disconnect the patient from the machine as soon as possible and protect the cannulae from clotting by flushing with normal saline.

Cannulae provide ideal intravenous access and should be preserved if possible. Note also, the increased likelihood of needle damage to the vascular access, and check frequently.

The differential diagnoses include cerebral haemorrhage, hypoglycaemia, delerium tremens, and a variety of metabolic and electrolyte derangements.

8.3 Haemolysis

Definition, causes and occurrence

Haemolysis refers to the 'breakdown of red blood cells and the release of haemoglobin' (Anderson 1994, p 725). Mild haemolysis is not uncommon in the dialysis population and common causes include:

- Red cell trauma due to:

  a) either the use of high blood flow rates that result in excessive negative arterial pressure, or

  b) over occlusion of the peristaltic roller pump due to failure to adequately maintain machines, or not ensuring that the blood pump segment of the extracorporeal circuit matches the occlusion programmed for the peristaltic roller pump.

- Increased fragility of the red cell that is common to all patients with end stage renal failure.

- The presence of trace levels of chemicals in the dialysate where oxidative injury causes haemoglobin to clump together as 'Heinz bodies'.

Life-threatening haemolysis that occurs during the dialysis procedure itself always represents a medical emergency. Such haemolysis is usually due to contamination of the dialysate, or to inadequately rinsed bloodlines and/or dialysers in units that reuse equipment. Prior to the use of haemodialysis machines that monitored the dialysate conductivity and temperature, hypotonic dialysate and overheated dialysate were causes of haemolysis. Dialysate contaminants known to cause haemolysis include formaldehyde, sodium hypochlorite (bleach), chloramines, copper and nitrates.

Signs, symptoms and management

Severe haemolysis presents with shortness of breath, chest tightness, back pain that is often severe and cramp like, and local pain and burning at the cannulation site if chemical contamination of the blood lines or dialyser has occurred. Cardiac arrest can follow rapidly if severe contamination has occurred.

Dialysis should be stopped immediately and *no attempt to return the blood should be made.* Any such attempt will exacerbate the situation by infusing additional haemolysed blood into the patient. Full emergency support should be prepared and the patient should receive oxygen through a cannula or mask to maximise the oxygen content of the remaining intact red blood cells. Many patients will require additional urgent dialysis to remove the potassium that leaked from the damaged cells. Some will require blood transfusion and they all should be hospitalised for observation for a twenty four-hour period because cell destruction can continue for several hours.

The classic sign of haemolysed blood is the colour change known as 'port wine staining'. This is usually best observed in the venous blood lines, especially if a light source is available to shine behind the lines. It is due to the loss of haemoglobin to the plasma. If there is time, take blood samples from both the venous and arterial blood lines, and from the dialysate inflow and outflow lines if it is possible to stop the dialysate flow as soon as the problem is recognised to determine the source of the contamination.

8.4 Membrane reactions

As discussed in Chapter 3, a number of adverse reactions can occur as a result of the patient's blood coming into contact with the extracorporeal circuit, especially the dialyser membrane. As most of these reactions have already been discussed, only 'blood gas' abnormalities are reviewed here.

Blood gas abnormalities

Hypoxaemia during haemodialysis occurs as a result of:

1. Using acetate dialysate. Hypocapnia occurs as a result of the diffusion of CO_2 across the dialyser membrane and into the dialysate. Because plasma CO_2 does not rise sufficiently to stimulate normal respiration, adequate oxygenation does not occur.

2. The sequestration of neutrophils in pulmonary capillaries, described as an 'intrapulmonary diffusion block' (Bregman et.al. 2001, p 166), reduces the surface area available for gaseous exchange.

In most patients this transient hypoxaemia causes no symptoms, but the regular use of intranasal oxygen can be beneficial for patients with underlying respiratory disorders or ischaemic cardiac disease, (Mujais 1996, p 696).

8.5 Air embolism

Causes and frequency

Air usually enters the extracorporeal circuit in patients with peripheral vascular access through a breach in the arterial portion of the circuit before the blood pump. As this portion of the circuit usually reflects a negative or subatmospheric pressure, any breach in the circuit at this point allows air to be drawn into the lines. Because the pressure profile in the circuit after the blood pump is positive, a breach in the circuit forces blood out of the lines.

These factors also apply to patients who have a central venous catheter inserted during the dialysis procedure, but there is the additional risk of the catheter being accidentally dislodged and falling out. Should this occur when the patient is upright, inspiration results in a negative pressure in the thoracic cavity and the associated danger of air being drawn into the circulation. This can also occur during catheter insertion or removal—and during connection to, or disconnection from—the extracorporeal circuit, if the catheter is disconnected without the catheter limbs being occluded.

The symptoms associated with the presence of air in the circulation vary from nothing to immediate cardiorespiratory collapse (Mujais et al. 1996, p 704). The exact amount of air required to cause cardiorespiratory arrest is probably small. Some studies suggest that '1 ml/kg may be fatal' (Mujais et.al. 1996, p 704).

Modern haemodialysis machinery is equipped with protective devices to ensure patient safety should air enter the extracorporeal circuit. Australian standards require machines to alert the operator with an audible and visual alarm, stop the blood pump, the venous line clamp must occlude the blood line and ultrafiltration reduced to its minimum value (Australian Standard 3200.2.16:1999, p 11). While the incidence of air embolism is small, technical and operator errors can still occur, and no haemodialysis equipment should be operated if the air detector cannot be armed.

The signs and symptoms of air embolism vary with the position of the patient:

> *In the sitting position, air will flow along the venous system to reach the central circulation and then will backflow into the cerebral venous system. The patient will transiently be aware of the sound of the air in his vessels and then will lose consciousness and develop seizures. In recumbent patients, air will reach the right atrium and the right ventricle, with the developing air/blood foam occluding the right ventricular outflow tract and the pulmonary vascular bed. Chest pain and shortness of breath occur, followed by cardiovascular collapse.*

(Mujais et al. 1996, p 704).

Management

Immediate management involves stopping the blood pump and placing the patient head down and on the left hand side. This position traps the air in the apex of the right ventricle and minimises frothing. As with haemolysis, *do not attempt to return blood*. Mechanical means of reducing the volume of infused air involve aspirating the air with a centrally inserted catheter, or reducing the effect of the air bubble with hyperbaric oxygen. Mechanical ventilation with normobaric oxygen can be helpful in centres that do not have access to hyperbaric oxygen (Mujais et al. 1996, p 704–705). During management, move the patient as little as possible.

The haemodynamic changes that result from air embolism include pulmonary vasoconstriction and pulmonary oedema, physical pulmonary obstruction to the microvasculature with permeability change. In addition, the presence of air in the blood activates platelets and complement (Mujais et al. 1996, p704–705).

8.6 Seizures

Predisposing haemodialysis factors

Seizures are said to occur in < 10% of patients undergoing maintenance haemodialysis, the occurrence is much higher in the ARF and ESRD populations (Swartz 1993, p 113). Seizures usually occur during haemodialysis or shortly after and careful observation is recommended for the first day after treatment. According to

Swartz (1993, p 114) there are a number of predictable characteristics associated with haemodialysis that can precipitate seizures. These include; uraemic toxicity, dialysis disequilibrium, rapid alterations in the acid-base status, hypoxaemia, haemodynamic instability, heparinisation (if intracranial bleeding has occurred), rapid transfusion (especially in children), and the dialytic removal of anticonvulsant drugs.

The association between transfusion and seizure activity in children is thought to occur because of either a rapid increase in blood viscosity or to the citrate used as an anticoagulant in blood products. While the use of erythropoietin has reduced the need for transfusions, it is also associated with seizure activity if the haemoglobin and therefore the haematocrit are increased too quickly.

Predisposing patient factors

It is also possible to identify certain patient groups who are predisposed to seizures. According to Swartz (1993, p 114) these include:

1. A history of seizure activity.

2. The presence of a primary CNS lesion.

3. Young age.

4. Microvascular disease:

   i)   malignant hypertension

   ii)   atheroembolism

   iii) haemolytic uraemic syndrome.

5. Myocardial infarction, severe cardiomyopathy.

6. Metabolic encephalopathy:

   i)   severe uraemia

   ii)   hepatic encephalopathy

   iii) sepsis

   iv)   drug intoxication.

7. Laboratory findings:

    i)   hypoglycaemia

    ii)   hyper/hypo tonicity

    iii)   marked acid-base disturbance

    iv)   low serum calcium and/or magnesium

    v)   hypoxaemia or severe anaemia.

Paediatric patients are especially prone to seizures during dialysis (Mujais et al. 1996, p 714). Using a dialyser and blood lines that are appropriate for the child's weight and body surface area can minimise the risk of seizures in children. Special aspects of paediatric dialysis are addressed later in Chapter 6.

Secondary central nervous system disorders that share cerebral involvement that can precipitate seizure activity, and renal involvement,(which frequently requires dialysis, also need to be considered. According to Ali and Pirizda (1999, p 427), these include:

1. Polyarteritis nodosa, with mononeuritis multiplex and central nervous system vasculitis.

2. Systemic lupus erythematosis, with neuropsychiatric disease, cerebral infarcts, myelitis and neuropoathy.

3. Wegener's granulomatosis, with granulomatous inflammation and peripheral neuropathy.

4. Thrombotic thrombocytopaenic purpura, with cerebral oedema, seizures, and fluctuating focal deficits.

5. Rheumatoid arthritis, with CNS vasculitis, cervical myelopathy and neuropathy.

6. Hypertensive encephalopathy, with headache, seizures, altered sensorium and coma.

7. Autosomal polycystic kidney disease, with cerebral aneurysms.

Therapeutic considerations

Predialysis interventions, and alterations in the dialysis prescription are the mainstay of therapeutic interventions designed to minimise seizures and were discussed in Chapter 1 of this section.

8.7   Cardiac arrhythmias

Overview

Ventricular dysfunction is often the cause of arrhythmias in dialysis patients. Conditions such as coronary artery disease, left ventricular hypertrophy, pericarditis and dilated cardiomyopathy are recognised as being specific contributors (Harnett et al. 1999, p 242). Arrhythmias also occur in patients with normal cardiac function where acid-base and/or electrolyte disorders are extreme. Rapid reduction of serum potassium, hypotension, and stopping antiarrhythmic medication also contribute to the problem.

Cardiac disease is common in the dialysis population and accounts for approximately 40% of overall deaths (Parfrey et al. 1996, p 990). It is not surprising that many patients develop an arrhythmia at some stage. While most of these are of little clinical importance, some require pharmacological intervention. Cardiac arrest accounts for approximately 9% of sudden deaths, with ventricular fibrillation being the most common cause (Harnet et al. 1999, p 242).

These figures relate to the end stage renal failure population in general and not to deaths that occur during the dialysis procedure itself. However, the electrolyte and fluid shifts that occur during dialysis predispose many patients to rhythm disorders, especially those patients undergoing dialysis during some other acute illness.

Arrhythmias related to digoxin

Arrhythmias that are associated with the use of digoxin occur most frequently due to hypokalaemia (Rutsky 1993, p 116) that is the result of inappropriately low potassium in the dialysate concentrate, or to intracellular shifts in potassium.

Many patients take digoxin preparations for congestive cardiac failure (CCF) before commencing dialysis (Rutsky 1993, p 117). CCF is frequently due to either fluid volume expansion and an increase in cardiac preload, or to hypertension causing an increase in after load—many patients experience both. Review of these patients at the commencement of dialysis might enable some to discontinue digoxin medication as both the volume expansion and hypertension often respond to ultrafiltration. If dilated cardiomyopathy is present, persistent problems with an increase in afterload might respond to vasodilatory drugs, thus avoiding the use of digoxin (Rutsky 1993, p 117).

Patients with acute renal failure who required unexpected dialysis could be taking digitalis preparations and the opportunity to review their medications can be overlooked.

Arrhythmias unrelated to digoxin

Arrhythmias occurring in patients not receiving digitalis are usually due to underlying cardiac disease but hypokalaemia can potentiate rhythm disturbances. Most patients can tolerate a potassium dialysate of 2 mmol/l. The use of this lower dialysate potassium is especially important in patients with atrioventricular block or impaired atrioventricular junctional conduction where hyperkalaemia can aggravate these disturbances (Rutsky 1993, p 117).

According to Rutsky (1993, p 117), haemodialysis is also associated with factors known to increase myocardial oxygen consumption such as tachycardia, as well as decreasing myocardial oxygen delivery e.g. anaemia, hypoxaemia and hypotension. All of these factors have the potential to cause arrhythmias.

Diabetes and cardiac dysfunction

In the diabetic patient, large and small vessel disease, as well as cardiac dysfunction, are thought to occur as a result of the cross linkage of collagen fibres. Cross linkage is in turn due to the glycosylation of collagen (Harnett et. al.1999, p 243). Other risk factors for cardiac disease in diabetics include hyperlipidaemia, hypertension (Harnett et. al. 1999, p 243) and hypercholesterolaemia (Nicholls 2001, p 606) all of which accelerate the atherosclerosis common in end stage renal failure, especially in diabetic patients.

The most common cause of morbidity and mortality in diabetics is cardiovascular disease (Mahgoub and Abd-Elfattah 1995, p 59) this is of particular concern because of the 'marked prevalence of silent ischaemic heart disease' that occurs in diabetics (Parfrey and Lamiere 2001, p 286). The term 'silent infarct' refers to the fact that the person is unaware of ischaemic pain due to autonomic neuropathy and does not seek treatment. Without treatment the cardiac pathology progresses and often proves fatal.

References

In text references

Ali, I., Pirizda, N, 1999, 'Complications associated with dialysis and chronic renal insufficiency', in *Principles and Practice of Dialysis,* Henrich, W. (ed), 2nd ed., William and Wilkins, Maryland.

Anderson, K., 1994, *Mosby's Dictionary,* Mosby, Sydney.

Australian standard 3200.2.16:1999, 'Medical and electrical equipment: particular requirements for haemodialysis, haemodiafiltration and haemofiltration equipment', Standards Association of Australia, Sydney.

Biasioli, S., 2000, 'Neurological complications of dialysis', in *Complications of dialysis,* Lamiere, N., Mehta, R., (eds.), Marcel Dekker, New York.

Bregman, H., Daugirdas, J., Ing, T. 2001, 'Complications during hemodialysis' in *Handbook of Dialysis,* Daugirdas, J., Blake, P., Ing, T. (eds.), 3rd ed., Lippincott Williams and Wilkins, Philadelphia.

Hansen, S., 1992, 'Patient assessment in acute haemodialysis', J CNNT, vol.2, no., 1, pp 17–9.

Harnett, J., Foley, R., Parfrey, P., 1999, 'Left ventricular dysfunction in dialysis patients', in *Principles and Practice of Dialysis,* Henrich, W. (ed), 2nd ed., William and Wilkins, Maryland.

Kaufman, A., Polascheggi, H., Levin, N., 1993, 'Common clinical problems during hemodialysis', in *Dialysis Therapy*, Nissenson, A., Fine, R, (eds.), 2nd ed., Hanley and Belfus, Philadelphia.

Leunissen, K., Kooman, J., van der Sande, 2000, 'Acute dialysis complications', in *Complications of Dialysis,* Lamiere, N., Mehta, R. (eds.), Marcel Dekker, New York.

Lysaght, M., 1995, Evolution of Haemodialysis Membranes in *Dialysis membranes: structure and predictions,* Bonomoni, V., Berland, Y. (eds.), Karger, Sydney.

Mahgoub, M., Abd-Elfattah, A., 1995, 'Diabetes mellitus and cardiac function,' in *Molecular and Cellular Biochemistry,* vol. 180, nos. 1–2, pp 59–64.

Mujais, S., Ing, T., Kjellstrand, C., 1996, 'Acute complications of haemodialysis', in *Replacement of Renal Function by Dialysis,* Jacobs, C., Kjellstrand, C., Koch, K., (eds.), 4th ed., Kluwer Academic Publishers, Boston.

Parfrey, P., Lamiere, N., 2001, 'Cardiac disease in haemodialysis and peritoneal dialysis patients,' in *Complications of Dialysis,* Lamiere, N., Mehta, R., Marcel Dekker, New York.

Parfrey, P., Foley, R., Harnett, J., 1996, 'Organic and metabolic complications: cardiac', in *Replacement of Renal Function by Dialysis,* Jacobs, C., Kjellstrand, C., Koch, K., (eds.), 4th ed., Kluwer Academic Publishers, Boston.

Rutsky, E., 1993, 'Arrhythmias in hemodialysis patients', in *Dialysis Therapy*, Nissenson, A., Fine, R, (eds.), 2nd ed., Hanley and Belfus, Philadelphia.

Sherman, R., 1988, 'The pathophysiological basis for hemodialysis-related hypotension', *Seminars in Dialysis*, vol. 1, no. 2, pp 136–142.

Solez, K., Nadjafi, I., Zafarmand, A., Collins, A., 1996, 'Planning of dialysis for disasters', in *Replacement of Renal Function by Dialysis,* Jacobs, C., Kjellstrand, C., Koch, K., (eds.), 4th ed., Kluwer Academic Publishers, Boston.

Spence, A., Mason, E., 1987, *Human Anatomy and Physiology*, (3rd ed.) Benjamin Cummings, Sydney.

Swartz, R., 1993, 'Haemodialysis associated seizure activity', in *Dialysis Therapy*, Nissenson, A., Fine, R, (eds.), 2nd ed., Hanley and Belfus, Philadelphia

Wakim, G., 1969, 'The pathophysiology of the dialysis disequilibrium', Mayo Clinic Proceedings, vol. 44, pp 406–429.

Woods, F., 1998, 'Trends in haemodialysis technology', Paper presented on behalf of Fresenius Medical Care, Melbourne, Victoria, December 1998.

Recommended reading

Perazella, M., 1999, 'Approach to patients with intradialytic hypotension: a focus on therapeutic options', Seminars in Dialysis, vol. 12, no., 3, pp 175–181

Epstein, A., Kay, G., Plumb, V., 1989, 'Considerations in the diagnosis and treatment of arrhythmias in patients with end stage renal disease', *Seminars in Dialysis*, vol. 2, no. 1 (Jan–Mar), pp 31–37.

CHAPTER NINE

Assessment of therapy

Introduction

During the 1960's and early 1970's when haemodialysis was in its infancy, the majority of patients with end stage renal failure were dialysed three times a week for between six and eight hours per session. As dialyser efficiency increased, membrane surface area was reduced and treatment times were shortened accordingly. The advent of dialysers with an ultrafiltration coefficient greater than 10 ml/hour/mmHgTMP led to the use of what became known as 'high flux' or 'high efficiency' dialysis. When this was combined with blood flow rates of up to 500 ml/min. treatment times were further decreased, often to less than three and one half-hours per session. There is an ever-increasing search for additional funding in health care and these short treatment sessions enabled dialysis to be used for the maximum number of patients over the shortest period of time.

However, not all countries adopted the shortened programs and when morbidity and mortality rates were compared amongst a number of countries it became apparent that those using the shortest treatment times had the highest rates of morbidity and mortality. This study suggested that there were probably a number of factors involved in providing 'optimum' dialysis and the search for ways by which this could be determined commenced. They are known by such terms as 'dialysis prescription' and 'dialysis dose'. This chapter will address the factors that, at the time of writing, appear paramount in the provision of adequate dialysis.

9.1 Historical perspective

Background

A review of the morbidity and mortality rates for patients receiving maintenance dialysis in a variety of countries showed that patients in the United States of America

(U.S.A.) had a higher death rate than other countries (Depner 1999, p 79). This unacceptably high mortality rate led to the eventual recognition that solute clearance, and not membrane size, as had previously been thought, was one of the most significant factors in patient survival.

In 1974 the National Institutes of Health convened the National Cooperative Dialysis Study (NCDS) to evaluate methods that could be used to determine the amount of dialysis that was required to keep a patient essentially free of the 'clinical consequences of renal failure' (Harter 1983, p S 107). Nine dialysis units throughout the U.S.A. participated in the study that involved dividing patients in to four groups:

Group 1:   Long dialysis time (4.5 to 5 hours) with a low serum urea.
Group 2:   Long dialysis time (4.5 to 5 hours) with a high serum urea.
Group 3:   Short dialysis time (2.5 to 3.5 hours) with a low serum urea.
Group 4:   Short dialysis time (2.5 to 3.5 hours) with a high serum urea.

Low urea was defined as a midweek predialysis blood urea nitrogen (BUN) of 60–80 mg/dl with a 'time averaged concentration' of 50 mg/dl * and high was defined as midweek predialysis level between 110 and 130 with a 'time averaged concentration' of 100 mg/dl)(Hakim 1990, p 822). This relates approximately to serum urea levels of 21(5–28 (5 mmol/l and 39.5–40.5 mmol/l respectively. Time averaged concentrations are (again approximately), 18–35(5 mmol/l respectively. In the USA serum urea is given in mg/dl. The author made the conversions to mmol/l.

To convert urea nitrogen given in mg/dl (as measured in the U.S.A.) to mmol/l (as for SI units), multiply by 0.357. To convert creatinine to µmol/l multiply by 88.4

* The use of 'time averaged concentration' of urea (TAC urea) corrects for the fluctuations of serum urea levels seen in dialysis-dependent people and is a more accurate reflection of the 'uraemic environment', specific for a given patient.

All patients participating in the NCDS study had their daily protein intake controlled to 0.8 gm/kg/day for the group with a low BUN and 1.4 gm/kg/day for the group with a high BUN (Harter 1983, p S 107).

The findings of the study were:

1. Fewer hospitalisations at the end of one year for groups 1 and 3 (longer dialysis and lower BUN) than for groups 2 and 4 (shorter dialysis and higher BUN).

2.   Increased cardiovascular morbidity for groups 2 and 4.

3.   Increased prevalence of GIT disorders for groups 2 and 4.

There was no difference in the mortality rate between the four groups during the six months of the study, but in the year following the completion of the study nine of thirteen reported deaths occurred in patients from groups 2 and 4.

From these data, the authors concluded that, in the presence of adequate dietary protein a low TAC urea was the most important factor in preventing high rates of morbidity and mortality. Later analysis of the data showed that longer dialysis was also an independently significant factor. The higher death rates for groups 2 and 4 following the study indicated that improved dialysis adequacy could not readily undo the damage caused by initial inadequate treatment.

Many other studies have been conducted over the past decade and consideration of the combined findings of this research resulted in the development of best practice standards by several countries. Quantification of the amount of dialysis required and the amount that is delivered is now standard practice for many units.

9.2   The kinetics of urea generation and removal

Why measure urea?

Urea is a substance of low molecular weight that diffuses easily across biological membranes. Because it is dissolved in total body water it is dispersed evenly across all body compartments. Once equilibration occurs the measurement of serum urea is considered to be representative of urea distribution in other body compartments (Depner 1994, p 1522). This is known as a single-pool model.

Dual-pool models consider urea to be distributed in two primary areas, the intravascular compartment and the extravascular compartment. During dialysis, and for a short period after, there is a lag time during which the extracellular urea levels will be lower than those within the cells. Once equilibration between both compartments occurs, serum urea levels taken some hours after dialysis will be higher than levels taken immediately after dialysis. During conventional dialysis the single-pool model is satisfactory. Dual- or multiple-pool analysis becomes important when high efficiency/high flux dialysis is used because these treatments result in greater disparity between the intra and extravascular compartments. In turn, this results in a greater level of urea rebound after treatment and a higher Kt/V is usually required if conventional treatment times are reduced or if the number of treatment sessions is decreased (Haraldsson 199 pp 1849–1850).

The term 'kinetic modelling' describes the construction of a mathematical model that enables the study of a substance from the time it is introduced into the body until it is excreted. Modelling the kinetics of urea enables analysis of nitrogen intake and excretion to be analysed. Such a model provides a useful marker for the study of protein intake, catabolic status and nutrition because urea is the primary metabolite generated from protein catabolism, (Terrill 1990, p 86).

Using the observation that uraemic symptoms are usually absent with a glomerular filtration rate of 10% of normal, early studies indicated that the removal of urea should at least approximate this minimal glomerular filtration rate (Teschan, in Hakim 1990, p 824). When this figure is normalised to the volume of distribution (V) of the 'average' man, dialytic urea clearances should approximate 100 litres/week. This represents a Kt/V of 1.0. Subsequent studies indicated that this figure, the 'dialysis dose', was somewhat conservative and the Caring for Australians with Renal Impairment Guidelines (CARI) recommend a Kt/V of 1.2.

The term Kt/V relates dialyser clearance (K) and the time of dialysis (t) to the volume of urea distribution (V). In the 'average' 70 kg man, 60% of body weight is water; therefore the average distribution of urea is into 60 litres of water. There are some problems with these 'averages' that are discussed later. Thus, the time (t) that a dialyser has to achieve a given urea clearance (K) is individualised to the volume of urea distribution (V) for each patient. The resulting figure represents an index (1.2 is the aim) that in turn represents the 'adequacy of dialysis'.

Why is this important? The NCDS found that high levels of urea, especially TAC urea, were associated with an increase in morbidity and mortality. The cardiovascular, gastrointestinal and neurological systems were found to be particularly vulnerable and it was noted that once damage had occurred to these organs it was not easily reversed. Once recognised, it was considered prudent to maximise the quality and quantity of each patient's life by commencing dialysis with an adequate prescription.

The formula for determining dialyser clearance (litres/hr) is shown in Figure 2.9.1.

$$Qb \times [(Cb_{in} - Cb_{out}) \div Cb_{in}] \times (60 \div 1000)$$

Key: Cb in is the concentration of urea entering the dialyser (mmol/l)
Cb out is the concentration of urea leaving the dialyser (mmol/l)
Qb is blood flow rate
The blood ports on the arterial and venous lines are used to obtain samples.

Figure 2.9.1: The formula used to calculate dialyser clearance rates.

Urea generation: It is well documented that many patients with end stage renal failure are malnourished. The NCDS found that inadequate nutrition was the second major contributor to mortality and morbidity. A variety of methods, including food diaries, anthropometric measurements and measurement of serum albumin levels, have been devised in an attempt to measure nutritional status, but they all have deficiencies.

The target protein intake is generally set at 1.2 g/kg/ideal body weight (IBW) with a range between 0.8 and 1.4. Patients with a dietary protein intake < 0.8 g/kg/IBW are considered malnourished and those with an intake > 1.4 g/kg/IBW are at risk of becoming uraemic. Sargent et al. (1978) who were amongst the pioneers in the development and use of urea kinetic modelling, suggested that the urea kinetic model could be extended to measure a given patient's protein intake. Dietary protein intake is linked directly to urea generation and this in turn is linked to the protein catabolic rate (PCR). PCR is usually measured in grams per day and protein intake is measured in g/kg. To enable the comparison of 'like' units the normalised protein catabolic rate is used (nPCR). Calculations can be undertaken using computerised programs or manual calculations. Manual calculation of the urea generation rate can be determined as follows:

a)   Subtract the urea level postdialysis (C_2) from the urea level prior to the commencement of the next dialysis (C_3).

b)   Divide this figure by the number of hours from the end of previous dialysis and the start of the next, i.e. the interdialytic time (Id).

c)   Multiply this figure by the volume of body water (V). Remember this is an ~ of 60% of body weight.

d)   Multiply this by 24 (the number of hours per day).

The equation is written as: $[(C_3 - C_2) \div Id] \times V \times 24$ (Terrill 1990, p 87).

Protein intake can then be determined using the following formula:

(urea generation x 0.175) + (weight in kgs x 0.2)

For patients with residual renal function, calculate the urinary urea for the 24 hours between dialyses, add this figure to the urea generation rate and then proceed using the formula given for calculating urea generation (Terrill 1990, p 87). The figure 0.2 incorporates nitrogen generated from non-urea sources, and the 0.175 converts mmols of urea to grams of protein.

9.3   Determining the dialysis prescription

Factors to consider

There are a number of patient-specific and treatment-specific variables that need to be considered when determining the amount of dialysis required for a given patient. Patient-specific considerations include volume for urea distribution (total body water), the urea generation rate, residual renal function, fluid accumulation and solute compartmentalisation. Treatment-related variables include dialyser clearance, which will be affected by the type of dialyser chosen, and the flow rates for both blood and dialysate, the duration of dialysis and its frequency (Depner 1999, p 81). Patients with diabetes, or who are pregnant, may need additional dialysis because of increased catabolism.

The current trend towards providing higher doses of dialysis has resulted in average urea levels falling below the safe figure initially recommended by the NCDS. Despite the shift away from protein restriction, less emphasis is now placed on adjusting the dialysis dose in accordance with urea generation rates (Depner 1999, p 81).

Residual renal function, even as low as 2ml/min, can make a significant contribution to overall urea removal (Depner 1999, p 81). The practice of decreasing dialysis time in accordance with the contribution to urea removal varies from unit-to-unit. Some nephrologists make no allowance, with the rationale that residual function will soon disappear. Others alter treatments, for example to 2 x 5 hour sessions or 3 x 3 hour sessions. Although a patient receiving thrice-weekly dialysis may have the same K^t/V as a patient receiving twice-weekly dialysis, they are receiving very different doses of dialysis. Gotch suggested that the K^t/V for a twice-weekly dialysis should be 1.8; this corresponds to a K^t/V of 1.0 for dialysis that occurs three times a week (Blake and Daugirdas 1994, p 626). It is possible to calculate the contribution of residual function to the K^t/V index, and the interested reader is referred to Terrill (1990).

The practice of using V, although convenient and currently still practiced, is a guide only. While the concentration of urea in body fluids is thought to be a primary contributor to toxicity, 'concentration is a function of generation and removal' (Depner 1999, p 81), and as such does not depend on the V. If generation and removal are equal, V becomes irrelevant in determining the prescription. It is interesting to note that, while interdialytic fluid gain increases the need for fluid removal, it actually decreases the diffusive requirement for dialysis. This is due to both a dilutional effect, and the fact that fluid removal increases solute removal (Depner 1999, p 81), but does not mean that you should encourage large fluid gains.

Deciding on the amount

According to Depner (1999, p 81) 'the amount of dialysis required to keep patients healthy and relatively symptom free is probably greater that the amount required to keep them alive for a year'. The NCDS showed that low average TAC urea and proving adequate nutrition were two of the most important features in the reduction of morbidity and mortality. When this knowledge is combined with the minimum dialysis requirement, expressed as a K^t/V of 1.0 'adequate' dialysis is probably being delivered. The aim however should be for a K^t/V of 1.2 (CARI Guidelines 2000). However, because other, as yet unidentified, toxins contribute to the uraemic syndrome, adequate dialysis is probably not occurring in a symptomatic patient.

The extremely good survival rates for Charra's haemodialysis population in Tassin, France revealed the length of each dialysis session to be an important indicator of adequacy, despite the fact that dialysis was given using acetate-based dialysate and cuprophan membranes. Charra et al's much-quoted 1992 study has important implications for the future of dialysis, especially with the continuing push towards shorter treatment times and more efficient membranes.

Urea removal: Urea removal can be calculated by biochemical analysis of either the blood or dialysate.

1. Analysis of the dialysate focuses on the urea present in the dialysate effluent and can be done by collecting the effluent and calculating the urea content, which is difficult and impractical at best. Alternatively, specifically designed tools that calculate K^t/V and urea reduction ration (URR) in real time can be used. The latter has the theoretical advantage of not exposing the blood compartment

while 'simultaneously focusing upon the amount of urea removed rather than the amount remaining (Basham & Agar 1997, p733).

2. Analysis of the blood is usually done in one of two ways:

    a) Via measurement of K^t/V that has already been discussed at length.

    b) Via measurement of the URR, also known as percentage (of) reduction of urea (PRU).

URR is calculated as follows:

[(Predialysis urea - postdialysis urea) ÷ predialysis urea] x 100.

Kerr et al. (1993 p 152) have shown that this calculation compares favourably with formal calculations of K^t/V, and is a quick and reliable method of assessment.

K^t/V of 1.2 equates to a URR of 65%. The current practice in the UK favours the analysis of blood samples and URR is used more frequently because of its ease (Renal Association Standards, 2002).

1. Problems and pitfalls

Traps for new players

For starters, both K^t/V and URR describe the clearance of urea for a given time period. When used to estimate protein intake, they only examine what has happened from one dialysis to the next. If patients know that they are to have a 'kinetic model' performed, chances are that they will adhere strictly to their prescribed diet and fluid regimen. K^t/V analysis (or the estimation of URR) will therefore reveal 'what should be happening' as opposed to 'what is really happening'.

1. The 't' part of this equation, time spent on dialysis, often does not incorporate nondiffusive events such as the time that the blood pump may have stopped due to arterial or venous pressure alarms, or the time spent in 'housekeeping' or the 'time out' that the machine takes out to perform its automated 'self-checks' in relation to the accuracy of fluid removal. Some haemodialysis machines add the 'nondiffusive time' automatically to the total treatment time, while others do not, which allows the dialysis nurse the option of adding it to the total treatment time.

2. Volume of distribution is another variable. Sixty percent of body weight is a convenient and average figure for the V of urea, however the question, should

allowances be made for the difference in V for males and females and/or for the differences that occur in people who have more or less body fat, arise. Males, on average, have a higher proportion of lean tissue to fatty tissue than do females. This means that males have a higher percentage of body weight as water than females because lean tissue contains more water than fatty tissue (Smith 1991, p 26).

3.   Dialyser clearance figures provided by the manufacturer are also only a guide and the invitro clearance figures they provide are only accurate to +/- 10%. The use of 'invitro' as opposed to 'invivo' measurements can make a significant difference to clearance data, and are recognised as possible sources of inaccuracies. It is suggested that, prior to initiating dialysis-adequacy studies, individual clearance figures for each patient (invivo clearance data) should be determined.

4.   Recirculation of blood also affects clearance studies. Two types of recirculation need to be considered.

   a)   Recirculation occurring in the vascular access will reduce clearance for all solutes and occurs when blood that has already been 'dialysed' is returned to the arterial needle prior to being returned to the central circulation. Most nephrologists agree that recirculation is excessive when it exceeds 10%, and it may be preferable to revise the vascular access, or the placement of cannulae before considering a change in either dialysis time or dialyser. Increasing the blood flow rates is not always the answer for poor clearances. In some instances it will only result in an increase in the recirculation rate.

   b)   Cardiopulmonary recirculation occurs when dialysed blood is returned to the central circulation and after passing through the heart and lungs it is returned to the access limb. This is a normal event, but it can result in apparently poor clearance figures. To prevent cardiopulmonary recirculation confusing the results, it is suggested to either wait for a short period of time (~ 30 seconds) or reduce the blood flow rate, prior to collecting blood for the systemic sample. Sherman and Kapoian (1999, p 64) suggest that the following method should be used when collecting blood for recirculation studies:

      1.   Set the blood pump to the desired speed for at least three minutes.

      2.   Collect venous and arterial blood samples.

      3.   Reduce blood pump speed to between 120 and 150 ml/min. for at least 10 seconds, and then stop the pump.

4. Place a clamp above the arterial port.

5. Collect systemic sample from the arterial port.

6. Determine the recirculation rate (%R); %R = (s - a) ÷ (s - v).

Current suggestions for improving the dose of dialysis that is delivered include haemodiafiltration (discussed in Chapter 3), short daily dialysis (for 2 to 2$^{1}/_{2}$ hours per day), nocturnal daily dialysis (for 6 to 10 hrs/night) and the use of two dialysers in tandem (Powers et al. 2000).

There are several other problems with the interpretation of Kt/V but the ones discussed here are the principal ones especially as far as nursing assessment is concerned. Modelling for Kt/V measures the dose of dialysis that was provided. Although it correlates with outcomes, the correlation is not linear, neither is it perfect, but it does provide a guide to treatment, and a 'stop gap method of assuring dialysis adequacy in the absence of knowledge about the critical toxins removed' (Depner 1999, p 82).

References

In text references

Basham, L., Agar, J., 1997, 'Time spent on dialysis: The paramount consideration in dialysis adequacy? *Dialysis and Transplantation*, vol. 26, no.11, pp 739, 743–749.

Blake, P., Daugirdas, J., 1996, 'Quantification and prescription general principles' in *Replacement of Renal Function by Dialysis*, Maher (ed.), 3rd ed., Kluwer Academic Publishers, Boston.

CARI Guidelines, 2000, 'Caring for Australians with renal impairment', a joint project between the Australian and New Zealand Society of Nephrology and the Australian Kidney Foundation, Excerpta Medica Communications, Sydney.

Charra, B., Calemard, E., Ruffet, M., Chazot, C., Terrat, J., Vanel, T., Laurent, G., 1992, 'Survival as an index of adequacy of dialysis', *Kidney International*, vol. 41, pp 1286–1291.

Depner, T., 1994, 'Assessing adequacy of haemodialysis: urea kinetic modelling, *Kidney International*, vol. 45, pp 1522–1535.

Depner, T., 1999, 'Approach to haemodialysis kinetic modelling', in *Principles and Practice of Dialysis*, Henrich, W. (ed), 2nd ed., William and Wilkins, Maryland.

Gotch, F., 1990 'Kinetic modelling in haemodialysis' in *Clinical Dialysis*, 2nd edition Nissenson, A, Fine, R., Gentile, D., (eds.), California, Appleton and Lange.

Hakim, R., 1990 'Assessing the adequacy of dialysis', Kidney International, vol. 37, pp 822–832.

Haraldsson, B., 1995, 'Higher Kt/V is needed for adequate dialysis if treatment time is reduced', *Nephrology, Dialysis and Transplantation*, vol. 10. pp 1845–1851.

Harter, H., 1983, 'Review of significant findings from the National Cooperative Dialysis Study', *Kidney International*, vol. 23, Suppl. 13, pp S 107–S112.

Kerr, P., Argiles, A., Canaud, B., 1993, 'Accuracy of estimations in high flux haemodiafiltration using percentage reduction of urea: incorporation of urea rebound', *Nephrology, Dialysis and Transplantation*, vol. 8, no. 2, pp 149–153.

Powers, K., Wilkowski, J., Helmandollar, A., Koenig, K., Bolton, W., 2000 'Improved urea reduction ration and Kt/V using two dialysers in parallel', *American Journal of Kidney Disease*, vol. 35. no. 2, pp 266–274.

Renal Association Standards (3e), 2002, *Treatment of Adults and Children with Renal Failure*.

Sargent, J., Gotch, F., Boral, M., Piercy, L., Spinozzi, N., Schoenfeld, P., Humphries, M., 1978, 'Urea kinetics: a guide to the nutritional management of renal failure, *American Journal of Clinical Nutrition*, vol. 31, pp 1696–1702.

Sherman, R., Kapoian, T., 1999, 'Re-circulation in the haemodialysis access', in *Principles and Practice of Dialysis*, Henrich, W. (ed), 2nd ed., William and Wilkins, Maryland.

Smith, K., 1991. 'Fluids and electrolytes: a conceptual approach', Churchill Livingstone, London.

Terrill, B., 1990, 'Urea kinetic modelling', *Renal Educator*, vol. 10, no. 4, pp 86–88.

Teschan P., Ginn, H., Bourne, J., Ward, J., 1977 'Neurobehavioural problems for adequacy of dialysis', *Trans American Society for Artificial Internal Organs*, vol. 23, pp 556–560.

Recommended reading

Bergstrom, J., 1993, 'Nutrition and adequacy of dialysis in haemodialysis patients', *Kidney International*, vol. 43, Suppl. 41, pp S 261–S 267.
Levin, N., Gotch, F., Bednar, B., Gallaher, N., Peterson, G., 1991, 'Kinetics and quality assurance: prescription therapy through kinetic modelling', *ANNA Journal*, Vol. 18, no 3. pp 269–279.

Powers, K., Wilkowski, J., Helmandollar, A., Koenig, K., Bolton, W., 2000, 'Improved urea reduction ratio and Kt/V using two dialysers in parallel', *American Journal of Kidney Disease*, vol. 35. no. 2, pp 266–274.

SECTION THREE

Haemofiltration

Introduction

Haemofiltration is a process that relies on ultrafiltration to remove excess body water, and on convective solute transport to remove metabolic waste products and accumulated electrolytes.

Haemofiltration, in a variety of forms, has been available to treat renal failure for the last three decades, but the process has only recently been employed on a large scale to treat both acute and chronic renal failure. In some parts of the world, automated haemofiltration is the standard thrice-weekly treatment for patients with end stage renal failure. In other areas, it is only available in its continuous form as a treatment for acute renal failure in critical care environments. Either way, it offers options that minimise many of the side effects of conventional haemodialysis for both the acute and chronically ill.

1.1 Overview of haemofiltration

Historical perspective

Although haemofiltration has been available for the treatment of renal failure since the 1970's (Stansfield 1988, p 1), it is only in the last decade that it has become accepted as a valid treatment for both acute and chronic renal failure (Mehta 1996, p 81). Initially these therapies evolved in an attempt to improve the outcomes of patients with acute renal failure. Many of these patients had multiple organ failure, often complicated by septicaemia and gastrointestinal bleeding (Sigler and Teehan 1993, p 143). Conditions such as these frequently render patients haemodynamically unstable and therefore unsuitable for 'conventional' dialysis for the following reasons:

1. Patients with acute renal failure often poorly tolerate the sudden shifts in fluid and electrolyte balance that occur with haemodialysis, especially if inotropic support is required to maintain blood pressure.

2. Peritoneal dialysis, although considered a 'gentler' form of treatment, is also poorly tolerated by patients with compromised cardiopulmonary status, and is unsuitable for patients who are in a catabolic state, or who have undergone recent abdominal surgery.

Although the advantages of convective solute removal for the correction of uraemia was described during the 1970's, it was not until the advent of low resistant haemofilters that the technique could be used to allow the continuous removal of fluid and metabolic waste. This treatment commenced with the use of ultrafiltration for the emergency removal of fluid from patients with pulmonary oedema, and was followed by its use as an adjunct to treatment with end stage renal failure. Finally, it was introduced as a renal replacement therapy in intensive care units for patients with acute renal failure (Kaplan 1996, p 390). These initial therapies used a system that was powered by the patient's arterial blood pressure. Known as continuous arteriovenous haemofiltration, the technique is described in Section 2 of this chapter.

Transport principles

Early articles on haemofiltration often referred to the procedure as 'artificial glomerular filtration' (Stansfield 1988, p 3), because, in principle, it is similar to normal glomerular function. In the normal kidney, water and small solutes are freely filtered at glomerular level, and the excess is reabsorbed in the renal tubule. With haemofiltration, water and solutes are also freely filtered across the filtration membrane in accordance with membrane porosity and molecule size. In those treatments that require it, the excess fluid is replaced via an appropriate infusion into the extracorporeal circuit.

Haemofiltration is a generic term that refers to a number of techniques, all of which share similar principles, but which have been modified to treat a variety of conditions. These different modifications are described fully later in the chapter. Before proceeding to these sections, it will be helpful to discuss the similarities involved.

Solute removal occurs according to 'high volume ultrafiltration'. This means that as fluid moves across the semipermeable membrane, solute accompanies it according to the principle of convection, sometimes referred to as 'solute drag'. Some treatments are used for fluid removal only, while others are used as renal replacement therapies. For haemofiltration to be effective as a renal replacement therapy, sufficient fluid must cross the membrane to 'drag' accumulated solute and metabolic waste products in quantities that will keep plasma solute levels in a normal or 'safe' range. This requires the removal of large volumes of fluid (often exceeding 50 litres) and therefore requires the simultaneous replacement of most of this fluid and many of the electrolytes. If fluid removal only, is required, the amount is determined by the patient's fluid volume and proposed infusion requirements, and replacement fluid is not required.

As with all extracorporeal therapies designed to remove a component in the plasma, the pore size (sieving coefficient) of the membrane will determine the dalton size of the substance removed. For haemofiltration membranes, the sieving coefficient is up to 50 000 daltons (Price 1991, p 241). This is far in excess of that of haemodialyser membranes, but still less than that of the glomerular basement membrane.

Fluid replacement

For those therapies requiring fluid replacement, the fluid selected should be similar to 'non uraemic plasma'. This may be supplied by using a combination of isotonic fluids usually selected for standard intravenous fluid use, or the use of a replacement product manufactured specifically for use in haemofiltration. Increasingly, intermittent therapies, which are discussed in Section 3, use 'on line' production of a replacement fluid manufactured from a mix of water and dialysate concentrate that has been subjected to a filtration process that renders it suitable for infusion into the extracorporeal circuit.

The fluid may be infused 'prefilter' into the arterial portion of the extracorporeal circuit where it achieves 'predilution' of the extracorporeal blood. Alternatively, it is given 'post filter' into the venous portion of the extracorporeal circuit where it achieves 'post dilution' of the extracorporeal blood. According to Whittaker (1989, p149) predilution has a number of advantages:

1. The prefilter haematocrit is lowered, resulting in decreased blood viscosity and a reduced likelihood of clotting.

2. Blood flow through the filter is enhanced, and ultrafiltration is maximised due to the decrease in oncotic pressure.

The major disadvantage is the increased amount of replacement fluid that is required, because approximately one third will be removed with the ultrafiltrate.

Post dilution avoids this problem, but should be avoided in patients with a high haematocrit, as the risk of clotting will be increased (Whittaker 1989, p 149).

Circuit maintenance

The extracorporeal circuit is subject to problems similar to those seen in haemodialysis. Anticoagulation is required for most patients and may be systemic or regional. Some patients, especially those with impaired coagulation, are treated without anticoagulation. As mentioned above, coagulation, especially in the dialyser, can be prevented, or at least reduced, by infusing replacement fluid prior to the filter.

In automated therapies, devices to monitor arterial pressure, venous pressure, and air in the circuit should be present and activated in a manner similar to haemodialysis. Those therapies that include the use of dialysate delivered in an automated manner should also be subjected to the same monitoring as haemodialysis (Australian Standard 3200.2.16:1999, p 11).

Patient- or machine-generated circuitry?

Patient-generated (passive) circuitry: Haemofiltration can be undertaken without electronically operated equipment. In its simplest form, an artery and a vein are cannulated, and the cannulae are then connected to the arterial and venous portions of the extracorporeal circuit. The haemofilter is then placed between these two portions of the circuit. Blood flow is generated in accordance with the patient's cardiac output, and ultrafiltration occurs according to the pressure gradient that is generated when blood flowing into the filter is opposed by the venous pressure resisting its return. The haemofilter is placed in an upright position with the filtrate and venous ports uppermost. Ultrafiltrate is collected in a device that accords with current infection control standards, and anticoagulant, if required can be administered in increments.

Machine-generated (active) circuitry: If control of blood flow is required, a blood pump, with the attendant alarms mentioned above, can be used. If control of ultrafiltration is required, a pump can be connected to the filtration port and set to remove the desired amount of fluid for a given amount of time. Ultrafiltration control is usually only employed when a blood pump is used.

If a diffusion gradient is required, a 'dialysate' can be introduced into the filtrate compartment, using a counter current flow as for haemodialysis. It is usual to control the flow rate into, and out of, the haemofilter. To really complicate the picture, a combination of haemofiltration, providing convective solute transport, and dialysis, providing diffusive solute transport, can be used. This process is called haemo*dia*filtration.

Terminology

The nomenclature surrounding the various continuous therapies has caused much confusion. There was little consensus of opinion before 1996 about the terms that should apply to the various treatments. Mehta (1996) used terminology that has been accepted by the medical fraternity and is used in this chapter. The author has found the following explanation to be a convenient way of explaining the terminology and associated acronyms:

Continuous therapies are represented by the upper case 'C', while automated therapies are preceded by an 'A'.

If renal replacement therapy is *not* required (fluid only is being removed in accordance with the patient's volume status and expected intravenous infusion requirements), the ultrafiltration that occurs is represented by an upper case 'UF' (or 'U' in articles dated prior to 1996).

Patient-generated circuits are represented by an upper case 'A.V' (arteriovenous), indicating the cannulation of an artery ('A') and a vein ('V').

Machine-generated circuits do not require arterial pressure to generate blood flow, so arteries do not require cannulation. A double-lumen catheter is inserted into a suitable central vein, and this 'venovenous' flow pattern that follows is represented by a 'VV'.

Haemofiltration (convection only) is used when the upper case 'H' follows. If dialysis (diffusion) is being used, it is represented by the letter 'D', and if both haemoperfusion *and* dialysis are being performed simultaneously, haemo*dia*filtration is in use, and is indicated by the use of the upper case 'HDF' The use of these three terms indicates that renal replacement therapy is being undertaken.

1.2 Continuous therapies

Ultrafiltration

When glomerular filtration is sufficient to achieve satisfactory clearance of metabolic waste and keep electrolyte levels within acceptable limits, fluid removal alone may be all that is required. Known as slow continuous ultrafiltration (SCUF), or sometimes, continuous arteriovenous ultrafiltration (CAVU). CAVU is simple, and is used when fluid volume expansion is large, and considerable amounts of intravenous fluids are required.

Ultrafiltration was introduced in 1980 (Price 1991, p 240) and is seldom employed at the time of writing, because few intensive care patients with acute fluid problems retain sufficient renal function to achieve satisfactory solute clearance. Patients with the nephrotic syndrome who need to mobilise and remove large volumes of fluid may respond to several days of SCUF, especially if continuous fluid removal is required and the response to diuretic therapy is limited by a general decline in renal function (Gruskin et al. 1992, p 845–846).

Renal replacement therapies

The preference of the nephrologist or the intensive care physician, the familiarity of staff with the procedures available, the haemodynamic and electrolyte status of the patient, and the equipment available, determine the choice of therapy.

Some medical practitioners prefer patient-generated (AV) systems because the patient's cardiac output and venous pressure determine the rate of ultrafiltration. This means that the patient is 'in charge' of the rate of fluid removal in much the same way as occurs during normal glomerular filtration. Because these therapies approximate normal physiological processes, they are generally considered to be suitable for use in patients with multiple problems. However, a mean arterial pressure in excess of 70 mmHg is required to maintain satisfactory blood flow throughout the circuit, and to prevent stasis and subsequent clotting (Price 1991, p 240). If suitable arterial access cannot be established, or if the mean arterial blood pressure is low, these therapies cannot be established and machine-generated (VV) circuits are preferred.

Suitable percutaneous double-lumen venous access is not difficult to establish, and provides the benefits of controlled blood flow at a predetermined rate. However, the benefits of a patient-generated system are lost and the approximation to normal physiology is compromised. Patient mobility can also present difficulties; arterial access can be difficult to maintain in an ambulant patient, and VV techniques can be compromised if frequent trips to the operating suite or diagnostic areas are required because they interrupt the therapy.

Most patients in acute renal failure cared for in an intensive care unit are hyper-catabolic with a daily urea generation that precludes satisfactory treatment with intermittent haemodialysis (Mehta 1997, p 85). The slow continuous therapies are preferred for these patients because they remove urea and other electrolytes in a manner similar to the way they accumulate—*slowly* and *continuously*. Haemofiltration (H) alone may not maintain urea levels at a suitably low level because convection is the only transport mechanism available with haemofiltration. While larger molecules are cleared effectively with the use of convection, smaller molecules, those <300 daltons in size, rely on diffusion for removal. Therefore, haemofiltration may not be adequate. In these cases dialysate introduced into the filtration compartment can be beneficial. The use of dialysate and diffusion can completely replace convection (HD), or it can be added to complement the convective solute transport already occurring, in which case both diffusion and convection are used (HDF).

The use of pumps to control the removal of ultrafiltrate, or to control both the inflow and outflow of dialysate, or dialysate and ultrafiltrate in HDF, is the choice of individual units. It is increasingly common for such control to be used when blood pumps control the blood flow rate.

1.3 Intermittent therapies

The future for patients with end stage renal failure

Earlier discussion addressed many of the long term problems for patients with end stage renal failure, and the limitations of haemodialysis as a treatment. Standard dialysis membranes achieve satisfactory clearance of small molecules, but are unable to remove substances in the middle molecular range. Dialysers with larger sieving coefficients are able to remove these middle molecules and provide a better treatment option for patients who demonstrate the signs and/or symptoms associated with the accumulation of these molecules. Even so, the standard thrice-weekly treatment, even with the use of these membranes, is insufficient for the complete relief of symptoms for a number of patients.

The answer to many of these problems may be provided by the use of automated (A) and intermittent (I) forms of haemofiltration (H) or haemodiafiltration (HDF.). The technology is now available to 'compress' the convection provided by CVVH, and the diffusion and convection provided by CVVHDF, into a standard four or five-hour treatment appropriate for patients with end stage renal failure. At the time of writing intermittent haemodiafiltration (IHDF) appears to be the treatment of choice by renal units who have the technology available (Unpublished survey of Australian renal units, Fresenius Medical Care 1999).

This adequately removes small molecules via diffusion and allows larger molecules to be removed by high volume ultrafiltration. Using this combination, up to forty or fifty litres of fluid can be removed per treatment session. It follows, that concomitant fluid replacement, minus the amount required to return the patient to their base weight by the completion of therapy, is required. This is most economically achieved via the use of 'on line' production of replacement fluid.

This is achieved by subjecting water treated in the accepted manner for haemodialysis to filtrate through a fine micron filter. After the addition of standard dialysate concentrate, a second filtration occurs, and the haemofiltration machine then proportions the 'treated' dialysate. A preset amount will be delivered to the dialysate compartment to provide the diffusive component for the treatment, while a second preset amount is delivered into the extracorporeal circuit to provide replacement fluid for the haemofiltration component of the treatment. Filter changes and microbiological assessment must be done in accordance with the machine manufacturer's instructions to prevent infusion of contaminated fluid into the patient.

According to Canaud et al. (1993, pp S 296–299) this form of therapy should:

> ... provide high efficiency performances for both small and large molecular weight solutes in a relatively short time, ... improve haemocompatibility of the dialysis system ... [and] optimise fluid and electrolyte removal in order to increase cardiovascular stability particularly for the elderly and high risk patients.

Health care ethics and distributive justice

Canaud et al. (1993) also state that, as well as providing for greater patient stability, treatments such as IHDF are expected to be affordable for our health economic system. The money assigned by the State and Federal Governments to the provide health care is finite, and the ethical principle of 'justice' that presides over the distribution of treatments funded by the health care dollar has many components.

Two questions that often arise when allocating scarce resources are:

1. Which treatments should be made available? (e.g. haemodiafiltration versus conventional dialysis).

2. Which patients should receive the treatment, once it has been made available? (e.g. the older patient who is symptomatic and who receives the most immediate benefit, or the younger, asymptomatic patient, in whom the development of symptoms could be prevented).

Current contenders agree that, while there are no hard and fast rules, community input into decisions about the allocation of these resources is required.

References

In text references

Australian standard 3200.2.16:1999, 'Medical and electrical equipment: particular requirements for haemodialysis, haemodiafiltration and haemofiltration equipment'.

Canaud, B., Kerr, P., Argiles, A., Flavier, J., Stec, F., Mion, C., 1993, 'Is haemodiafiltration the dialysis modality of choice for the next decade? *International Society of Nephrology*, vol. 43, Suppl. 41, pp S296–299.

Gruskin, A., Baluarte, H., Dabbagh, S., 1992. 'Haemodialysis and peritoneal dialysis, in *Pediatric Kidney Disease*, Edelmann, C., (ed), 2nd ed., Little Brown and Co., Boston.

Kaplan, A., 1996, 'Continuous arteriovenous haemofiltration and related therapies', in *Replacement of Renal Function by Dialysis*, Jacobs, C., Kjellstrand, C., Koch, K., (eds.), 4th ed., Kluwer Academic Publishers, Boston.

Mehta, R., 1996, 'Continuous renal replacement therapies in the acute renal failure setting: current concepts', *Seminars in Dialysis*, vol. 4, no 2., Suppl. 1, pp 81–92.

Mehta, R., 1997, 'Continuous renal replacement therapies in the acute renal failure setting: current concepts', *Advances in Renal Replacement Therapy*, vol. 4, no. 2, Suppl 1, pp 81–92.

Mitchell, A., 1992, Original illustration drawn for the Intensive Care Unit, Heidelberg Repatriation Hospital.

Price, C., 1991, 'Continuous renal replacement therapy: the treatment of choice for acute renal failure', *ANNA Journal*, June, vol. 18, no. 3, pp 239–244.

Stansfield, G., 1988, *'Haemofiltration in perspective'*, Booklet based on a lecture given at the EDTNA, Brighton, Gambro Pty. Ltd., Lund, Sweden.

Sigler, M., Teehan, B., 1993, 'Slow continuous renal replacement therapies: CAVH, CVVH, CAVHD, CVVHD,' in *Dialysis Therapy*, Nissenson, A., Fine, R, (eds.) 2nd ed., Hanley and Belfus, Philadelphia.

Whittaker, A., 1989, 'Continuous ultrafiltration therapy', in *Advanced Technology in Critical Care Nursing*, Clochesy, J., (ed.), Aspen, Maryland.

Recommended reading

Ashton, D., Mehta, R., Ward, D., McDonald, B., Aguilar, M., 1991, 'Recent advances in continuous renal replacement therapy: citrate anticoagulated continuous arteriovenous haemodialysis', *ANNA Journal*, vol. 18, no 3, pp 263–267, 329.

National Health and Medical Research Council, 1993, 'Ethical Considerations Relating to Health Care Resource Allocation Decisions', Report of the Australian Health Ethics Committee.

Price, C., 1991, 'Continuous renal replacement therapy: the treatment of choice for acute renal failure', *ANNA Journal*, June, vol. 18, no. 3, pp 239–244.

Plasmapheresis and haemoperfusion

Introduction

There are a number of extracorporeal treatments that can be used for patients with renal impairment, as well as for patients with other disease processes. Some of these treatments are required on a permanent basis while others are used for limited periods only. Some are performed in dialysis units, others in critical care settings, or in oncology or neurology wards. Some treatments are curative, while others are only palliative.

Originally, most of these therapies were undertaken in dialysis units and were a routine part of the work undertaken by dialysis nurses. However, they are now being performed with increasing frequency, in the specialty areas that relate to the original disease process, and it is important that dialysis nurses do not lose the knowledge of how, and why, these extracorporeal treatments are performed.

2.1 Apheresis

Terminology

Apheresis is a Greek word meaning to separate, or to take out, and is the name used to describe the technology associated with the separation of blood into its numerous constituents, followed by the manipulation of one or more of these parts (Rodwig 1999, p 363).

Apheresis is divided into two primary categories:

1. Cytapheresis, where blood is separated into its cellular components. The desired component is then collected and the remaining cells and plasma are returned to the patient.

2. Plasmapheresis, where the plasma is separated from formed blood elements and removed. The cellular components are then returned to the patient.

Cytapheresis is used to collect healthy cells from volunteer donors for later transfusion in patients with a variety of disorders relating to the 'formed' blood elements. Granulocytes are used for patients with aplastic anaemia and leukaemia, reticulocytes for patients with thalassaemia major, and platelets for use with patients who have polycythaemia vera or idiopathic thrombocytopaenia (Rodwig 1999, pp 369–371). One recent advance with cytapheresis used with increasing frequency, is the collection of stem cells for preservation and later autotransfusion in patients who undergo bone marrow ablation to treat malignancy (Rodwig 1999, p 370). A modification of the cytapheresis technique is used for patients with chronic leukaemia to remove excess leukocytes and prevent the vascular sludging and stasis that occurs when the leukocyte count is excessive.

Plasmapheresis is used to collect plasma from healthy individuals, and for the subsequent transfusion of the plasma into patients who require plasma supplementation. For example, hypovolaemia due to injury, hypoproteinaemic states such as the nephrotic syndrome, and tissue injury due to burns.

Plasma exchange, sometimes termed 'therapeutic plasma exchange' or TPE, refers to the transfusion of plasma into patients undergoing therapy designed to remove their own plasma, which will be replaced with plasma collected from healthy people. Plasma for transfusion is collected from health volunteers who attend an outpatient setting similar to that in which whole blood is collected by institutions such as the Red Cross Blood Bank.

The involvement of dialysis nurses in apheresis procedures is almost exclusively limited to plasma exchange. Therefore, the other techniques will not be discussed further. However, the interested reader is referred to the recommended reading in the reference section at the end of the chapter.

Treatment methodology

As with the treatment modalities discussed in previous chapters, specifically designed software and hardware has been developed to effect the various apheresis therapies. All the precautions relevant to other extracorporeal therapies also apply to patients undergoing apheresis.

Current separation techniques are divided into two categories:

1. Centrifuge separation. When blood is centrifuged, specific formed blood elements or plasma can be collected. Each substance separates according to its molecular weight after anticoagulation and centrifugation.

    When this principle is applied to large volumes of blood passing through an extracorporeal circuit and centrifuge bowl, separation in accordance with density allows specific elements to be drawn off individually. The remainder is reinfused into the donor if the process is for collection and later use, or the patient, if the procedure is for therapeutic purposes.

    Centrifuge separation can be further divided into intermittent and continuous collection, but these techniques are beyond the scope of this text. Interested readers should consult specific texts dealing with blood bank practices.

2. Membrane separation. This method uses a filter similar to that used for haemofiltration but the membrane is much more porous than the membrane used for either haemodialysis or haemofiltration. As blood passes through the 'plasma' filter, the highly porous membrane allows plasma to pass through it and into the filtrate compartment from where it is collected. Electrolytes and, perhaps more importantly, clotting factors are also 'lost' to the filtrate. Therefore, electrolytes and occasionally clotting factors should be present in any replacement fluid used. The use of replacement fluids is discussed later in this chapter.

Anticoagulation is required irrespective of the separation technique used for plasma collection/exchange. Patients undergoing plasma exchange/removal who have a pre-existing coagulation disorder are occasional exceptions. Heparin is the anticoagulant of choice for patients undergoing therapeutic plasma exchange in haemodialysis units for therapeutic plasma exchange conducted in haemodialysis units. Sometimes sodium citrate, as either ACD 'A' or ACD 'B', is used, especially with machines specifically designed for its use. When the procedure is undertaken for donor collection and subsequent recipient transfusion, 4% sodium citrate is used.

Citrate achieves its anticoagulant effect by binding with calcium. It is infused at the site usually reserved heparin infusion and is a regional anticoagulant that requires reversal with a calcium infusion to avoid systemic hypocalcaemia. Patients should be monitored for the early signs of hypocalcaemia. If the early signs are not recognised, life-threatening cardiac arrhythmias can occur (Ismail et al. pp 242–243).

When using citrate anticoagulation the infusion rate should not exceed the body's ability to metabolise citrate. High blood flow rates should be avoided, especially in small patients (Ismail et al. 2001, p 243). For blood flow rates recommended for use with various ACD 'A'/ blood ratios, and for further information relating to the use of ACD 'A' and ACD 'B' refer to the preceding text. When using citrate in any form, be sure to carefully read the instructions for use. The main difference between the types of citrate available is the amount of sodium citrate and citric acid in the preparation.

Therapeutic application

Therapeutic plasma exchange is used to remove high molecular weight substances in clinical conditions where these substances are thought to contribute to the development of the disease. According to Gurland et al. (1996, pp 472–473) well-acknowledged disease mediators include:

1. Uraemic toxins.

2. Endogenous and exogenous poisons, especially those that are highly plasma-bound (Rodwig 1999, p 373).

3. IgG and IgM autoantibodies, which are seen in autoimmune diseases such as Goodpasture's syndrome, myasthenia gravis and immune thrombocytopaenia.

4. Circulating immune complexes that cause damage due to their deposition in tissue. Such diseases include the various forms of vasculitis, and SLE (Rodwig 1999, p 373).

5. Low density lipoproteins, such as those seen in patients with type 11 hyperlipidaemia.

6. Paraproteins, which are seen in diseases such as multiple myeloma and cryoglobulinaemia.

Rodwig et al. (1999, p 373) includes the removal of inflammatory mediators such as fibrinogen and complement, and platelet aggregating factors to this list.

Therapeutic plasma exchange is based on the principle that, if a disease mediator is circulating in the plasma, the removal of the plasma and replacing it with a disease-free substitute should alleviate the condition. Plasma exchange does not cure the disease, but allows time for the body's own homeostatic mechanisms to overcome the disease, or for symptoms to be alleviated. Concomitant immunosuppressive drug therapy is often used, especially when antibodies or immune complexes are involved in the disease process. Treatment is often intensive, given daily, and short term, as with an acute presentation of Guillian-Barre syndrome, or regular and long term as with type 11 hyperlipidaemia.

Diseases for which plasma exchange can be used have been divided into four categories:

Category 1. Standard, accepted treatment, which includes disease such as cryoglobulinaemia, Goodpasture's syndrome, Guillain Barre-syndrome, myasthenia gravis, post transfusion purpura, thrombotic thrombocytopaenic purpura.

Category 2. Sufficient evidence exists to suggest benefit, especially as an adjunct therapy. Diseases in this category include chronic inflammatory demyelinating polyneuropathy, haemolytic uraemic syndrome, cold agglutinin disease, rapidly progressive glomerulonephritis, and pemphigus vulgaris.

Category 3. There is inconclusive evidence of benefit and an uncertain 'risk/benefit' ratio. Diseases include ABO incompatibility, multiple sclerosis, and progressive systemic sclerosis.

Category 4. Lack of evidence in controlled trials. Diseases such as AIDS, aplastic anaemia, lupus nephritis, transplant rejection, rheumatoid arthritis, and schizophrenia are included in this category.

(Rodwig 1999, p 372).

The efficacy of the procedure depends on the amount of plasma exchanged and is reduced by the need to replace plasma as it is removed. A routine plasma exchange is between two and four litres, with the amount being determined by the patient's plasma volume. It is usual to exchange between one and one and one half volumes per treatment (Price and McCarley 1993, p45). Procedure efficacy also depends on the volume of distribution of the pathogenic substance. Large immunoglobulins such as IgM are limited to the intravascular compartment and are removed well during plasma exchange. Smaller immunoglobulins, such as those intended to deal with tissue antigen (IgG), are not limited to the vascular compartment, and are less efficiently removed.

Replacement fluids

To avoid potential life threatening complications, separated plasma should be replaced isovolumetrically and iso-oncotically (Gurland et al. 1996, p 476). In other words, volume-for-volume, and contain physiologically normal levels of albumin.

Albumex 4 is the usual replacement fluid (20g albumin in 500 mls), and is usually administered via a peripheral vein on a volume-for-volume basis. Care should be taken when replacement is through a centrally placed catheter because most albumin-containing solutions do not contain potassium and cardiac arrhythmias can occur if potassium-poor fluid is delivered directly into the heart (Gurland et.al. 1996, p 476).

If central fluid replacement is required, 200 ml of Albumex 20 (20g albumin in 100 mls) can be mixed with Hartmann's solution (800 mls) (personal experience). Care should be taken to avoid hypocalcaemia when acid citrate dextrose (ACD) is used as the anticoagulant. In some countries plasma protein fraction (PPF) is be used. While it has the advantage of containing potassium, it has been associated with hypotensive reactions and is no longer available in Australia for this reason.

Plasma replacement solutions are heat sterilised therefore, the risk of viral disease transmission is eliminated. However, heat sterilisation destroys clotting factors, and should not be used for patients with bleeding disorders. Patients with coagulation disorders, who are at risk of bleeding, should have their plasma volume replaced with fresh frozen plasma (FFP).

Alternative techniques

Plasma exchange can be combined with haemoperfusion, haemodialysis, cytapheresis or a 'second step' plasma separation process that further divides plasma according to protein density. Plasma exchange can be done for patients with concomitant problems or for patients with disorders of selected protein types. 'Plasma fractionation' is the name used to describe these therapies and is divided into three broad groups:

1. **Cascade filtration**: After the initial separation of intravascular components into formed elements and plasma, the plasma is subjected to a second passage through a filter with a membrane designed to divide it into high and low molecular weight fractions. The low molecular fraction, primarily albumin, is returned to the patient. The high molecular weight faction, primarily pathological proteins, is discarded. The process is varied for patients with

hyperviscosity syndromes such as hypercholesterolaemia and macroglobulinaemia. While cascade filtration does not result in the exact separation of molecules into groups that allow for removal with no 'overlap', it does usually reduce the need for plasma replacement (Gurland 1996, p 479).

2. **Precipitation:** High levels of low-density lipoproteins (LDL) have a direct correlation with the development of arteriosclerosis. Plasma exchange is now accepted as a valid treatment for LDL conditions (Bosch 1996, p 414). Conventional plasma exchange removes potentially antiatherogenic high-density lipids, among other things. One method to avoid their removal is to subject the separated plasma to further heparinisation (Gurland 1996, p 479) and acidification (B Braun, 1995) to reduce the pH. The low pH enables the plasma-heparin complex to precipitate and be removed. The remaining plasma is reinfused after the pH has been normalised. This process is known as Heparin-Induced LDL Precipitation (HELP), and is now used in a number of units as routine therapy for familial hypercholesterolaemia.

3. **Immunoadsorption:** When using this technique, filtered plasma is passed through an adsorption column containing a 'ligand' capable of binding a specific protein. Either an antibody/antigen or chemical (Rodwig 1999, p 373) mediates the process. Immunoadsorption has been used for the removal of cytotoxic antibodies in potential renal transplant recipients, and IgG or complexes in idiopathic thrombocytopaenia, chemotherapy-induced haemolytic uraemic syndrome, and thrombotic thrombocytopaenic purpura (Rodwig 1999, p 373). One aspect of developing immunoadsorptive technology is aimed at removal of enough cytotoxic antibodies to enable the survival of transplanted kidneys.

Photopheresis: This is a technique that combines photochemotherapy, the use of specific light sensitive chemotherapy, with leukoplasmapheresis, the separation of leucocytes from other plasma constituents. Before undergoing the treatment the patient ingests a drug, psoralen, which binds to DNA in nucleated cells. After the separation of cells and plasma, the leucocytes are exposed to ultraviolet light to activate the psoralen and prevent replication. The modified cells are returned to the patient, and induce an immune response to the abnormal lymphocyte clone, and decrease the immune response the patient is able to mount against a given antigen (Rodwig 1999, p 374).

It was originally used in the early 1990's to treat cutaneous lymphoma and is currently being researched as a possible preventive treatment for cardiac and renal transplant rejection (Gurland 1996, p 479).

Risks of apheresis

Remember that plasma exchange/phareresis encompasses procedures that exposures health professionals to blood and body fluids. Gloves, protective eye wear and protective clothing should be worn during all procedures that have potential for the transmission of these fluids between patient and carer. Many of these procedures involve the use of replacement fluid that was collected from multiple donors, and carries an inherent risk for the transference of disease. Fresh frozen plasma is not heat sterilised, and therefore carries an additional risk factor for both the staff that prepare the treatment and the patient who receives it.

The treatment itself is considered to be a relatively safe procedure. Most of the complications are similar to those occurring in all extracorporeal therapies. Complications specific to plasma exchange include citrate toxicity, hypovolaemia, allergic responses to replacement fluids, depleted clotting factors, hypocalcaemia if citrate is used as an anticoagulant, and transfusion-related infection.

2.2 Haemoperfusion

Overview of poisoning

For the past thirty years extracorporeal therapies have been employed to remove toxic substances directly from the blood stream (Lorch and Garella 1999, p 490). Extracorporeal therapy is particularly helpful when a potentially poisonous substance has been ingested and wholly or partially absorbed from the gastrointestinal tract.

Other methods used to remove poisons include:

1. Forced diuresis, which is now recognised as only being of value when the kidney can excrete the poison in an unchanged state.

2. Alkalinisation of the extracellular fluid—with overdose of tricyclic antidepressants, or the urine, with overdose due to salicylate or long acting barbiturate poisoning—is used with substances that are excreted by the kidney where increased tubular ionization enhances elimination.

3. Gastric lavage was once widely practiced, but is now rare because it is thought to increase the absorption of some drugs.

4. The introduction of charcoal directly into the stomach is still considered valuable because the nonspecific adsorptive properties of charcoal-assist removal, even when the toxic agent is unknown (Lorch and Garella 1999, p 490).

Extracorporeal methods of removing poisons include:

1. CAVH, especially when the ingested substance released slowly from its reservoir, as with paraquat poisoning.

2. Plasma exchange.

3. Exchange blood transfusion.

4. Resin haemoperfusion, developed especially to increase the removal of lipid soluble substances.

5. Charcoal haemoperfusion.

6. Haemodialysis with lipid dialysate formed by emulsifying soybean milk and aqueous dialysate. There is little benefit over standard haemodialysis or haemoperfusion.

7. Haemodialysis with ultrafiltration. Again there is no real benefit over standard dialysis or haemoperfusion).

Plasma exchange has been discussed and will not be reviewed further. The remainder of this section is primarily concerned with the use of charcoal haemoperfusion.

Choice of therapy

The principles governing the removal of solute from the blood of uraemic patients undergoing haemodialysis are the same as those that govern the removal of toxins from the blood of patients who ingested poisons. Haemodialysis is, therefore, usually implemented when poisoning is due to substances that have a low molecular weight, a small volume of distribution, and minimal protein-binding. The impact of membrane size, sieving coefficient and blood flow rate are the same as for dialysis. At the time of writing, no studies were identified about the use of high flux membranes and poison removal (Lorch and Garella 1999, p 492). If cascade therapy is unavailable, haemodialysis is usually employed when the patient has concurrent renal failure, or marked fluid, electrolyte or acid base disturbance. Haemoperfusion is the treatment of choice for patients who ingested toxins with a high molecular weight, a large volume of distribution, are fat soluble or are highly protein-bound.

Principles of haemoperfusion

Haemoperfusion refers to the use of an extracorporeal circuit that enables the removal of toxins via *direct* contact between the blood and an a*d*sorbent material. The sorbent material used is rendered biocompatible by the use of a polymer membrane that coats the surface of the particles. The membrane is semipermeable, enabling the movement of substances from the blood to the sorbent. The material is then 'housed' in a container similar to that used for conventional dialysis, but there are no dialysate ports.

Vascular access and anticoagulation are required, as for haemodialysis. Particular care should be paid to the manufacturer's instructions for the safe priming and preparation of the device. Some haemoperfusion devices require priming with a glucose solution because glucose is able to occupy binding sites on the sorbent material. If a glucose solution is not used to fill these sites during priming, a precipitous fall in the patient's blood glucose levels will occur when therapy is commenced.

The extracorporeal circuit is similar to that used for haemodialysis and, in many instances, the same software and machinery are used. Pressure monitoring for arterial and venous access is required, as is monitoring for, and protection against, the accidental infusion of air.

During haemoperfusion blood percolates through a cartridge filled with activated charcoal or other material coated with a semipermeable membrane. The removal of toxins is not dependent on a diffusion gradient (remember that no dialysate is used), but occurs in accordance with 'the avidity of the charcoal for the toxin, ... and the toxin's binding to plasma proteins' (Lorch and Garella 1999, p 492). The function of the semipermeable membrane is to ensure that the sorbent material is contained and not released into the patient's circulation as occurred during the early use of charcoal, which caused 'charcoal emboli', and to prevent the adsorption of substances such as platelets and red blood cells, rather than to facilitate toxin removal. The semipermeable nature of the material used for coating ensures that toxins are able to move from blood to sorbent.

The most frequently used sorbent is carbon that has been subjected to 'activation'; a process 'induced by controlled oxidation in air, carbon dioxide or steam' (Winchester 1989, p 440) and which is used to increase the surface area of the sorbent.

Toxins removed by haemoperfusion

Haemoperfusion is most frequently used to remove drugs or chemicals ingested either deliberately or accidentally. It has also been attempted, with varying success, for a number of other conditions. Gurland et al. (1996, pp 488–493) describe them as:

1.   Uraemia, where the 'cascade use' or 'in series' use of both dialyser and haemoperfusion cartridges enhances total clearance. This was of most clinical benefit prior to the advent of high flux dialysers that are able to remove a greater spectrum of solute.

2.   Immunoadsorption, where antigen or antibody-coated carrier particles designed to adsorb specific immunogenic proteins are contained in the haemoperfusion device.

3.   Hepatic encephalopathy.

4.   Schizophrenia.

5.   Psoriasis.

   The results of controlled trials are limited and controversial for the last two conditions. More information about toxin removal by haemoperfusion can be found in the articles n the recommended reading list at the end of the chapter.

Complications

The problems associated with particle embolisation have been overcome by using the encapsulation techniques discussed earlier in this section. These encapsulation techniques have also reduced, but not eliminated, thrombocytopaenia associated with platelet adsorption. Transient leucopoenia also occurs and is thought to be due to mechanisms similar to those seen with haemodialysis.

   Problems specific to haemoperfusion include:

1.   Hypoglycaemia and hypocalcaemia due to the adsorption of glucose and calcium by the sorbent cartridge.

2.   Hypothermia due to the extracorporeal exposure of blood to atmospheric temperature.

3. Alterations in the coagulation status of the patient, including:

a) increased risk of coagulation as a result of:

i) exposure of blood to incompatible substances

ii) the production of platelet aggregates in patients with liver disease, especially those with hepatic coma.

b) increased risk of coagulation because adsorption of coagulation factors, especially fibrinogen, occurs.

(Gurland et al. 1996, p 487–488).

It is also possible for cartridges to become 'saturated', especially when long term continuous therapy is used. Regular monitoring of serum levels for the toxin being removed, and timely replacement of the cartridge will avoid compromising the treatment.

References

In text references

Australian Red Cross Blood Services, 1997, *Blood Product Tissue Policy*, Prepared by the Australian Red Cross Blood Services, Victoria.

B. Braun Mediothec, 1995, Melsungen AG, Carl Braun Strabe, 15 D–34212 Melsungen, Germany.

Bosch, T., 1996, 'Lipid apheresis: from a heroic treatment to routine clinical practice', *Artificial Organs*, vol. 20, no. 5, pp 414–419.

Gurland, H., Samtleben, W., Lysaght, M., Winchester, J., 1996, 'Extra-corporeal blood purification techniques: plasmapheresis and haemoperfusion', in *Replacement of Renal Function by Dialysis*, Jacobs, C., Kjellstrand, C., Koch, K., (eds.), 4th ed., Kluwer Academic Publishers, Boston.

Ismail, N., Neyra, R., Hakim, R., 2001, 'Dialysis in infants and children' in *Handbook of Dialysis*, Daugirdas, J., Blake, P., Ing, T., (eds.), 3rd ed., Lippincott Williams and Wilkins, Philadelphia.

Lorch, J., Garella, S., 1999, 'Hemodialysis and hemoperfusion for poisoning', in *Principles and Practice of Dialysis*, Henrich, W. (ed), 2nd ed., William and Wilkins, Maryland.

Price, C., McCarley, P., 1993, ' Technical considerations of therapeutic plasma exchange as a nephrology nursing procedure', *ANNA Journal*, February, vol. 20, no. 1, pp 41–46.

Rodwig, F., 1999, 'Apheresis', *in Modern Blood Banking and Transfusion Practices*, Harmening, D., (ed.), 4th ed., Davis Company, Philadelphia.

Winchester, J., 1989, 'Haemoperfusion', in *Replacement of Renal Function by Dialysis*, Maher J (Ed.), 3rd ed., Kluwer Academic Publishers, Boston.

Recommended reading

Chen, W., Yeh, J., Chiu, H., 1999, ' Experiences of double filtration plasmapheresis in the treatment of Guillain Barre Syndrome', *Journal of Clinical Apheresis,* vol. 14, pp 126–129.

Deshpande, G., Meert, K., Valentini, R 1999, 'Repeat charcoal hemoperfusion treatments in life threatening carbamazepine overdose, *Paediatric nephrology',* vol. 13, no. 9, pp 775–777.

Furuyoshi, S., Nakatani, M., Taman, J., Kutsuki, H., Takata, S., Tani, N., 1998, 'New adsorption column (Lixel) to eliminate beta 2 microglobulin for direct haemoperfusion', *Therapeutic Apheresis,* vol. 2, no. 1, pp 13–17.

Kawasaki, C., Nishi, R., Uekihara, S., Hayano, S., Otagiri, M., 2000, ' Charcoal hemoperfusion in the treatment of phenytoin overdose', American Journal of Kidney Disease, vol. 35, no.2, pp 323–326.

Kutsuki, H., Takata, S., Yamamoto, K., Tani, N., 1998, 'Therapeutic selective adsorption of anti-DNA antibody using dextran sulphate cellulose column (Selsorb) for the treatment of systemic lupus erythematosis', *Therapeutic Apheresis,* vol. 2, no. 1, pp18–24.

Mahalati, K., Dawson, R., Collins, J., Bell, W., McCrae, K., Martin, J., 1999, 'Persistent pre-eclampsia post partum with elevated liver enzymes and hemolytic uraemic syndrome', *Journal of Clinical Apheresis,* vol. 14, pp 69–78.

Mertins, P., Schonfelder, T., Handt., S., Kierdorf, H., Marschall, H., Busch, N., Heintz, B., Sieberth, H., 1998, 'Long term extra-corporeal bilirubin elimination: a case report on cascade resin plasmaperfusion', *Blood Purification,* vol. 16, no. 6, pp 341–348.

Nilsson, I., Berntorp, E., Freiburghaus, C., 1993, 'Treatment of patients with factor IX inhibitors', *Thrombosis and Haemostasis,* Vol. 17, no. 1, pp 56–59.

Price, C., McCarley, P., 1993, ' Technical considerations of therapeutic plasma exchange as a nephrology nursing procedure', *ANNA Journal,* February, vol. 20, no. 1, pp 41–46.

Price, C., McCarley, P., 1994, ' Physical assessment for patients receiving therapeutic plasma exchange', *ANNA Journal,* June, vol. 21, no.4, pp 149–153, 201.

Splendiani, G., Zazzaro, D., Di Pietrantonio, P., Delfino, L., 2000, 'Continuous renal replacement therapy and charcoal plasmaperfusion in treatment of amanita mushroom poisoning', Artificial Organs, vol. 24, no. 4, pp 305–308.

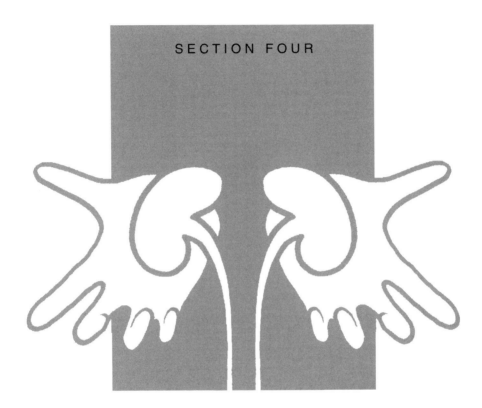

SECTION FOUR

CHAPTER ONE

Anatomy and physiology

Introduction

It is now nearly 200 years since the transport characteristics of the peritoneal membrane were first recognised and studied. These beginning experiments revolved around either the movement of substances from within the peritoneal cavity and their transport into the blood, or their removal from the blood and into the peritoneal cavity. The visceral peritoneal membrane of animals was amongst the membranes used during early experiments with haemodialysis. Although it was only during the last two decades that peritoneal dialysis was recognised as a suitable treatment for end stage renal failure, it has rapidly been accepted, and offers considerable advantages over haemodialysis, especially for people who value mobility in their work and leisure activities.

1.1　A brief history of peritoneal dialysis

How it all started

The following review of the development of peritoneal dialysis is summarised from Drukker (1989, pp 475–15). Modern peritoneal dialysis originated from the technique of peritoneal lavage, a therapy first undertaken in 1744. The following process appears to have been used:

Christopher Warrick, an English surgeon, was asked to attend to a lady who was bed ridden as a result of an accumulation of several liters of ascitic fluid. A trochar was inserted into the lady's abdomen and 36 pints (sic) of fluid was withdrawn. As may be expected, the ascitic fluid soon reappeared, and 14 days after the initial procedure the lady again sought the services of the surgeon. Following his initial paracentesis, Mr. Warrick had studied ascitic fluid in an attempt to determine its source, in order to effect a cure. He was prepared therefore, when the lady's condition recurred. This time he withdrew 20 pints (sic) and replaced the fluid, volume for volume, with equal parts of water drawn fresh from the Bristol River and a Bordeaux wine. Jane Roman, the lady concerned, 'collapsed, and … went into an alarming condition.' Mr Warrick suggested a second attempt, and after obtaining the patient's consent, he repeated the procedure, but doubled the proportion of wine to water. The patient again collapsed, but again recovered after some time and considerable concern for the surgeon. However, this time the ascites did not recur. Presumably, the peritoneal membrane had suffered sufficient chemical sclerosis to cause the 'ruptured lymphatics to close their mouths' as was Mr. Warrick's initial intent.

After this experiment, subsequent procedures were modified to include the insertion of two trochars, one to drain the abdominal fluid and one to introduce a fluid that was used in a manner similar to that used with contemporary peritoneal lavage. The introduction of this solution called 'medicinal liquor', was titrated to prevent patient discomfort when large amounts of fluid were withdrawn. There is no mention in the text of any modifications to the composition of the fluid used for this lavage.

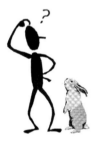

Mr. Warrick's work with this form of *intermittent* peritoneal lavage is essentially the same as the *continual* form that was subsequently used to treat uraemia. The next major step forward in the study of the peritoneal membrane came during 1877 when a German physician, Wegner, observed that infusing cold saline into the peritoneal cavity of a rabbit was followed by a fall in body temperature. He later observed that the use of a short 'dwell' time resulted in the appearance of 'concentrated sugars' in the saline. Wegner's work was confirmed by English physiologists.

Starling and co-workers (1894–95) soon discovered that the use of hypotonic solution was followed by the absorption of some of the fluid over a period of hours. Later experiments by Orlow in Germany confirmed that the reverse was also true; that the use of hypertonic fluid resulted in a transfer of body water to the infusate.

Later, work by Clarke showed that the absorption of fluid from a saline solution was followed by the diffusion of smaller ions from the body into the peritoneal cavity and that adding glucose to make the infusate 'hypertonic' could prevent the initial absorption of fluid. Clark also noted that the rate of fluid absorption could be increased by warming the infused fluid or the abdominal wall, and slowed by either cooling the solution or the abdominal wall. Later studies showed that an increase in intestinal motility enhanced absorption and decreased motility hindered it.

After these experiments, the peritoneal membrane was recognised as being capable of 'bi-directional' flow and was more permeable than the membranes that were currently being studied for haemodialysis (Drukker 1989 p 478). As a 'living membrane' it was subject to inflammation that would further increase its permeability, allowing the passage of protein molecules.

Early peritoneal dialysis

After several experiments with the use of intraperitoneal saline to 'normalise' the plasma of uraemic animals, Dr G. Ganter, a German clinical investigator, is credited with the first attempts to use peritoneal dialysis in humans when two patients were treated with a single infusion of saline into the peritoneal cavity. Although neither patient recovered fully, both showed a transient improvement in their respective conditions. Several years of unsuccessful experiments using intermittent and continuous methods in both humans and animals followed.

In 1946 Howard Frank, Arnold Seligman and Jacob Fine reported the survival of a patient suffering from severe sulphathiazol-induced uraemia treated with four days of continuous peritoneal lavage. Their success prompted a review of the available literature, which interestingly, revealed several reported 'cures', primarily in patients with acute, reversible renal lesions. This opened the floodgates for further serious investigation into the clinical application of peritoneal dialysis, with the emphasis on the sodium and glucose concentration of the dialytic fluid and the addition of buffering agents. The use of continuous versus intermittent therapy was debated, different catheter styles were developed, and clearance studies increased the awareness of the importance of flow rates.

Thus far, treatment was restricted to patients with acute renal failure. The first success with a patient suffering from end stage renal failure occurred in 1959 when an American lady survived for six months using an intermittent therapy when ever she became 'uraemic', approximately weekly. This success was followed by research into catheters suitable for long term use, the use of 'automated cyclers' (1962), and the reuse of the dialysing solution using closed loop reverse osmosis recycling (1972), adsorbent cartridges (1974) or extracorporeal recirculation using dialysers designed for haemodialysis (1976).

Peritoneal infection was a major factor that slowed the acceptance of peritoneal dialysis as a suitable treatment for end stage renal failure. Peritonitis has been responsible for many patient deaths over the years and many more patients were changed to haemodialysis as a treatment option on account of the risk of peritonitis.

More references to the development of peritoneal dialysis as a treatment for renal failure can be found in subsequent chapters.

1.2 Anatomy and physiology

Anatomy

The peritoneal membrane is the largest serous membrane in the human body. It derives its name from the Greek word, 'peritonaion' which means 'to stretch around' (Wild 1998, p 248), and it is usually described as consisting of two principal components:

1. The parietal peritoneum that covers the inner abdominal wall.

2. The visceral peritoneum that lines the intraperitoneal organs.

   Approximately 10% of the peritoneal membrane is parietal and 60% is visceral. In the male the membrane is continuous, and in the female it is open where the ends of the Fallopian tubes enter the pelvic cavity (Krediet 1996, p 146). The peritoneal membrane also forms the mesentery that provides the support structures for bowel loops and other pelvic and abdominal organs. The membrane covering these structures makes up the remaining 30% of surface area. These membrane supports are called mesenteries and are given specific names depending on the organs they support, e.g. mesocolon, mesovarium and mesoappendix. The two layers of membrane lie in close proximity and are usually only separated by approximately 100 ml of fluid that provides lubrication, allowing the membranes to move across each other without causing friction and pain. During peritoneal dialysis this 'potential' space becomes an 'actual' space when it is filled with dialysis solution.

   The peritoneal membrane consists of three layers:

1. The mesothelium, the luminal side of which is covered with microvilli. These microvilli enable the membrane to increase its surface area in non uraemic individuals who are *not* undergoing peritoneal dialysis. The cells are polygonal in shape and lie in an overlapping layer on the basement membrane. Tight junctions separate the cells.

2. The interstitium that consists primarily of bundles of collagen fibres. Fibroblasts, mast cells and macrophages are present and are considered normal.

3. The capillary endothelium that is usually continuous in nature with occasional fenestration.

Studies describing the m² surface area of the peritoneal membrane are limited, and those that have been published vary widely (Krediet 1996, p146). There is general consensus that the surface area is ~ 1.2m². It is thought that different parts of the membrane are responsible for different rates of solute transport, and that the portion covering the liver (10% of the visceral portion) could be of particular importance because of its close proximity to the liver sinusoids (Krediet 1996, p147).

The ratio of peritoneal surface area to body weight in the newborn is approximately twice that of the adult (Krediet 1996, p 146–147). This is one of the several reasons why peritoneal dialysis is suggested as the treatment of choice for children requiring dialysis.

The arterial blood supply for the parietal peritoneum is via the arteries of the abdominal and pelvic walls and its venous and lymphatic drainage is via the local veins that eventually join the caval vein and thoracic duct. The visceral areas receive their blood supply from the organs that they cover, and venous drainage is also via these local vessels that eventually join the portal vein. The main site for lymphatic drainage of the peritoneal cavity is via the stromata or subdiaphragmatic gaps in the mesothelium (Krediet 1996, p147). From there it passes into the anterior mediastinal lymph nodes and eventually to the right lymphatic duct.

Lymphatic drainage is a 'one way' system and is responsible for returning fluid and protein to the systemic circulation. During peritoneal dialysis a number of anatomical changes are apparent, especially in the mesothelial cells:

1. These cells 'have a more cubic form, and the number of cells per unit of surface area' are increased, leading to a lengthening of the intercellular junctions (Krediet 1996, p 147).

2. The numbers of microvilli are reduced, thus reducing the ability to increase surface area.

3. Occasional degeneration to the surface, with 'blebs and blisters' apparent during electron microscopy (Krediet 1996, p 147).

4. A reduction in the number of micropinocytotic vesicles.

5. The collagen bundles of the interstitial layer are distributed irregularly, and fibrosis is known to occur.

6. The capillary basement membrane 'reduplicates', resembling the alterations seen in vessels of patients with diabetes mellitus.

Krediet (1996, p 149) summarises the morphology that accompanies 'uncomplicated' peritoneal dialysis as:

> '... reactive changes are present in the mesothelium. The cells can show signs of degeneration, but also of high metabolic activity. The collagen in the interstitial tissue is irregular and reduplication of the capillary basement membrane occurs'.

Physiology of solute movement

The easiest way to visualise solute removal during peritoneal dialysis is to consider the process of diffusion. Solute will move along its concentration gradient until equilibrium has been reached. Haemodialysis occurs *outside* the body, requires *direct* access to the blood compartment, and uses the *artificial* membrane of the haemodialyser. Peritoneal dialysis is almost the opposite. It occurs *inside* the body, uses a *natural* membrane, the peritoneal membrane, and requires *in*direct access to the blood compartment.

As with haemodialysis, diffusion is the most important consideration with solute removal, with convection contributing to a lesser extent. Unlike haemodialysis, where countercurrent flow between dialysate and blood ensures maximal diffusion for the entire treatment and where consistent ultrafiltration rates maximise convection, both diffusion and convection slow once equilibration between the solute content of the intraperitoneal fluid and the blood is approached, and cease once it has been reached. To keep solute removal at its ideal rate for each patient, a 'prescription' (or ideal time) for changing the dialysate, must be determined for each person and will be discussed fully in later chapters.

In many ways it is more difficult for solute to move across the peritoneal membrane during peritoneal dialysis than it is during haemodialysis. There is a 'triple barrier' to solute removal in haemodialysis, whereas peritoneal dialysis presents a total of five barriers some of which are more of an obstacle than others (Krediet 1996, p150).

The three main obstacles appear to be the capillary endothelium, the interstitial tissue and the mesothelial cell. Stagnant fluid layers or areas of slower flow on either side of the membrane offer minimal resistance. The most significant is the capillary endothelium and the least significant appears to be the interstitium.

Solute movement has been explained by what is known as the 'three pore model' (Rippe 1993 9 S 35). Separating the capillary endothelial cells are both large and small pores. Large pores, also known as desmosomes, form probably < 0.1% of the transport capacity, and occur where the irregular edges of cellular plasma membranes are separated by areas of extracellular fluid. With a radius of between 25 and 35 nanometers (Spence and Mason, 1983, pp 60–61) they allow the movement of macromolecules, including plasma proteins. Small pores, also called gap junctions' are thought to be the equivalent of interendothelial clefts, and, with a radius of between 2 and 4 nanometers (Spence and Mason, 1983, p 61), they allow the transport of smaller molecules such as sodium, urea, and creatinine.

The recent proposal of the existence of very small, transcellular ultra pores completes the picture. These pores traverse the cell membrane, and are primarily responsible for the water removal that occurs during ultrafiltration.

Transport considerations:

1. The peritoneal membrane, like all cells, has a negative charge but unlike the negative charge on the glomerular endothelial cell it does not appear to hinder the transport of negatively charged molecules. Although some charge selectivity is demonstrated, the overall effect appears negligible (Krediet 1996, p 150).

2. Under basal circumstances, only approximately one quarter of the peritoneal capillaries are perfused. Once a dialysate solution is introduced into the peritoneal cavity an increase in blood flow, especially to the splanchnic organs, occurs (Krediet 1996, p 151). Without the presence of dialysate, the peritoneal blood flow is approximately 100 ml/min. Once dialysate is introduced, blood flow increases to approximately 200 ml/min.

3. Because diffusion takes place when a concentration gradient is present, and convection is maximal when ultrafiltration rates are highest, providing optimal gradients for both of these mechanisms contributes to the overall solute removal. Small solute clearance (urea, sodium, and potassium) is primarily dependent on diffusion, especially when the osmolality of the dialysate solution is low. Macromolecules (proteins, Beta 2 microglobulin) are restricted by the surface area of the peritoneum and by the size of the molecule. It is not clear at present whether the principal mechanism is restricted diffusion or hydrostatically induced convection via the large pores (Krediet 1996, p 152).

The movement of intraperitoneal solute from the peritoneum and into the blood seems to be diffusion-dependent. An example of this can be seen with the diffusion of lactate, the buffer supplied with peritoneal dialysis solutions, where the absorption rate is approximately 82% of the infused concentration over a four-hour 'dwell' time. The movement of larger molecules such as blood cells, bacteria, and some medications, appears to be reliant on uptake by the diaphragmatic lymphatics (Krediet 1996, p 160).

Physiology of water movement

As with solute movement, keeping the conceptualisation of water movement simple is the easiest way to remember what happens. Osmosis refers to the movement of water molecules from the area of lowest solute concentration towards the area of highest solute concentration. Similarly, this process can be viewed as the *diffusion* of water molecules from the area of highest concentration of water molecules to the area of lowest concentration of water molecules. Whichever interpretation you prefer (both are correct), water movement slows once equilibration approaches and ceases once it has been achieved.

Adding electrolytes to the dialysate fluid is designed to promote the diffusion of these substances *from* blood *to* dialysate. Thus the dialysate concentrations of sodium, chloride and magnesium are lower than serum concentrations. Calcium concentrations vary, and are discussed in Chapter 3. This promotes the movement of these solutes from blood to dialysate. The exception is lactate, a buffer, which is small enough to diffuse rapidly *from* dialysate *to* blood, thus correcting the metabolic acidosis that often occurs in patients with end stage renal failure. So far, there is no sustained increase in osmolality, and therefore no incentive for water to move from blood to dialysate. Water movement is achieved by adding an osmotically active agent that has limited absorptive capacity because of its size and which will be tolerated reasonably well by the peritoneal membrane, to the dialysate. Exceptions to the limited absorption and tolerance will be discussed in later sections.

Glucose is the usual osmotically active substance used. It is available in strengths of 0·55%, 1·5%. 2·5% and 4·25% and provides osmotic activity of 298 mOsmols/L (similar to that of non uraemic plasma), 346mOsmols/L, 396 mOsmols/L and 485 mOsmols/L respectively (Palmer 1999, p33). The higher the percentage of glucose, the greater the osmotic gradient and potential for fluid removal.

Fluid removal during peritoneal dialysis is a combination of water transport from the peritoneal capillaries into the peritoneal cavity, transcapillary ultrafiltration, and fluid loss from the peritoneal cavity into the peritoneal capillaries, a combination of transcapillary *backfiltration*, and fluid uptake by the lymphatic system (Krediet 1996, 161).

The net volume of ultrafiltration during a given dwell time is therefore the combination of transcapillary ultrafiltration, minus transcapillary backfiltration plus lymphatic absorption. Mathematically this is expressed as:

(transcapillary ultrafiltration) – (transcapillary backfiltration + lymphatic absorption).

The permeability of the peritoneal membrane for small solutes and therefore its ability to normalise electrolyte levels and to remove metabolic waste products, and for glucose and therefore its ability to maintain the osmotic gradient required for sustained fluid loss, are both measurable. Known as the 'Peritoneal Equilibration Test' (PET), these measurements enable the nurse to determine the appropriateness of peritoneal dialysis as a renal replacement therapy for a given patient, and to modify the peritoneal dialysis regimen to suit the transport characteristics of each patient's peritoneal membrane. This test will be discussed in Chapter 3.

References

In text references

Drukker, W, 1989, 'History of peritoneal dialysis', *in Replacement of Renal Function by Dialysis*, Maher, J., (ed), 3rd ed, Kluwer Academic Publishers, Boston.

Krediet, R., 1996, 'Peritoneal anatomy and physiology during peritoneal dialysis', in *Replacement of Renal Function by Dialysis*, Jacobs, C., Kjellstrand, C., Koch, K., Winchester, F., (eds.), 4th ed, Kluwer Academic Publishers, Boston.

Palmer, B., 1999, 'Dialysate composition in hemodialysis and peritoneal dialysis', in *Principles and Practice of Dialysis*, Henrich, W. (ed), 2nd ed., William and Wilkins, Maryland.

Rippe, B., 1993, 'A three pore model of peritoneal transport', Peritoneal Dialysis International, vol. 13 (Suppl 2), pp S35–S38.

Spence, A., Mason, E., 1983, *Human Anatomy and Physiology*, Benjamin Cummings, Sydney.

Wild, J., 1998, 'Peritoneal dialysis' in *Renal Nursing* (appendix), Smith, T., (ed.), 2nd ed., Bailliere Tindall, Sydney.

Recommended readings

Nagy, J., 1996, 'Peritoneal cell biology', *Kidney International*, vol. 50, S 56, November, pp S 2–S 11.

Initiation and maintenance of therapy

Introduction

For peritoneal dialysis to be successful as a treatment for end stage renal failure it requires careful assessment of the patient's ability to perform the procedure, as well as an estimation of the probable suitability of the peritoneal cavity. It also requires the selection of an appropriate catheter, the correct placement of the catheter and skilled management of the exit site and the catheter during the weeks after it is inserted. Ideally, peritoneal dialysis is selected in time for the patient to receive education about the care of their catheter and for selecting and inserting the catheter *prior* to the need for dialysis.

Once treatment commences, its successful continuance is a constant challenge to all members of the health care team. While sound patient education and regular follow up influence many of the factors that impact on the success of peritoneal dialysis, many of these factors, such as loss of filtration capacity, still remain beyond the control of either staff or patient.

2.1 Peritoneal access

Beginning principles

Haemodialysis requires *direct* access to the blood supply. Ideally, the access should be in the form of either a native or graft fistulae that requires the placement of fistula needles each treatment. Peritoneal dialysis also requires access to the blood supply, but the access is *indirect*. It would be impossible to place needles into the peritoneal capillaries.

Access to the peritoneal membrane is gained through a specially designed catheter that acts as a conduit for instilling and draining dialysis fluid. Diffusion of solute and water from the peritoneal capillaries into the dialysate occurs between instillation and drainage. There must be sufficient membrane available for peritoneal dialysis to effectively replace renal function. The membrane transport characteristics should be suitable and the correct catheter must be chosen and inserted in a sterile manner.

The catheter can be placed using one of the following methods:

1. Trochar insertion is rarely used in contemporary practice. It is associated with a high incidence of fluid leakage, difficulty in creating a subcutaneous tunnel and exit site at the selected area and puncture of pelvic organs. It is usually only used when acute catheter placement is required (Ash and Daugirdas 2001, p 313; Wild 1998, p 261).

2. Laparoscopic insertion is well accepted but requires a general anaesthetic and muscle relaxation. An abdominal puncture is performed using a trochar, gas is instilled to distend the abdomen and a laparoscope is used to facilitate placement of the catheter. Suturing the catheter to the bladder mucosa to prevent it migrating is rarely possible using this procedure

3. Peritoneoscopic insertion is a modification of laparoscopic insertion and is usually performed in radiology under local anaesthetic. After the introduction of a cannula, the peritoneal cavity is expanded with air and the peritoneoscope is introduced at the same time as the catheter and catheter guide. The use of a fluoroscope enables the catheter to be indirectly visualised as it is introduced. As with laparoscopic insertion, suturing the catheter to the bladder mucosa is difficult. The guide and cannula are withdrawn after the catheter is placed satisfactorily.

4. Laparotomy where the abdominal cavity is opened and the catheter is placed under direct vision. The catheter can be sutured to the bladder mucosa depending on the surgeon's preference. A subcutaneous tunnel and exit site are created. It is preferable to dress the abdominal wound and the exit site separately so that the abdominal wound can be inspected without unnecessarily disrupting the dressing to the exit site.

The exit site should be dressed in a manner that secures the catheter according to the direction of its natural lie to prevent it moving during healing. If the catheter does move during the two-week post operative period, epithelialisation of the subcutaneous tunnel and healing of the exit site will be delayed and the likelihood of infection increased. Ideally, the catheter should exit the subcutaneous tissue in a caudal (down ward) position to prevent the accumulation of skin cells and other debris in the sinus. With the exception of the 'Lifecath' the end of the catheter should be located as close as possible to the Pouch of Douglas.

Location of the exit site: Determining the location of the exit site is an important feature of comfortable and functional catheter placement and is usually the responsibility of the peritoneal dialysis nurse. The exit site should be located approximately 5 cm away from the midline and at least 2 cm from surgical scars. The abdomen should be observed with the patient sitting and standing to ensure skin folds are avoided and the site is away from the patient's preferred 'belt line'.

Once a suitable site has been selected the nurse should ensure that the patient can see the area from a recumbent position and reach it with both hands without pulling on the catheter. Eyesight should be assessed to ensure the patient can see the catheter clearly on the side that has been selected. Finally, the site should be marked with a semipermanent marker so that it can be easily identified during surgery.

Although the surgeon will determine the catheter length, it is helpful to remember that the length of the intraabdominal portion generally corresponds with the distance between the upper margin of the symphysis pubis and the umbilicus. The patient should be lying flat when the measurement is undertaken (Baxter Health Care Corporation 1997 p 4).

Catheter design

Acute catheters: Catheters designed for acute placement are usually made from a rigid material, often Teflon, and can be either straight or curved. They have multiple perforations at the distal end and a connection facility at the proximal end. They are inserted over a metal stylet and designed for short term use only, usually three to five days. Infection rates are high, leakage of peritoneal fluid is a common problem and there is a risk of puncturing the abdominal or peritoneal organs during insertion. Rigid catheters are rarely used and will not be discussed further. More information can be found in the historical references in Chapter 1 or to other articles listed as recommended reading.

Chronic catheters: All catheters currently used have three sections:

- an internal portion lying below the peritoneal membrane

- a transmural portion traversing the peritoneal membrane, the preperitoneal fat, muscle and fascia, subcutaneous fat and skin.

- an external portion visible above the skin surface.

(Wild 1998, p 259).

All catheters are made from soft silicon rubber, usually have a longitudinal radio-opaque strip and have one or two dacron cuffs. The usual internal and external luminal diameters are 2·67 mm and 4·75 mm respectively. A fast flow design with an internal diameter of 3·2 mm and an external diameter of 5·49 mm has recently become available. Catheters are available in a variety of lengths to suit adult, paediatric or neonatal patients and have either coiled or straight internal portions. The tip of the internal portion has multiple perforations to facilitate the inflow and outflow of dialysate, while the transmural and external portions have no perforations. If accidental perforation occurs the patient is at risk of peritoneal, subcutaneous, or exit site infection. The external portion can be straight or angled at the point of exit to facilitate caudal positioning.

The most popular catheter in Australia is the straight Tenckhoff catheter. Other catheters include the curled Tenckhoff catheter, the 'Curl-cath', either 'pig-tailed' or straight, the Missouri Swan Neck catheter designed for left and right-sided placement and the Toronto Western Hospital catheter (Dombros et al. 1997, p 251). The 'Lifecath', mentioned earlier in the chapter, is now rarely used.

The swan neck, presternal, or 'bathtub' catheter is a relatively new design and features a presternal section tunnelled through the subcutaneous tissue of the chest wall, and tailored to fit each patient. The presternal portion is then connected to the intraperitoneal portion of the catheter. The exit site is located on the upper chest wall, which allows the patient to bath, hence the popular name of 'bathtub' catheter. The swan neck catheter is especially suitable for obese patients who have multiple skin folds, patients with abdominal stomas that can leak and contaminate the exit site and paediatric patients because the exit site is located away from the nappy area (Baxter 2000).

2.2 Initiation of therapy

Preoperative care

Good planning for the choice of therapy, early catheter implantation, and thorough patient education all contribute to the successful initiation of therapy. They also allow for healing of the peritoneal incision, the abdominal wall, the subcutaneous tunnel and the exit-site prior to the commencement of therapy.

Preoperative care of the patient includes:

1.   Removing excessive abdominal hair or according to unit policy, and preparing the abdomen with an appropriate skin preparation, chlorhexidine or povidone iodine are common choices.

2.   Choosing and clearly marking the exit site. These procedures are often done earlier, but are commonly included as part of the preoperative checklist completed prior to the patient leaving the ward.

3.   Ensuring the bowel and bladder are empty.

4.   Administering prophylactic antibiotics in some units. According to Gocal et al. (1998, p 16) the results of studies that investigated the effectiveness of preoperative antibiotic administration differ. Some show a decline in postoperative infection rates while others show no change.

(Wild 1998, p 260–261).

Intraoperative care

The insertion techniques commonly used to place catheters have already been reviewed. The other important part of intraoperative care involves the dialysis nurse. In some hospitals it is common practice for a peritoneal dialysis nurse to either accompany the patient to theatre, or to be present in the theatre suite at the time of the first bag exchange to ensure that dialysate inflow and outflow occur without obstruction, and to check the peritoneal incision for leaks before the abdomen is closed. Alternatively, the surgeon will flush the catheter with twenty to thirty ml of 0·9% sodium chloride and cap the catheter for later use.

Postoperative care

Protection of the peritoneal cavity: Most peritoneal dialysis units have regimens that describe a slow initiation of treatment described as catheter 'break-in'.

After the peritoneal catheter is inserted, continuous lavage of the peritoneal cavity is undertaken ideally using an automated therapy until the effluent becomes clear and free of postoperative bloodstaining. This process can take a few hours and is almost always completed by the first postoperative day. Some units instil an anticoagulant (usually heparin) in an amount that corresponds to the intraluminal volume of the catheter. The catheter, subcutaneous tunnel and exit site are then left untouched for a period of up to two weeks unless signs and/or symptoms of infection indicate that the dressing should be removed. Once therapy commences, small volumes of dialysis fluid are instilled, often with the patient in a recumbent or sitting position. Gradually this 'fill' volume is increased until the patient can tolerate two litres or more, as is prescribed. The patient should then be encouraged to become mobile but coughing and exercise should be avoided for the first few weeks.

Modifications to the break-in procedures are required if immediate dialysis is needed. Some units prefer to adhere to the recommended break-in procedure, and insert a temporary vascular catheter in order to perform haemodialysis until the peritoneal catheter can be used.

Observation and protection of the exit site

The importance of correctly locating the exit site, immobilising the catheter and the need for a separate dressing for both the abdominal incision and the exit site has already been discussed.

Infection at the exit-site and subcutaneous tunnel are major contributors to catheter loss and the early detection and effective treatment of infection are second only to their prevention in maintaining effective therapy. In the past, exit sites were considered to be either ' infected' or 'not infected'. Such classification was very broad and subjective, which led to misdiagnosis and mismanagement. In response, Twardowski (1996) developed an exit site classification that consisted of 5 categories. The differentiation of infected sites from uninfected sites is essential to Twardowski's classification, which is based on the presence of characteristics such as erythema, discharge, tenderness, oedema and the presence of granulation tissue.

Evaluation involves several steps:

1. Taking a thorough history from the patient or reliable family member.

2. Inspecting the exit site in good light, palpating the tunnel and observing any tenderness and induration.

3. Examining the exit site for discharge and taking a swab for culture and sensitivity if discharge is present.

4. Comparing the findings with those of the previous examination.

Please see Appendix A for an adaptation of Twardowski's 1996 peritoneal dialysis catheter exit site classification guide.

In 1993, Moncrief et al. described a method of inserting catheters that does not involve the initial creation of an exit site. The catheter features:

> ...a 2.5 cm subcutaneous dacron cuff that is tapered on each end and has a 1 cm peritoneal cuff ... the external segment of the catheter is buried in the subcutaneous tissue for 3–8 weeks, allowing tissue ingrowth in a sterile environment
>
> (Baxter 2000).

After four to six weeks a small incision is made and the external portion of the catheter is drawn through the incision and connected to an adaptor (Ash and Daugirdas 2001, p 313).

Treatment of an infected exit site: Standard treatment includes cleansing with an appropriate, nonirritant solution, frequent dressing changes, systemic antibiotic therapy, releasing the superficial dacron cuff if it has either extruded or is thought to be the source of the infection and nasal swabbing and treatment using Mupirocin if nasal carriage of staphylococcus aureus is thought to be the source of the infection.

Some controversy exists about using cleansing agents. Both povidone iodine and hydrogen peroxide are cytotoxic, and are known to cause tissue damage (Lineaweaver et al. 1985 pp 269–270). Although povidone iodine has been shown to decrease the number of infections (Luzar et al. 1990), it is probable that an antibacterial soap altered to suit each patient's skin type would do equally well (Gokal et al. 1998, pp 19–20).

In one study (Ahmed et. al.1997), 31% of catheters developed exit site infections within the first year of implantation and one half of these required replacement within the first year. These same authors described a treatment for exit site infection that involved using a bone curette to scrape the exit site and sinus tract 'until bleeding and adequate debridement occurred'. They reported that 83% of their patients were infection-free at completion of treatment.

2.3 Patient selection

Cognition and learning

All aspects of successful home dialysis require the patient or carer to have sufficient cognitive capacity to learn specific techniques and to remember what they have learned. They also require the patient to be sufficiently motivated to reproduce the results of the education sessions on a regular basis without modifications or short cuts that eventually compromise their treatment.

End stage renal failure is a chronic illness and the 'rewards' for compliance that apply in the treatment of acute illness do not apply. The end stage renal failure patient will never receive the reward of good health no matter how strictly they adhere to the treatment protocol. The best that they can hope for is to minimise the signs and symptoms that accompany uraemia.

It has long been recognised that adequate renal function is required for normal mentation. In 1839 Addison wrote that:

> ...*dullness of intellect peculiar to uremia and intended to shew (sic), that, in recent as well as chronic disease of the kidney, the cerebral disorder is not unfrequently (sic) the most prominent, and occasionally the only symptom present.*
>
> (cited in Brown and Brown 1995, p 244).

In end stage renal failure, the neuropsychological alterations that occur range from subtle early changes that can be easily missed, to gross abnormalities that is alarming to family and carers alike. According to Brown and Brown, uraemic encephalopathy occurs once renal failure declines to 10% of normal. It appears rapidly in patients with acute renal failure and evolves more slowly in people with chronic renal failure. Cognitive ability, psychomotor activity and personality are all affected, with 'anorexia, nausea and asterixis [occurring] first, followed by vomiting, restlessness, myoclonus, seizures and coma' (1995, p 244).

The changes in mentation that occur are due, at least in part, to:

1. Neurotoxicity due to ammonia retention.

2. The accumulation of as yet unidentified uraemic toxins in patients undergoing peritoneal dialysis who have fewer changes in mentation than those undergoing haemodialysis.

3. Hyperparathyroidism with changes in visuomotor and visuospatial function, attention, and nonverbal problem solving.

4. Anaemia that affects the 'speed and accuracy of information processing'.

5. Nonspecific changes relating to electrolyte dysregulation. Low cation levels lead to 'neuromuscular irritability and elevated concentrations lead to flaccidity'. Lethargy, delirium, or comas are possible in both situations.

6. Low serum albumen that correlates closely with the length of delirium. The precise mechanism is unclear at present.

(Brown and Brown 1995, pp 244–249)

Neuropsychological testing prior to commencing dialysis education can assist in identifying and treating disorders such as depression as well as providing the nurse with an outline of any learning deficits that exist, and therefore a guide to teaching that is specific for each patient. Since the acceptance of more patients onto end stage renal failure programs that have a limited capacity to absorb them, many of these patients are now required to wait until renal function has declined to 5 ml/min. prior to starting dialysis. In view of the relationship between impaired mentation and glomerular filtration rate, commencing education at this time can prove frustrating to both the patient and the nurse.

As well as commencing education while the patient is still uraemic, a second mistake is to prepare reading material that is aimed at an educational level that suits the teacher and not the patient. According to Duffy (1988, p 114) 'over 50% of health care clients are unable to read instructional materials written at fifth grade level'. Reading and understanding literature are compounded when the patient has a disease that is known to cause cognitive impairment. Some patients are educated to a high level and respond to material written at an appropriately higher level.

People who are illiterate in either their own language, or the language of the country they live in, are often unprepared to admit that they cannot read and do not want health professionals to know that they cannot comprehend written material. Nurses should be aware that excuses such as having left their glasses at home, discrepancies between performance following verbal rather than written instructions and errors when attempting to follow simple signs can indicate an inability to read. Nurses should use tact and sensitivity if they suspect a person cannot read and are attempting to determine their level of understanding of instructions. Specific literacy tests are available (Duffy 1998, p 116, Doak et al.1996 pp 27–39). It is still possible to teach a patient to successfully manage their own care at home, despite their inability to read.

The impact on carers and society

Health care professionals often assume that family members of the person requiring dialysis will willingly assume the role of carer. While this assumption is often the case initially, the reality of caring for a chronically ill person, albeit a loved one, soon becomes apparent. This is especially so when the unwell person is dependent on a 'life support' system such as dialysis for their survival.

The following quotation is from a paper written by Campbell (1998 pp 98–108) addressing the role of family members of patients suffering from end stage renal failure.

> They move in and out of the dialysis and transplant scene like actors on a stage. They are viewed by renal care professionals alternately as blessings, Godsends, and problem solvers or as nuisances, troublemakers, and pests. They are seen at the patient's bedside in hospital rooms, with patients in clinic or office examination rooms, dropping patients off for treatment, pushing wheelchairs, and assisting patients. Mostly though, they are seen waiting. Endless hours of waiting … never the stars, always in the role of supporting actors, they are treated in every conceivable manner from invisible 'necessary evils' to trusted and valued vital necessities … they are the family caregivers of thousands of end stage renal disease patients nationwide.

So—next time you feel annoyed by the presence and persistence of a carer, or frustrated by a patient's apparent inability to retain the information that you have so carefully prepared and possibly repeated many times, reflect on the possible reasons why it occurs. Remember also, your own needs in relation to providing care for long term patients who are chronically ill, especially that you too, need to receive care.

References

In text references

Ahmed, Z., Choudhury, D., Lee, J., Girgis, H. 1997, 'The role of curettage in the care of persistent exit-site infection in CAPD patients', *Peritoneal Dialysis International,* vol.17, no. 2, pp 195–197.

Ash, S., Daugirdas, J., 2001, 'Peritoneal access devices', in *Handbook of Dialysis*, Daugirdas, J., Blake, P., Ing, T., (eds.), 3rd ed., Lippincott Williams and Wilkins, Philadelphia.

Baxter Health Care Pty. Ltd., 2000, 'PD access management', paper presented at the 19th Annual Peritoneal Dialysis Conference, Melbourne, Australia.

Baxter Health Care Pty. Ltd., 'Peritoneal Dialysis Catheter Exit-site Classification Guide', Adapted, in part, from Twardowski, Z., Prowant, B., 'Classification of Normal and Diseased Exit Sites', *Peritoneal Dialysis International*, S 3, 1996.

Baxter Health Care Pty. Ltd., 'Exit site care and catheter management: best demonstrated practice', *Peritoneal Dialysis Catheter and Complications Management,* Baxter Health Care Pty. Ltd., Sydney, Australia.

Brown, T., Brown, R., 1995, 'Neuropsychiatric consequences of renal failure', *Psychosomatics,* vol. 36, 3, pp 244–253.

Campbell, A., 1998, 'Family caregivers: caring fro ageing end-stage renal disease partners', *Advances in Renal Replacement Therapy,* vol 5, no 2, pp 98–108.

Duffy, M., 1988, 'Selecting educational materials for patients with limited reading abilities', *ANNA Journal,* vol. 15, no. 2, pp 114–117.

Doak, C., Doak, L., Root, J., 1996, *Teaching Patients with Low Literacy Skills.* (2nd edn.). Lippincott, Philadelphia.

Gokal, R., Alexander, S., Ash, S., Chen, T., Danielson, A., Holmes. C., Joffe, P., Moncrief, J., Nichols, K., Piriano, B., Prowant, B., Slingeneyer, A., Stegmayr, B., Twardowski, Z., Vas, S., 1998, 'Peritoneal dialysis catheters and exit-site practices toward optimum peritoneal access', *Peritoneal Dialysis International,* vol. 18, pp 11–33.

Lineaweaver, W., Howard, R., Soucy, D., McMorris, s., Freeman, M., Crain, C., Robertson, J., Rumley, T.,1985, 'Topical antimicrobial toxicity', *Archives of Surgery,* no. 120, pp 267–270.

Luzar, M., Brown, C., Balf, D., Issad, B., Monnier, B., 1990, 'Exit site care and exit site infections in Continuous Ambulatory Peritoneal Dialysis (CAPD): results of a randomised multicenter study', *Peritoneal Dialysis International,* no. 10, pp 25–29.

Moncrief. J., 1993, 'The Moncrief-Popovich catheter: a new peritoneal access technique for patients on peritoneal dialysis', *ASAIO J.* pp 39–62.

Twardowski, Z., Prowant, B., 1996, 'Classification of normal and diseased exit sites', *Peritoneal Dialysis International,* vol. 16, Suppl 3, pp S32–S50.

Wild, J., 1998, 'Peritoneal dialysis' in *Renal Nursing* (appendix), Smith, T., (ed.), 2nd ed., Bailliere Tindall, Sydney.

Recommended reading

Ibels, L., Venus, P., Watts, R., Wilson-Stevens, V. 1997, 'Peritoneal dialysis catheter management and exit-site care: an Australian survey of current practice', *Nephrology,* vol. 3, pp 143–148.

Nissenson, A., 1996, 'Assessing the effects of peritoneal dialysis on the health-related quality of life of the adult patient', *Peritoneal Dialysis International,* vol. 17, Supp 3, pp S32–S34.

Briton, C., 2000, 'Themes on hope and living with a life-threatening illness', *Australian Social Work,* March, vol. 53, no.1, pp 51–55.

Callahan, E., Carrol, S., Revier, Sr. P., Gilhooly, E., Dunn, D., 1996, 'The sick role in chronic illness: some reactions' *Journal of Chronic Illness,* vol.19, pp 883–897.

Roberts, M., 1998, 'Peritoneal access devices', in *Symposium on the History of Dialysis*, Nephrology, vol. 4, pp 242–245.

Wellard, S., 1998, 'Constructions of chronic illness', *International Journal of Nursing Studies,* vol. 35, pp 49–55.

Treatment : modalities, modifications and measurement

Introduction

In 1975 Robert Popovich and Jack Moncrief described the concept of Continuous Ambulatory Peritoneal Dialysis (CAPD), and shortly thereafter commenced their first patient on this form of therapy. Although Intermittent Peritoneal Dialysis (IPD) had been used successfully prior to this time, its application was limited by high rates of peritonitis, and CAPD soon became the favoured method of treatment. Most centres prescribed what became known as the 'standard' treatment prescription—two litre exchanges four times per day. There was little appreciation of the importance of residual renal function, or the need for more exchanges and/or higher volumes for people with larger dialysis requirements. High rates of peritonitis continued, causing a loss to haemodialysis of about 20% annually. Several significant advances have occurred during the past decade. They include the development of different treatment possibilities, individualised treatment prescriptions and the concept of 'flush before fill' bag change procedures designed to decrease peritonitis rates.

3.1 Choice of therapy

General principles

Peritoneal dialysis requires a number of 'cycles' to be performed each day. Each cycle has three 'phases':

- A 'drain' phase where the used dialysate is drained from the peritoneal cavity.

- A 'fill' phase where fresh dialysate is introduced into the peritoneal cavity.

- A 'dwell' phase where the fluid remains in the peritoneal cavity, and during which time the majority of the fluid and solute removal (dialysis) occurs.

The drain and fill phases are undertaken in sequence with the dwell phase, and take approximately twenty minutes. The dwell phase separates the fill and drain phases in any one cycle, and varies in length according to the type of dialysis being performed. The dwell phase can be anywhere between 10 minutes for acute renal failure and 10 hours for continuous ambulatory peritoneal dialysis.

Solute moves from the peritoneal capillaries into the peritoneal cavity during the dwell phase. The movement occurs in accordance with the solute concentration of the dialysate. Water also leaves the capillaries in the dwell phase and enters the peritoneal cavity in accordance with the osmotic gradient created by the glucose in the dialysate. Although a small amount of solute and water removal occurs during the fill phase and continues during the drain phase, most of the dialysis occurs in the dwell phase and most treatment modifications involve altering the length of this phase.

The dialysate is provided in sterile plastic bags, usually polyvinyl chloride, similar to those used for intravenous fluid, and are known as 'bags' or 'pacs'. You might hear staff refer to 'bag' or 'pac' exchanges; this simply means that the patient is draining out the used dialysate, or effluent, and replacing it with fresh solution. Once regular therapy commences, the peritoneal catheter is connected to a short fluid transfer set, between 15 and 20 cm long, designed to be changed approximately every six months unless accidental damage such as a puncture occurs, in which case the transfer set is changed immediately. Between each bag exchange a cap that usually contains a bacteriocidal agent protects the free end of the transfer set. During bag exchanges the cap is removed and the transfer set is used as a conduit to drain the used dialysate and to replace it with fresh solution.

The majority of units now employ some variation of what is known as a 'flush before fill' technique to perform the bag exchanges. The flush before fill bag exchange method requires the transfer set to be joined to a Y connection device, where one end is continuous with an empty bag to receive the dialysate effluent and the other is continuous with a bag containing fresh dialysate solution. Both the bags, and the Y set, are packaged as single use, sterile, disposable units. After the dialysate effluent drains into the empty bag, and prior to introducing the fresh dialysate solution into the peritoneal cavity, a small amount of the fresh solution (about 100 ml) is used to flush the connection between the fluid transfer set and the Y set. This process is designed to ensure that organisms accidentally transferred to the fluid transfer set during connection are flushed out into the dialysate effluent and not into the peritoneal cavity.

The Peritoneal Equilibration Test

Developed by Twardowski in 1987, the Peritoneal Equilibration Test (PET) is a standardised test designed to measure the equilibration rates for various solutes over a four-hour dwell time (Wild 1998, p 253). The PET measures the permeability of the peritoneal membrane and enables a decision based on clinical data, to be made about the suitability of a given treatment program.

After a PET, the peritoneal membranes are classified as high, high average, low average, or low transporters. These terms reflect the rate at which creatinine, which is a gauge of solute movement and glucose that determines fluid movement, move from blood to dialysate and dialysate to blood respectively. If creatinine diffuses readily from blood to dialysate, it can be presumed that other small molecular weight solutes will also move just as readily. Because glucose transport occurs in the opposite direction to creatinine, from dialysate to blood, the smaller the amount of glucose absorbed from the dialysate, the higher the osmolality and the greater the capacity for fluid removal.

Clinical application: The low transporter reaches creatinine and glucose equilibration slowly. This means, that although it takes longer for solute to cross the membrane and solute clearance rates are lower, glucose will also travel slowly, maintaining the osmotic gradient that enables fluid removal. These patients have the highest ultrafiltration rates, but experience poor solute clearance. They might do best with 'high dose dialysis', where overnight cycling peritoneal dialysis and one or two day time exchanges can achieve the required solute clearance. Because these patients have high ultrafiltration rates, high dose dialysis regimens require a dialysate with a low glucose content to avoid dehydration. An alternative treatment is to provide long 'day time' dwell times where the slow transport of solute can be maximised (Wild 1998, 253). In situations such as this, dialysate solutions containing higher dextrose concentrations will maintain fluid loss. If solute clearance remains poor, these patients often require transfer to haemodialysis (Prowant and Schmidt 1991, p364).

High transporters are the opposite—because creatinine moves quickly, most solute removal occurs early in the dwell phase, but glucose is also absorbed quickly, causing the osmotic gradient that supports fluid loss to rapidly dissipate. These patients do best with short dwell times (Wild 1998, p 253-254), and can benefit from a 'dry' period at night. The dry period prevents the reabsorption of water and the lack of solute removal that occurs when equilibration between blood and dialysate has been reached early in the dwell phase.

Patients with high average, good solute transport and average ultrafiltration, and low average transport rates, average solute transport and good ultrafiltration, usually do well on most standard peritoneal dialysis prescriptions (Prowant and Schmidt 1991, p363).

Once the transport characteristics of the peritoneal membrane are known, it is possible to assess the patient's response to therapy using computerised software that removes much of the guesswork previously associated with treatment modifications. Factors such as lifestyle choices, ultrafiltration rate, residual renal function, serum biochemistry, total body water, dietary protein intake, lymphatic uptake of dialysate, metabolic generation rate, and mass transfer coefficents are entered into a computer. Once data entry is completed, treatment targets are entered and the dialysis response to a number of different peritoneal dialysis regimens can be determined.

Treatment options

Continuous Ambulatory Peritoneal Dialysis (CAPD)

CAPD is designed to be performed manually by the patient and between four and five bags are exchanged during waking hours. The daytime cycles are short, between three and four hours, with a longer nighttime dwell. Fill volumes vary between two and three litres. The timing of exchanges is not critical, provided that the daytime ones start early, finish reasonably late, and that the exchanges in between are fairly evenly spaced.

It is possible to introduce an extra exchange during sleeping hours for CAPD patients who need increased clearances. Commencing the bag exchange process, but not proceeding to the manual drain phase can achieve the additional bag exchange. The prepared dialysate is placed onto a simple device that has been pre-programmed to commence a drain and fill phase at a predetermined time. Such devices are relatively economical to purchase, are able to be stored during waking hours and the procedure is easily learned by most patients.

1.   Continuous Cyclic Peritoneal Dialysis (CCPD)

CCPD is almost the opposite of CAPD, except that, because the frequent exchanges are performed at night, a machine is required. It is therefore, one of the automated therapies. Typically, between five and seven exchanges are performed overnight and the patient can be 'wet' (with fluid remaining in the peritoneal cavity) or 'dry' (no fluid remains in the peritoneal cavity) during the day. CCPD has an advantage over CAPD, in that an increased number of exchanges can be completed without the inconvenience that this would cause for the CAPD patient. It also allows more free time during the day.

2.   Intermittent Peritoneal Dialysis (IPD)

IPD is selected infrequently, but it does provide a treatment alternative for people, particularly the elderly, who are not suited to haemodialysis, and who are no longer able to perform either CAPD or CCPD. IPD is usually performed in the hospital setting. One of the automated forms of therapy, it is conducted for between twelve and twenty hours at a time and is required every two to three days (Wild 1998, p 270). The 'peak and trough' effect for water and solute loss is similar to that seen during haemodialysis and the length of time required for each treatment session makes it an unpopular choice. However, it offers an alternative for people with no other options who do not want to discontinue therapy.

3.   Tidal Peritoneal Dialysis

During tidal peritoneal dialysis only a part of the fill volume is ever drained at any one time. By initially introducing a fill volume of, for example, two litres and then draining only one and one half litres plus the ultrafiltrate, a residual amount of dialysate always remains in the peritoneal cavity. This ensures that diffusion and ultrafiltration never fall to the extent that they would if the peritoneal cavity were completely emptied. According to Twardowski (1990 M 584), this can increase clearances by up to 20%. Leaving some fluid in the peritoneal cavity also helps to decrease the discomfort some people experience when the peritoneal cavity is completely drained (Wild 1998, p268).

3.2 Choice of dialysate and delivery apparatus

Conventional dialysate solutions

As discussed in Chapter 1, the composition of the dialysate is designed to create a concentration gradient that will encourage the movement of solute from either blood to dialysate, or from dialysate to blood. For metabolic waste products like urea and creatinine the movement will always be from blood to dialysate, and for electrolytes such as sodium, potassium, magnesium and chloride, the movement will be also from blood to dialysate. Buffer, either lactate or bicarbonate, is designed to move in the opposite direction, i.e. from dialysate to blood. The only electrolyte that is routinely varied is calcium, to allow for movement either way, in accordance with the patient's blood chemistry. The lower calcium strengths allow the increased use of calcium-containing phosphate-binders without the risk of hypercalcaemia (Sorkin 1993, p 158). One example of available solution strengths is shown in Table 4.3.1.

Table 4.3.1: Solute values commonly available in dialysate solutions.

Electrolyte	PD1 (mmol/L)	PD2 (mmol/L)	PD4 (mmol/L)
Calcium	1.0	1·75	1·25
Sodium	132	132	132
Chloride	96	96	96
Magnesium	0.5	0·5	0·5
Lactate	40	40	40
pH	← 5.5	5.5	5.5 →
Glucose		As per prescription	

Lactate has long been used as a buffering substitute in peritoneal dialysate solutions because its absorption and metabolism results in the generation of bicarbonate ions in a one-to-one ratio, and it is well tolerated as long as hepatic function is normal (Palmer 1999, p 35). Because lactate is rapidly metabolised to bicarbonate, a high dialysate-to-plasma ratio of bicarbonate is maintained, ensuring continued absorption of lactate and therefore a continuing supply of buffer in all patients except those with high ultrafiltration rates. In the latter group of patients, the dilution of lactate in the peritoneal cavity reduces the diffusion gradient necessary for lactate absorption to occur and the supply of bicarbonate is correspondingly decreased (Palmer 1999, p 35–36). Acetate has also been used as an indirect source of buffer, but has been largely discontinued because of links connecting its use with the development of ultrafiltration failure, and sclerosing peritonitis (Palmer 1999, p 35).

Recent introductions

Bicarbonate as a buffering agent: As with modern haemodialysis, the direct use of bicarbonate for the normalisation of acid-base balance is a recent introduction. The use of bicarbonate with peritoneal dialysis has the same physiological advantages as haemodialysis, but is associated with two major disadvantages:

1. The high pH of solutions containing bicarbonate can result in the precipitation of calcium and magnesium ions. During haemodialysis, the bicarbonate-containing solution is separated from the acid solution containing the calcium and magnesium to prevent the precipitation of calcium and magnesium salts that occurs when the solution pH is high. The same would occur during peritoneal dialysis if calcium and magnesium were present in a solution with a high pH.

2. The heat sterilisation process used to ensure that peritoneal dialysis solutions are pyrogen-free results in caramelisation of the glucose unless the pH of the solution is acidic.

These difficulties can be overcome by using a dual bag system—one bag containing the bicarbonate and the other containing glucose, calcium and magnesium and the other necessary ions. The two bags are connected via a sealed section that can be broken by the patient, allowing the contents of both bags to be mixed immediately prior to use. Although limited in use at present, clinical trials have shown this system to be both safe and effective (Palmer 1999, p 36, Passlick-Deetjen and Jaeckle-Meyer, 1998 p 18).

A second new development, aimed specifically at removing the problems associated with heat sterilisation, is the use of filtration and not heat to ensure pyrogen-free solutions. This removes the risk of glucose caramelisation associated with solutions that do not have an acidic pH (Johnson 2000).

PVC free delivery systems: Di (2-ethylhexyl) phthalate (DEHP) is frequently used as a plasticiser to improve the flexibility of the polyvinyl chloride (PVC), which is widely used in the production of medical equipment, including the delivery systems used in peritoneal dialysis (Mettand et al. 1999, p S31). Because the DEHP is not chemically bound to the PVC, it is able to leach out of the plastic matrix, and is easily detected in the environment as well as in the organs of patients who are exposed to equipment containing DEHP (Mettand et al. 1999, p S31). Although little is known about the effects of retained plasticiser, studies indicate it could have a role in depressed phagocyte function and uraemic pruritus. These findings resulted in the production of PVC-free products by some suppliers of dialysis equipment. Although still in the introductory phase, initial multicentre evaluation of PVC-free equipment has been positive (Lambert et al. 1999).

Alternatives to glucose as an osmotic agent: As previously discussed, glucose, in a variety of concentrations, is the agent most frequently used to promote the osmotic gradient that enables fluid removal. However, the presence of glucose in the peritoneal cavity, and its systemic absorption, is associated with a number of undesirable effects, which include:

1. An increase in caloric intake and subsequent weight gain.

2. Hypertriglyceridaemia.   } Glucose absorption

3. Loss of appetite and subsequent protein malnutrition.

4. Depressed phagocyte function.   } Glucose contact

5. Loss of membrane function

Given these complications, a number of alternative substances have been tried including fructose, dextran and gelatine, but have been found to be either unsafe or ineffective as osmotic agents (Palmer 1999, p 34). Most recent studies have involved the use of amino acids, which have the additional benefit of opposing the amino acid loss characteristic of glucose containing dialysate, and glucose polymers. The main benefit of the amino acid solutions, for example Nutrineal, is improved nutritional status of the patient (Palmer 1999, p 34), while the main benefit of the glucose polymer solutions, for example Icodextrin, is the production of a sustained ultrafiltration rate for prolonged periods of time.

This sustained ultrafiltration (8–12 hours) is the result of what is termed colloid osmosis. This refers to water removal that continues because the size of the molecule used prevents rapid absorption (Wilkie and Brown 1997 p S 47). Solutions containing glucose polymers are thought to be of most benefit to patients who are high transporters, and can be used at night only, or in combination with traditional glucose-containing solutions during the day. The use of either solution will be of advantage to the diabetic patient because they prevent glucose absorption.

Additional benefits of glucose-free solutions are the preservation of the ultrafiltration characteristics of the peritoneal membrane in type 2 ultrafiltration failures, and a reduction in the production of advanced glycosylation end products (AGE), both of which will be discussed in Chapter 4.

Icodextrin hypersensitivity, where pruritus associated with a maculopapular rash occurs on the abdomen, hands, arms, legs and lower back, is a rare occurrence and resolves when dialysate containing Icodextrin is discontinued (Lam-Po-Tang et al. 1997, pp 82–84). The use of Icodextrin is not recommended for pregnant or lactating women, children under the age of 18 years, in acute renal failure, or where the peritoneum and/or abdomen are not intact.

Additions to the dialysate fluid

Insulin: When insulin is added to the peritoneal dialysis solution of diabetic patients it is absorbed along with glucose during the dwell phase and has the advantage of providing smoother blood glucose control than that achieved using intermittent injections (Wild 1998, p 273). An additional benefit is that insulin administered via the peritoneal route has a higher portion 'absorbed by the liver directly via the portal circulation, and thus resembles 'naturally' secreted insulin' (Rutecki and Whittier 1993, p 323). This also results in a decrease in peripheral insulin doses and can slow the accelerated atherogenesis seen in the diabetic patients (Rutecki and Whittier 1993, p 323).

The daily dose of insulin is usually higher than the doses required prior to commencing dialysis due to both glucose absorption and adherence of insulin to the dialysate delivery system. The daily insulin requirements are divided between each of the bags to be used during the 24 hours. The nighttime bag usually contains slightly less insulin than the daytime bags to prevent hypoglycaemia occurring overnight (Wild 1998, p 273). Patients who use APD or CCPD can use a combination of subcutaneous and intraperitoneal insulin.

A number of protocols for the administration of intraperitoneal insulin are available. Individual hospitals have protocols that are usually based on one of them, with or without modifications that accord with the preference of individual nephrologists. There are also units that believe that the risk of accidental contamination of the dialysate fluid by the patient is too great to allow the use of intraperitoneal insulin.

Antibiotics: Agents used to combat peritoneal infection are probably the most frequent addition to the dialysate and are discussed in Chapter 4.

Heparin: Heparin is usually added only after catheter insertion or during bouts of peritonitis. In both situations it is used to prevent blockage of the catheter by fibrin or blood and its use is by no means universal. Heparin is not absorbed across the peritoneal membrane and therefore, does not increase the risk of bleeding (Korbet and Kronfol 2001, p 338). Some units use a heparin-based solution to 'lock' the catheter following insertion and prior to using it.

Potassium: The addition of potassium should only be considered in patients who have low to normal serum potassium levels and in whom dietary or oral potassium supplementation cannot maintain normal serum levels. If peritoneal dialysis is used in an acute setting, serum potassium levels are usually maintained within normal limits with intravenous potassium supplements.

Cytotoxic drugs: Chemotherapeutic agents have been used to treat intraperitoneal malignancy but have been associated with chemical peritonitis (Terrill 1992).

Calcitriol: Few studies have been completed in this area. One prospective randomised study (Gadallah et al. 2000), found intraperitoneal calcitriol to be superior to pulse oral doses in 'lowering PTH and alkaline phosphatase levels and in resolving renal osteodystrophy, and that [intraperitoneal] calcitriol is associated with a lower incidence of hyperphosphatemia and elevated Ca x PO4 by product.

Streptokinase: Streptokinase has been used to treat relapsing peritonitis that does not respond to appropriate antibiotic therapy. Relapses are thought to be due to bacterial colonisation of the fibrin layer that adheres to the catheter. Streptokinase has proven useful as a treatment for peritonitis because it destroys the fibrin layer. Some patients develop a peritonitis-like syndrome between one to two days after therapy, which is thought to be due to the release 'of fibrin clot containing bacteria, leukocytes and debris from the colonised catheter into the peritoneal cavity into the peritoneum' (Nankivell et al. 1999, pp 20–22). Urokinase has also been used to achieve the same result.

3.3 Assessment of therapy

What is adequate therapy?

Early CAPD treatment involved routinely using 4 x 2 litre exchanges daily. This was similar to the routine use of four hours of haemodialysis, three times each week, in that there was little recognition that people of different body sizes could need different treatment prescriptions.

The conduct of the 1996 Canadian and United States of America (CANUSA) study into the efficacy of peritoneal dialysis revealed information similar to that revealed by the 1983 National Co-operative Dialysis Study into the efficacy of haemodialysis. In the vast majority of cases peritoneal dialysis patients under dialysed.

The CANUSA study questioned the previously held belief that a K^t/V of 1·7 and a creatinine clearance of 50 litres/week were sufficient to replace renal function (Oreopoulos 1998, p 361). Current CAPD and APD prescriptions, based on the findings of the CANUSA study, require a minimum K^t/V of 1·7, with an ideal K^t/V of 2. Corrected creatinine clearance should be 60 L/week for high and high average transporters, and 50 L/week for low and low average transporters (CARI Guidelines 2000, p19).

The CANUSA study also revealed the difference in outcomes for patients who retained residual renal function and those who did not. As a result of the study, CAPD 'lost its simplicity' (Oreopoulos 1998, p 362) and it is now recognised that successful peritoneal dialysis in the anuric patient requires a much higher peritoneal clearance rate than that required in the patient who retains even minimal renal function.

In addition, some studies indicate that the use of K^t/V should be employed with caution when used as a guide to the adequacy of treatment in peritoneal dialysis patients. This is because the glucose absorbed during bag exchanges often results in a 'body composition [that] often deviates from normal because of an increase in percentage body fat' (Wong et al. 1995, p 563).

How should 'adequate therapy' be achieved?

As a result of the CANUSA study, an 'Ad Hoc Committee on Peritoneal Dialysis' met during January 1996 to prepare a consensus statement that provided guidelines to achieve adequate clearances using peritoneal dialysis. This group concluded that:

> *[A]dequate clearance … can be achieved in almost all patients if the prescription is individualized according to the patient's body surface area, amount of residual renal function, and peritoneal membrane transport characteristics. Use of 2.5 to 3.0 L fill volumes, the addition of an extra exchange, and giving automated peritoneal dialysis patients a 'wet' day are all options to consider when increasing weekly creatinine clearance and K^t/V. Rather than specify a single clearance or K^t/V target, the recommended clinical practice is to provide the most dialysis that can be delivered to the*

individual patient, within the constraints of social and clinical circumstances, quality of life, life style and cost.

(Blake et al. 1996, p 448).

The same group stated that prescription management should be an integral part of everyday patient management, with peritoneal membrane transport characteristics, the amount of dialysis delivered, and the amount of residual renal function all being considered when adjustment to the dialysis prescription is required.

What other factors are important?

1. Burkart (1999, p163) cautioned that, while the CANUSA study is one of the most thorough studies as yet undertaken, and gives the best evidence that patient survival is related to solute clearance, the study has limitations. The study was based on the assumption that solute clearance remained stable over time, and that 'one unit … of clearance due to residual renal function is equal to one unit … of clearance due to peritoneal dialysis'.

    Because residual renal function is known to decrease once dialysis commences, as stated by Blake et al., regular estimates of the kidney's contribution to solute removal should be undertaken so that unrecognised under dialysis does not occur.

2. As with haemodialysis, the nutritional status of the patient is a major predictor of outcomes in the peritoneal dialysis population. The decrease in appetite that accompanies the uraemic syndrome and the strict control of protein intake that is required prior to the commencing dialysis, often result in a patient beginning treatment in a malnourished state. In addition, peritoneal dialysis is associated with problems different from those seen in the haemodialysis population.

    When the decreased appetite and early satiety that result from glucose absorption are combined with the loss of protein and amino acids to the dialysate, between 5–15, and 2–4 g/day respectively, the potential for protein malnutrition becomes a significant comorbid factor (Burkart 1999, p164). It should be noted that these losses increase during episodes of peritonitis. To prevent malnutrition, the CARI guidelines recommend a protein intake of 1.2 g/kg body weight and a total energy intake of 35 kcal/kg body weight. Additional protein is required if peritonitis develops.

3.4 Limitations of treatment

Considerations

Initial considerations as to the suitability of peritoneal dialysis for a given patient relate to the amount of peritoneal membrane that is available, the presence and severity of comorbid conditions, and the ability of the patient to perform the procedure in a safe and consistent manner. The majority of these factors has been addressed earlier in the chapter and will not be discussed further.

There is a growing body of opinion that all suitable patients should commence their renal replacement therapy with peritoneal dialysis. This is seen as the first step in an integrated approach to care, during which patients are transferred from one treatment modality to another in accordance with their treatment requirements (Biesen et al. 2000, p 116). It is also believed that residual renal function will be best preserved by implementing peritoneal dialysis as the treatment of first choice, thereby maximising the 'dose' of dialysis that is available to the patient prior to the loss of their residual renal function.

References

In text references

Biesen, W., Vanholder, R., Veys, N., Dhondt, A., Lameire, N., 'An evaluation of an integrated care approach for end stage renal disease patients', *Journal of the American Society of Nephrology*, vol. 11, pp 116–125.

Blake, P., Burkart, J., Churchill, D., Daugirdas, J., Depner, T., Hamburger, R., Hull, A., Korbet, M., Moran, J., Nolph, K., Oreopoulos, D., Schreiber, M., Soderbloom, R., 1996, 'Recommended clinical practices for maximizing peritoneal dialysis clearances', *Peritoneal Dialysis International*, vol.16, no. 5, pp 448–456.

Burkart, J., 1999, 'Adequacy of peritoneal dialysis' in *Principles and Practice of Dialysis*, Henrich, W. (ed), 2nd ed., William and Wilkins, Maryland.

CARI Guidelines, 2000, A joint project between the Australian and New Zealand Society of Nephrology and the Australian Kidney Foundation, Excerpta Medica Communications, Sydney.

Gadallah, M., Arora, N., Torres, C., Ramdeen, G., Schaffer-Pautz, A., Moles, K., 2000. 'Pulse oral versus intraperitoneal calcitriol: a comparison of efficacy in the treatment of hyperparathyroidism and renal osteodystrophy in peritoneal dialysis patients' *Advances in Peritoneal Dialysis,* vol. 16, pp 303–307.

Johnson, D., 2000, 'Biocompatibility', paper presented at the 19th Annual Peritoneal Dialysis Conference, Melbourne, Australia.

Korbet, S., Kronfol, N., 2001, 'Acute peritoneal dialysis prescription', *in Handbook of Dialysis*, Daugirdas, J., Blake, P., Ing,T. (eds.), 3rd ed., Lippincott Williams and Wilkins, Philadelphia.

Lambert, M., Lage, C., Kirchgessner, J., 1999, 'Stay-safe – a new PVC free system in long-term CAPD treatment', *EDTNA/ERCA Journal*, vol. 25, no. 3, pp 30–34.

Lam-Po-Tang, M., Bending, M., Kwan, J., 1997, 'Icodextran hypersensitivity in a CAPD patient', *Peritoneal Dialysis International*, Jan., vol. 17, no. 1, pp 82–84.

Mettang, T., Fischer, F., Dunst, R., Kuhlmann, U., Rettenmeier, A., 1997, 'Plasticizers in renal failure: aspects of metabolism and toxicity', *Peritoneal Dialysis International*, vol. 17, Suppl. 2, pp S31–S36.

Nankivell, B., Lake, N., Gillies, A., 1991, 'Intercatheter streptokinase for recurrent peritonitis in CAPD', *Clinical Nephrology*, vol. 35, no. 1, pp 20–23.

Oreopoulos, D., 1998, 'A backward look at the first 20 years', *Peritoneal Dialysis International*, vol. 18, no. 4, pp 360–362.

Palmer, B., 1999, 'Dialysate composition in hemodialysis and peritoneal dialysis', in *Principles and Practice of Dialysis,* Henrich, W., (ed.), 2nd ed., William and Wilkins, Maryland.

Passlick-Deetjen, J., Jaeckle-Meyer, I., 1998, 'Bicarbonate buffers in peritoneal dialysis', *Artificial Organs*, vol. 22, no. 1, pp17–19.

Prowant. B., Schmidt, L., 1991, 'The peritoneal equilibration test: a nursing discussion', *ANNA Journal*, vol. 18, no. 4, pp 361–366.

Rutecki, G., Whittier, F, 1993, 'Intraperitoneal insulin in diabetic patients on peritoneal dialysis', in *Dialysis Therapy*, Nissenson, A., Fine, R., (eds.), 2nd ed., Hanley & Belfus Inc.Philadelphia.

Sorkin, M., 1993, 'Peritoneal dialysis solutions', in *Dialysis Therapy*, Nissenson, A., Fine, R., (eds.), 2nd ed., Hanley & Belfus Inc.Philadelphia.

Terrill, B., 1992, 'Use of peritoneal dialysis technology to treat abdominal malignancy', Poster presentation, 11th Annual Peritoneal Dialysis Nurses Conference, Baxter Healthcare Pty. Ltd., Sydney, Australia.

Twardowski, Z., Nolph, K., Khanna, R., 1987, 'Peritoneal equilibration test', *Peritoneal Dialysis Bulletin*, vol. 7, no. 3, pp 138–147.

Twardowski, Z., Prowant, F., Nolph, K, Khanna, R., Schmidt, L., Stanalowich, R., 1990, 'Chronic nightly tidal peritoneal dialysis' American, Society of Artificial organs—Transactions vol 36:M 584–M 588.

Wild, J., 1998, 'Peritoneal dialysis' in *Renal Nursing* (appendix), Smith, T., (ed.), 2nd ed., Bailliere Tindall, Sydney.

Wilkie, M., Brown, C., 1997, 'Polyglucose solutions in CAPD', *Peritoneal Dialysis International*, vol. 17, Suppl. 2, pp S47–S50.

Wong, K., Xiong, D., Kerr, P., Borovincar, D., Stroud, D., Atkins, R., Strauss, B., 1995, 'Kt/V in CAPD by different estimations of V', *Kidney International,* vol. 48, pp 563–569.

Recommended readings

Diaz-Buxo, J., 1997, 'Peritoneal dialysis modality selection for the adult, the diabetic, and the geriatric patient', *Peritoneal Dialysis International,* vol.17, Suppl. 3, pp S28–S31.

Newman, L., Hanslik, T., Tessman. M., 1994, 'Cost effective automated peritoneal dialysis with average to low transport', ANNA Journal, vol.21, no. 5., pp 271–273.

Nolph, K, 1997, 'Factors affecting peritoneal efficiency in different treatment schedules' *Peritoneal Dialysis International*, vol.17, Suppl. 2, pp S98–S101.

Schmidt, L., Prowant, B., 1991, 'How to do a peritoneal equilibration test', *ANNA Journal*, vol. 18, no. 4., pp 368–369.

Complications of therapy

Introduction

Peritoneal dialysis is not generally considered to be a long term option to replace renal function, even though it is used by thousands of people throughout the world and recommended by many nephrologists as the treatment of choice for commencing dialysis therapy. Its limitations primarily relate to the number of treatment-related complications that can occur.

When broadly divided into those complications that relate to infection, and those that don't, infection is generally considered to be the major factor that limits peritoneal dialysis to a five-year treatment option. There are, however, a number of patients who manage on peritoneal dialysis for longer periods.

Although the flush before fill techniques discussed in Chapter 3 have resulted in a marked decrease in peritoneal-related infection rates over recent years, peritonitis is still considered to be the Achilles' heel of this form of dialysis.

4.1 Infective complications

Peritonitis

Peritonitis is a major cause of morbidity and mortality and has been described as the Achilles' heel of peritoneal dialysis. It is also significant because of the costs associated with diagnosis and treatment and the loss of productivity. According to Tzamaloukas and Fox (1999, p.556) CAPD-associated peritonitis should be regarded as a disease process different from that which is encountered in post surgical patients, because it is similar to the 'spontaneous bacterial peritonitis occurring in patients with cirrhosis of the liver, ascites, and portal hypertension'.

Organisms responsible: Normal skin or nasal organisms, such as staphylococcus epidermidis and staphylococcus aureus respectively, cause the majority of peritoneal infections. These organisms usually gain entry to the peritoneal cavity during bag exchanges. Infections caused by gram-negative species are also quite common. Other organisms, e.g. protozoa, fungi and proteus can also cause infection, but are less common. Tzamaloukas and Fox (1999, p.557) document these organisms as follows:

1. Gram-positive bacteria—coagulase negative staphylococci are the most common followed by staphylococcus aureus and streptococcus species. Enterococcal infections and those caused by the Neisseria and Diphtheroid species are less common.

2. Gram-negative bacteria—Escherichia coli and Pseudomonas species are the most frequently seen followed by Proteus, Acinetobacter, Klebsiella and Serratia species.

3. Fungi are responsible for less than 10% of infections.

4. Five percent of infections are caused by rare organisms such as, mycobacteria and protozoa.

The previously mentioned flush before fill technique used for most bag exchange procedures today is responsible for markedly reducing the peritonitis rate. However, when infections do occur, they tend to be of a more serious nature and involve organisms that are more difficult to treat.

Routes of entry: Organisms can enter the peritoneal cavity through five possible entry points:

1. Intraluminal, as a result of contamination during the bag exchange procedure. The most common organisms seen are staphylococcus epidermidis and staphylococcus aureus.

2. Periluminal, where infection is present in either the tunnel or the exit site allows organisms to gain entry by migrating along the catheter tract. Common organisms are staphylococcus epidermidis, staphylococcus aureus, pseudomonas, proteus and yeast.

3. Transmural, where infection occurs when organisms enter the peritoneal cavity through a perforation in the intestinal wall, or by migrating through the intestinal wall. The most common organism seen is Escherichia coli, with anaerobes and fungi occasionally seen.

4. Haematogenous, where organisms enter via the blood stream. Streptococcus and mycobacterium are the usual causative organisms.

5. Ascending infections are seen only in women and occur when organisms enter via the Fallopian tubes. Candida and pseudomonas are the most frequently seen organisms.

(Wild 1998, p 295–296).

Predisposing factors include a decrease in humoral and cell-mediated immunity and suppression of phagocytic and chemotactic responses that are the sequelae to chronic renal failure, the presence of dialysate that dilutes peritoneal macrophages and washes them out with each bag exchange, and the suppression of local leukocyte function by the high dialysate osmolality and low pH (Tzamaloukas and Fox 1999, p 560). Lactate also appears to decrease the function of peritoneal inflammatory cells, while the heat sterilisation process decreases the ability of leukocytes to adhere to endothelial cells (Tzamaloukas and Fox 1999, p 560).

Diagnosis: Various criteria for the diagnosis of peritonitis have been developed; most usually require two of the following symptoms to be present:

1. cloudy dialysate effluent with >100 white cells/microliter, more than 50% of which are neutrophils

2. diffuse abdominal pain

3. fever

4. nausea or vomiting.

Identifying the organism, either by gram stain, or culture confirms the diagnosis.

Treatment: Protocols vary between hospitals and a complete review of those in common use is beyond the scope of this text. Included in most protocols however, is the use of rapid flushing of the peritoneal cavity by performing two, or more bag exchanges in quick succession with no dwell time, a request for the patient to bring in the bag used prior to these flushes for culture and sensitivity and to commence broad spectrum antibiotic therapy until the organism has been identified and specific antibiotic therapy can be started.

However the ISPD Guidelines state that it is 'reasonable to delay initiation of antimicrobial therapy' in asymptomatic patients who present with cloudy dialysate effluent until the 'results of cell count, differential and gram stain are available' provided that these tests can be performed without delay (Kean et al. 2000). Performing two or three rapid exchanges when peritonitis is suspected is 'reported to be of symptomatic benefit, but does not appear to offer any other specific benefits (Kean et al. 2000 p 404). Consequently, some units do not advise patients to use rapid flushes unless they experience considerable abdominal discomfort, in the belief that the beneficial effect of intraperitoneal macrophages and antibiotics should be preserved in the patient without symptoms.

It is important for all patients to be taught the importance of contacting their hospital *immediately* they suspect that an infection is present, or whenever they suspect, or know, that they have deviated from the bag exchange or catheter care procedure taught by their hospital.

After an episode of peritonitis it is common to review patient's bag exchange technique. Any corrections that need to be made should be done so with tact, and the patient should not be made to feel either guilty or responsible otherwise next time they may not 'own up', and present only when severe peritonitis is well established.

Eosinophilic peritonitis: This is seen most frequently after catheter insertion and is thought to be due to an allergic reaction to the introduction of air at the time the catheter is inserted, or to the catheter itself. Treatment is not indicated, although some authorities recommend using corticosteroids for pain (Tzamaloukas and Fox 1999, p 561). Eosinophilic peritonitis usually presents with cloudy effluent and no other signs or symptoms. Although it is rarely associated with fungal or parasitic infections appropriate antibiotic therapy should be commenced in such cases (Leehey et al. 2001, p 377).

Eosinophilic peritonitis should not be confused with 'culture negative' peritonitis. Culture negative peritonitis is the term used when symptoms of peritonitis are present but no organisms are grown on culture. In these cases It is usual to commence broad spectrum antibiotics. If there is no clinical improvement after five days both cell count and culture are repeated. If the effluent remains culture negative unusual pathogens should be considered and/or catheter removal.

If peritonitis reoccurs within a short period, usually defined as four weeks, after apparent resolution of the infection and is due to the same organism, treatment may have been inadequate, organisms may have colonised the catheter, tunnel infection may be present, or, more seriously, there may be a peritoneal abscess. This is often termed 'relapsing peritonitis' and can lead to removal of the catheter.

Exit site and tunnel infection

Tzamaloukas and Fox (1999, p 571) suggest that exit site and tunnel infections should be discussed together because it is not always possible to distinguish clearly between the two. These infections are not as common as peritonitis, but unlike the reduction in peritonitis rates attributed to the flush before fill technique, the incidence of both tunnel and exit site infections has remained stable over recent years.

Tunnel infection does not respond well to antibiotic treatment and often requires temporary removal of the catheter (Wild 1998, p 305). The poor response is primarily due to the difficulty accessing pathogens in areas lined with epithelium that are, therefore, relatively isolated from the blood supply that transports antibiotics.

4.2   Noninfective complications

Short term

Catheter malfunction: This is a frequent complication of peritoneal dialysis and accounts for considerable morbidity, additional treatment costs and less frequently, to catheter loss.

Diaz-Buxo (1998, p 256) divides catheter malfunction into three groups:

1. Intraluminal obstruction resulting from fibrin plugs, blood clots or fungus balls.

2. Extraluminal, which result from omental wrapping, obstruction from adhesions and catheter kinking.

3. Catheter migration.

Catheter migration, which probably goes undetected in many cases, is often responsible for one way obstruction—either slow inflow or poor drainage. Migration can occur 'into the lesser sac of the peritoneal cavity or into compartments defined by viscera, the abdominal or pelvic walls, and adhesions' (Diaz-Buxo 1998, p 256). Pain associated with inflow in the latter instances is caused by distension of the cavity walls.

Removal of an intraluminal obstruction should first be attempted by compression of the dialysis fluid pac during inflow or by flushing the catheter with 0·9% normal saline either with, or without, heparin. If unsuccessful, allowing a heparin solution to 'dwell' in the catheter prior to aspiration or by a similar procedure using urokinase can be tried (Diaz-Buxo 1998, p 256). Recently, intraluminal brushing similar to that used with percutaneous haemodialysis catheters has met with some success (Tranter 2000).

Poor flow associated with omental wrapping may respond to an enema designed to stimulate peristalsis or to physical activity. If this fails, catheter manipulation using a variety of techniques may be required. Such techniques involve using a semiflexible wire and fluoroscopic control, the intraluminal insertion of a Fogarty catheter and laparoscopic or surgical repositioning. Catheter replacement is the last resort (Diaz-Buxo 1998, p 256).

Genital oedema: This complication only affects a small number of patients and there are two ways it can occur. The first is where dialysate tracks from the catheter incision site along a soft tissue plane. The second is where dialysate leaks through a patent processus vaginalus into either the scrotum or the labia (Bargmann 2001, p 402). In men, scrotal swelling can be associated with penile oedema (Leehey et al. 1994, p 365). Treatment usually involves bed rest and low volume exchanges. Persistent oedema may require temporary cessation of treatment and surgical repair if a patent processus vaginalus is present.

Hydrothorax: This problem is usually seen early after treatment commences, but in some cases it may not occur for several years. It is more common in women than men and right sided effusions are more common than left sided ones (Churchill 1996, p 613). The effusion is due to peritoneal dialysate leaking into the thoracic cavity through a defect that is often congenital in the diaphragm (Kaupke and Vaziri 1994, p 599). Treatment consists of stopping peritoneal dialysis if the leak is severe enough to cause respiratory distress and transfer to haemodialysis either permanently, or temporarily, while surgical repair is undertaken. The incidence of hydrothorax in children is estimated to be between 7% and 10% (Bunchman 2000, p 646).

Peritoneal fluid leaks: These occur when closure of the peritoneal cavity is incomplete and dialysate leakage is evident either onto the abdominal dressing, or into the tissue adjacent to the abdominal incision. Treatment usually requires a return to the 'break in' procedure. Occasionally the patient may need to return to theatre to ensure that the peritoneal membrane has been appropriately sealed.

Long term

Malnutrition: While peritoneal dialysis corrects, or at least minimises, the nutritional defects associated with end stage renal failure, the treatment itself is associated with specific nutritional problems as mentioned in Chapter 3. As well as those mentioned in there, the 'continuous supply of glucose and lactate provides an energy load that may induce or worsen hyperglycemia, hyperinsulinemia, or hypertriglyceridemia' (Churchill 1996, p 613).

The increased caloric load associated with glucose absorption contributes to weight gain usually plateaus after the first twelve to eighteen months of treatment (Churchill 1996, p 613). Weight gain can be associated with noncompliance with the dialysis prescription when young women recognise the association between weight gain and glucose absorption (personal observation).

Hernia: Hernias can occur through the abdominal incision made to place the catheter, a pre-existing defect in the abdominal wall or through the site of a previous surgical incision. They are due, primarily, to the increase in intra-abdominal pressure that results from the presence of two to three litres of fluid in the peritoneal cavity. For this reason hernias occur less frequently in the CCPD population than the CAPD population. Most hernias are asymptomatic and do not require treatment. However if they cause intestinal obstruction the symptoms can be severe. Schools of thought differ as to whether hernias should be repaired when they are symptomatic or as soon as they become apparent (Churchill 1996, p 613, Leehey 1994, p 364). As a general rule, small hernias should be routinely repaired because they are at the greatest risk of strangulation (Bargmann 2001, p 400).

Sclerosing encapsulating peritonitis: This rare condition, for which there is no satisfactory treatment, and which is associated with a very high mortality rate, is characterised by weight loss, abdominal pain, nausea and/or vomiting, and signs and symptoms of bowel obstruction (Churchill 1996, p 614). If the abdomen is opened, the small intestine is often encapsulated in a thick, fibrous membrane that is thought to cause the bowel constriction (Leehey et.al. 1994, p 366). Possible causes are using acetate as a buffering agent, recurrent peritonitis, using chlorhexidine as a sterilising agent during bag exchanges and beta blocking drugs (Churchill 1996, p 614). The latter was especially true for practolol, which was also associated with pericardial sclerosis, and which has now been withdrawn from use.

The incidence of sclerosing encapsulating peritonitis has diminished with the reduction in use of acetate in the dialysate and chlorhexidine during pac exchanges. The reduction in symptomatology associated with transplantation is thought to be due to decreased lymphokine activity, which is, in turn, associated with immunosuppression. The decrease in lymphokine activity implicates the irritant effect of the dialysate and is thought to be a key component in the development of sclerosing encapsulating peritonitis (Korbet and Rodby 1999, p 201–203).

The recent introduction of the anticancer drug Tamoxifen, which has been used successfully to treat retroperitoneal fibrosis, a condition similar to peritoneal sclerosis, could be a treatment option (Korbet and Rodby 1999, p 201–203). Peritoneal dialysis patients who develop sclerosing encapsulating peritonitis and who do not succumb, frequently require transfer to haemodialysis, because the associated peritoneal sclerosis prevents satisfactory water and solute transfer (Leehey et al. 1994, p 366).

Back pain: Lumbar lordosis becomes a problem when it is exaggerated by the presence of two or three litres of fluid in the peritoneal cavity. The weight of the fluid places a strain on the lower back that is exacerbated by weak abdominal musculature that often occurs elderly people, and with pre-existing vertebral disease. Treatment options include using lower exchange volumes, which may involve more frequent exchanges, CCPD, or transfer to haemodialysis (Churchill 1996, p 614).

Ultrafiltration failure: is also referred to as membrane failure and has been described as ' [c]linical evidence of fluid overload which persists despite restrictions of intake and the use of three or more hypertonic exchanges per day' (Mactier 1991, p 57). Peritoneal dialysis patients can sustain injury to the peritoneal membrane directly through the components of the dialysate e.g. glucose strength, method of sterilisation, and pH, or indirectly due to the effect of inflammatory substances or the generation of free radicals that affect cell morphology, maturation and function (Schreiber 1997, p S20). Three different types of membrane failure have been identified:

1. Type 1 failure, which is due to high permeability of the peritoneal membrane and subsequent high rates of glucose absorption that result in the loss of the osmotic gradient required for fluid removal. Type 1 failure can be managed successfully with short daytime exchanges and a 'dry' overnight period, or with dialysate containing an iso-osmotic glucose polymer as the osmotic agent.

2. Type 2 failure is due to loss of peritoneal surface area, which can occur with recurrent peritonitis. Patients with this problem usually require transfer to haemodialysis or intermittent, but regular, isolated ultrafiltration.

3. Type 3 failure is associated with excessive absorption of the dialysate by the lymphatic system.

(Coles and Williams, 1994, p S 14).

The diagnosis of type 1 failure is not difficult because the PET will classify the patient as a 'high transporter'. With type 2 failures the PET will classify the patient as a 'slow transporter', but a high dialysate glucose level does not result in the expected high UF rate. Type 3 failure should be suspected when a patient with normal solute transport has an unacceptably low UF rate (Oreopoulos and Rao 2001, pp 367–368).

Cuff extrusion: This term is used when the superficial cuff protrudes through, or is visible at, the exit site. The condition is seen when:

1. The cuff is located too close to the exit site during initial placement.

2. Exit site infection causes tissue retraction during healing.

3. The deep cuff becomes separated from the abdominal musculature, pushing the entire catheter outward. If this occurs the catheter requires replacement. In the first two cases, careful removal of the superficial cuff should be attempted.

4.3 Contraindications to commencing or continuing therapy

Overview

There are few absolute contraindications to the commencement of peritoneal dialysis as a renal replacement therapy. Those that do exist relate to severe reduction of the peritoneal surface area or to very low rates of water and solute transport. As discussed elsewhere in this chapter, the patient's cognitive, affective, and psychomotor skills are a primary consideration because a great deal of commitment and self-care is required. However, even patients with severe physical limitations can be helped to perform bag exchanges safely with the assistance of a variety of devices. Patients with a marked reduction in cognition can still undertake peritoneal dialysis with help, if they can be relied on to leave the connections alone and not pull dressings apart.

Relative contraindications

As listed by Churchill (1996, p 614), the relative contraindications to commencing peritoneal dialysis are:

1. **Obesity**, especially if it is severe, because it will result in a thick layer of adipose tissue that makes catheter implantation difficult and predisposes the system to leakage difficulties. The absorption of glucose causes additional weight gain and compounds the weight gain problems already discussed.

2. The presence of an **enterostomy,** although not proven to increase the likelihood of infection, is usually a strong argument against using peritoneal dialysis.

3. Patients with severe **obstructive pulmonary disease** are believed to be likely to develop breathing difficulties if peritoneal dialysis is commenced. This is due to the presence of two or more litres of fluid in the peritoneal cavity and the pressure it puts on the diaphragm, especially in the recumbent position.

4. There is concern about commencing peritoneal dialysis in patients with **intra-abdominal grafts** because of the possibility of graft. Although not proven, the presence of an intra-abdominal graft should be a consideration when selecting a renal replacement therapy.

5. **Diverticular disease** can predispose the patient to faecal peritonitis. Again, there is no proven relationship between the two, but as with the presence of an intra-abdominal graft, it should be considered when selecting treatment.

References

In text references

Bargman, J., 2001, 'Mechanical complications of dialysis' in *Handbook of Dialysis*, Daugirdas, J., Blake, P., Ing. T., (eds.), 3rd ed., Lippincott Williams and Wilkins, Philadelphia.

Bunchman. T., Maxvold, N., 2000, 'Complications of acute and chronic dialysis in children', in *Complications of Dialysis*, Lameire, N., Mehta, R., (eds.), Marcel Dekker, New York.

Churchill, D., 1996, 'Results and limitations of peritoneal dialysis', in *Replacement of Renal Function by Dialysis,* Jacobs, C., Kjellstrand, C., Koch, K., Winchester, F., (eds.), 4th ed, Kluwer Academic Publishers, Boston.

Diaz-Buxo, J., 1998, 'Management of peritoneal catheter malfunction', *Peritoneal Dialysis International*, vol.18, no. 3, pp 256–259.

Coles, G., Williams, J., 1994, 'The management of ultrafiltration failure in peritoneal dialysis', *Kidney International*, vol. 46, Suppl. 48, pp S 14–S 17.

Kaupke, C., Vaziri, N., 1994, 'Special problems pertaining to various organ systems: lungs and pleura', in *Handbook of Dialysis*, Daugirdas, J., Ing., T., (eds.), 2nd ed., Little Brown, Boston.

Kean, F., Bailie, G., Boeschoten, E., Gokal, R., Golper, T., Holmes, C., Kawaguchi, Y., Piraino, B., Riella, M., Vas, S., 2000, 'ISPD Guidelines/Recommendations: Adult peritoneal dialysis-related peritonitis treatment recommendations: 2000 update', *Peritoneal Dialysis International,* vol. 20 pp 396–411.

Korbet, S., Rodby, R., 1999, 'Causes, diagnosis, and treatment of peritoneal membrane failure' in *Principles and Practice of Dialysis,* Henrich, W. (ed), 2nd ed., William and Wilkins, Maryland.

Leehey, D., Gandhi, V., Daugirdas, J., 2001, 'Peritonitis and exit site infection', in *Handbook of Dialysis*, Daugirdas, J., Blake, P., Ing., T., (eds.), 3rd ed., Lippincott Williams and Wilkins, Philadelphia.

Leehey, D., Gandhi, V., Daugirdas, J., 1994, 'Peritonitis and exit site infection', in *Handbook of Dialysis*, Daugirdas, J., Ing., T., (eds.), 2nd ed., Little Brown, Boston.

Mactier, R., 1991, 'Investigation and management of ultrafiltration failure', *Advances in Peritoneal Dialysis*, vol. 7, pp57–62.

Oreopolous, D., Rao, P., 2001, 'Assessing peritoneal ultrafiltration, solute transport and volume status' in *Handbook of Dialysis,* Daugirdas, J., Blake, P., Ing, T., (eds.), 3rd ed., Lippincott Williams and Wilkins, Philadelphia.

Schreiber, M., 1997, 'Membrane viability in the long term peritoneal dialysis patient', *Peritoneal Dialysis International*, vol. 17, Suppl. 3, pp S19–S24.

Tranter, S., 2000, "What can you do with brush?' paper presented at the19th Annual Peritoneal Dialysis Conference, Melbourne, Australia.

Tzamaloukas, A., Fox, L., 1999, 'Infections in patients on continuous ambulatory peritoneal dialysis' in *Principles and Practice of Dialysis,* Henrich, W. (ed), 2nd ed., William and Wilkins, Maryland.

Wild, J., 1998, 'Peritoneal dialysis' in *Renal Nursing* (appendix), Smith, T., (ed.), 2nd ed., Bailliere Tindall, Sydney.

Recommended reading

Brunier, G., 1995, 'Peritonitis in patients on peritoneal dialysis: a review of pathophysiology and treatment, *ANNA Journal*, vol.22, no. 6, pp 575–584.

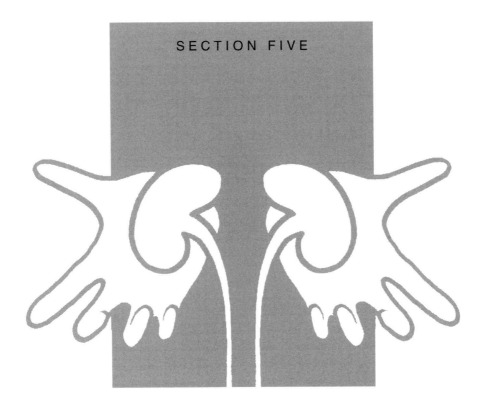

SECTION FIVE

The history of transplantation

Introduction

Many nephrologists consider a successful renal transplant to be the best available form of renal replacement therapy. Many patients have achieved this goal and the transplanted kidney functioned well for many years. For others, the transplant option was fraught with difficulties. For some it was fatal. For still others, a transplant remains elusive and the years of waiting cause considerable depression and a loss of hope.

Transplantation should be viewed as part of an integrated approach to care along with haemodialysis and peritoneal dialysis. It is a treatment, not a cure. This following brief review of the history of transplantation introduces the complexities and dilemmas that surround all organ transplants.

1.1   Overview of development

The first attempts

Although the concept of transplanting organs from one person to another dates back to Greek mythology, the first real consideration occurred in 1597 when the surgeon Gaspare Tagliacozzi was asked to transplant the nose of a slave onto the face of a nobleman whose own had been destroyed by syphilis (Fine 1984, p3). The request was refused because the surgeon recognised what he referred to as 'the singular character of the individual'; by which he meant the immunological reaction that occurs when the body recognises a foreign substance.

The first partially successful experimental organ transplant occurred in 1902 when Emmerich Ullmann transplanted the kidney of a dog from its normal anatomical position to vessels in the dog's neck and achieved some flow of urine (Hamilton 2001, p1). In the same year, Ullmann attempted, unsuccessfully, to graft a pig kidney into the elbow of a uraemic woman (Fine 1984, p 3). Many more experiments followed, including attempts to use animal kidneys in humans. Although these early experiments showed that transplants were technically possible few methods were available to study renal function. For this reason, and because the cause of rejection was not known, interest began to fade.

It was revived again in 1936 when a Russian surgeon, Voronoy, attempted to treat acute renal failure by transplanting a human kidney onto the recipient's thigh, a procedure he had attempted six times by 1949 (Allen and Chapman 1994, p2). All six attempts were unsuccessful, probably because the significance of prolonged warm ischaemic time was not recognised, and the importance of matching the blood groups of donor and recipient was not fully understood. Progress continued, and in 1946 a Boston group achieved renal function three days after transplanting a cadaveric kidney into the arm of a person with acute renal failure. The person recovered, and it is possible that the limited contribution made by the transplanted kidney assisted their recovery (Hamilton 2001, p 4).

True success did not occur until 1954 when a kidney was successfully transplanted from one identical twin to his brother. The transplanted kidney continued to function without immunosuppression for eight years, until the primary disease recurred and resulted in chronic renal failure for the recipient.

Immunosuppression

In 1906 Paul Ehrlich noted that when a mouse tumour was transplanted into a rat it grew for approximately eight days and then regressed (Fine 1984, p1). From this observation, Ehrlich concluded that each species of animal produced a substance that was needed for growth and concluded that the mouse tumour died because the rat could not provide the substance for tissue growth derived from a different species. The concept of immunity in transplant rejection was proposed in 1912 by James Murphy, who suggested that a 'small lymphocyte was … involved in tissue rejection' (Fine 1984, p 3). In 1943 Medawar described 'accelerated rejection' as rejection that occurred after repeated transplantation from the same donor. The accelerated rejection theory was followed by the concept of 'immunological tolerance' when Billingham, Brent and Medawar showed, that if fetal mice or chicken embryos were inoculated with donor tissue, transplantation of tissue from the same donor did not cause rejection after birth or hatching.

A successful kidney transplant in 1954 prompted attempts to suppress the immune system. The first occurred in 1959 when Hamburger used total body radiation to prevent rejection (Allen and Chapman 1994, p2). This form of immunosuppression blocked DNA synthesis in lymphocytes and their precursors, preventing cell replication (Kirkwood and Lewis 1983, p 80). However, total body radiation is a non specific form of immunosuppression that caused unacceptably high rates of mortality due to overwhelming infection, and it was soon abandoned.

Calne noted the immunosuppressive qualities of azathioprine (a 6-mercaptopurine analogue) in 1961 and those of corticosteroids in 1962. The first indication that renal transplantation could be a viable treatment for end stage renal failure occurred in 1962 when corticosteroids were combined with azathioprine to treat allograft rejection. At this stage, graft survival was about 50% for one year (Allen and Chapman 1994, p 4). However, the combination was not entirely successful, and the search for new and improved drugs continued. In 1967 antilymphocyte serum was introduced. Its use was based on the assumption that, if lymphocytes were responsible for rejection, one way to control them, but still leave other cells intact, might be to develop an antibody to the lymphocyte. This was achieved by injecting T lymphocytes into a horse after the horse's immune system had recognised the injected cells as foreign and raised antibodies against them. These antibodies could be purified and injected into the patient experiencing a rejection episode (Kirkwood and Lewis 1983, p82). The antilymphocyte serum method of immunosuppression also posed problems because serum is a protein and the patient could have a severe hypersensitivity reaction when their immune system recognised the horse serum as foreign. The first clinical use of cyclosporine occurred in 1978, followed by monoclonal antibodies, antibodies directed towards a specific target cell, in 1981. This introduced a new era in immunosuppression that places the emphasis on increased specificity.

Related milestones

Other major advances include the introduction of 'machine hypothermic perfusion' that enabled kidneys to be stored for up to 72 hours, in 1967. In 1968, criteria for brain death were developed and implemented by an Ad Hoc Committee of Harvard Medical School. The first prospective histocompatibility locus antigen matching of cadaver kidneys took place in Melbourne, Australia, in 1968, and cold storage of kidneys for 24 hours (Allen and Chapman 1994, p 3).

1.2 Terminology

Common terms and their meaning

Some of the frequently used terms relating to the type of transplant being undertaken are:

1. **Autograft:** tissue that is grafted back to the donor.

2. **Isograft:** a graft between syngeneic persons i.e. identical twins.

3. **Allograft:** grafting of tissue between members of the same species but of differing genetic makeup, previously referred to as a homograft.

4. **Xenograft:** grafting of tissue between species. It is also known as a heterograft.

The location of a transplant is referred to as either:

1. **Ipsilateral:** located on the *same* side of the recipient as it was in the donor i.e. left donor kidney placed in left side of recipient.

2. **Contralateral:** located on the *opposite* side of the recipient, as it was in the donor i.e. right donor kidney placed in left side of recipient.

3. **Heterotopic:** located in a position other than that which is anatomically normal. Transplanted kidneys are located in the right or left iliac fossa.

4. **Orthotopic:** located in the usual anatomical position (Roitt 1998, p 353).

References

In text references

Allen, R., Chapman, J., 1994, *A Manual of Renal Transplantation*, Edward Arnold, Melbourne.

Fine, R., 1984, 'Historical perspective of the treatment of ESRD in children', in *End Stage Renal Disease in Children*, Fine, R., Gruskin, A., (eds.), W. B. Saunders Company, Philadelphia.

Hamilton, D., 2001, 'Kidney transplantation: a history', in *Kidney Transplantation*, Morris, P., (ed.), 5th ed., Saunders, Sydney.

Kirkwood, E., Lewis, C., 1983, *Understanding Medical Immunology*, Wiley and Sons, Brisbane.

Roitt, I., 1998, *Essential Immunology*, 9th ed., Mosby, Sydney.

Recommended reading

Murray, J., Merrill, J., Harrison, J., 1958, 'Kidney transplant between seven pairs of identical twins', *Annals of Surgery*, no. 148, p343.

Terasaki, P., 1991, *History of Transplantation: thirty-five recollections,* UCLA Tissue Typing Laboratory, Los Angeles.

Recipient selection and preparation

Introduction

Although transplantation is accepted as the best available therapy for people with end stage renal failure, it is unfortunate that not all patients are suitable candidates. Despite the many advances that have occurred over recent years, the secrets of tissue typing have not been fully unravelled. This means that many patients wait for extended periods of time before being offered a transplant. For those who do have a transplant, nonspecific immunosuppression and tissue incompatibility can result in rejection. Technical mishaps can cause the transplant to become necrotic and require removal. Despite these difficulties, transplantation is a viable option and optimum preparation affords the best opportunity for success, despite the uncertainties.

2.1 General issues

Education

The educational preparation of potential transplant recipients is as important as the physical and emotional preparation. Many centres offer transplant education days as part of the preparation and ongoing care provided for their patients. Potential recipients and their families should be given the opportunity to discuss the available treatment options with all members of the health care team and then to go home and discuss the options in private and return with further questions and requests for clarification as often as necessary. Many centres also provide the opportunity for potential recipients to discuss the issues with patients who have already had a successful or unsuccessful transplant. Videos and books should be available and should supplement open and honest explanation of the possible risks as well as the potential benefits of transplantation.

Age is usually not a major consideration unless the person is very old, very young, or has a disease process that places them in a high risk category. If the risk of morbidity or mortality is increased for any reason, the risks should be explained to the patient and they should be encouraged to realistically compare these risks with the disadvantages of ongoing dialysis.

General medical and physical evaluation

The general examination should include:

1. A complete history and physical examination. Special attention should be paid to the presence of symptoms of cardiovascular, respiratory and gastrointestinal disease, a history of smoking and its subsequent diseases, prior malignancy, chronic infection and drug or alcohol use.

2. Serum biochemistry.

3. Full Blood Examination (FBE), coagulation profile and blood type.

4. Serological examination to determine Hepatitis A, B, C, and Human Immunodeficiency Virus (HIV) status, cytomegalovirus (CMV) titres, and the presence of sexually transmitted diseases and herpes simplex virus (HSV).

5. Chest X-ray.

6. Electrocardiogram,

7. Papanicolaou smear for women.

Thorough urological evaluation of all patients should be undertaken and ideally the lower urinary tract should be 'sterile, continent and compliant' prior to surgery (Kendrick 2001, p 134). Nephrectomy may be required for patients with severe reflux, polycystic kidneys that are extremely large, infected or causing pain or bleeding, when infected kidney stones are present and when heavy proteinuria or intractable hypertension is present. Although ureteric implantation into a diverted urinary tract is possible, for example, some congenital or acquired abnormalities of the lower urinary tract, implantation into the native bladder is preferred (Miller 1991, p 6, Kendrick 2001, p 134).

Further elective investigation should be undertaken if the general examination suggests any underlying pathology. Tissue typing and cytotoxic antibody status should be determined and will be discussed separately.

Psychiatric evaluation

Considerable controversy surrounds transplantation as a treatment option for patients with psychiatric or cognitive disorders. Most transplant units consider people with severe mental retardation who do not have a long life expectancy and who do not have an excellent social support system to be unsuitable for transplantation (Kendrick 2001, p 132, Murphy 2001, pp 365–379). Those who do have reasonable life expectancy and good support systems usually do as well as the general transplant population (Kendrick 2001, p 132). Patients who use either drugs of addiction or alcohol are also not considered to be suitable candidates for transplantation unless they successfully complete a treatment program (Kendrick 2001, p 132).

Psychiatric disorders exclude people in two principal areas:

1. Many patients are unreliable with respect to the self-administration of immunosuppressive drugs and there is considerable social and emotional drain on those people who form a part of their usual support systems.

2. Optimum graft survival is currently achieved using a regimen that includes long term corticosteroids. The potential to induce or exacerbate psychotic episodes is amongst the known side effects of this drug (Murphy 2001, p 365).

In addition to these factors, most other immunosuppressive drugs are associated with either central or peripheral neurotoxicity, a factor that places all patients at increased risk of developing a number of psychiatric symptoms (Murphy 2001, p 365).

Consideration should also be given to the cause of the patient's primary renal disease. Systemic diseases that have a known association with the central nervous system, particularly diabetes mellitus, hypertension, and systemic lupus erythematosus, can increase the risk of psychiatric symptoms when immunosuppressive therapy is commenced (Murphy 2001, pp 365-366).

Coexisting disease

Continuing improvement in intraoperative and postoperative care and the discovery of cyclosporine as an effective immunosuppressant has resulted in a relaxation of the criteria for transplantation used in earlier years. This has meant that many patients are now accepted for transplantation despite the existence of disease processes that would previously have excluded them. They were excluded because of the greater risk of death that was associated with their coexisting disease (Briggs 1994, p 43). From earlier reading, you will recall that few renal patients have disease affecting only their kidneys. Most, if not all, have multisystem disease that requires careful assessment and treatment if possible, prior to accepting them for transplantation.

Cardiac disease is the major cause of death in renal transplant recipients (Kendrick 2001, p139-140) and should be carefully evaluated prior to surgery. The presence of cardiac valve pathology may require prophylactic antibiotics, and ischaemic heart disease may require reversal with either coronary angioplasty or coronary artery bypass grafting (Allen and Chapman 1994, pp 13-14). Severe lung disease places the patient at increased risk of both infection and ventilator dependence post transplant.

Pulmonary function tests should be considered to determine whether transplantation is an appropriate option. Chronic respiratory diseases are considered to be contraindications for transplantation by some centres, others recommend treatment followed by a six to twelve month disease-free period before the transplant takes place. The two most problematic diseases are tuberculosis and bronchiectasis. Once tuberculosis has been effectively treated, the disease-free period should be followed with prophylactic antibiotics when immunosuppression is commenced. The presence of bronchiectasis requires individual assessment. If the disease is severe and recurrent, but limited to one area, lobectomy might be considered, but severe and recurrent generalised disease usually places the patient at too great a risk of overwhelming infection once immunosuppression commences (Allen and Chapman 1994, p 13, Kendrick 2000, p 141).

Active gastrointestinal disease is a contraindication to transplantation until it has been successfully treated. A past history of gastric or duodenal ulceration is no longer a contraindication because low dose steroid immunusuppression regimens and H2 receptor-blocking drugs has greatly reduced the risk of activating or perforating the ulcer. These complications were previously associated with high dose steroid therapy. Other gastrointestinal diseases that can be activated post transplant are pancreatitis, associated with the use of cortisone and azathioprine and cholecystitis that may be difficult to diagnose and treat post transplant (Kendrick 2000, p 14).

Primary renal disease

If there is a possibility that the patient's primary renal disease could recur in the transplanted kidney their educational preparation should include discussion about such a possibility. While is it not unknown for a second renal lesion to appear *de novo* in a transplanted kidney, or for the recipient to develop a systemic disease that leads to renal damage, it is uncommon. It is more common for renal impairment to occur when the original renal disease is of a type known to recur in transplanted kidneys. The most frequent of these are:

1. Glomerulonephritis, with mesangiocapillary type 11 (95%), mesangiocapillary type 1 (20–30%), IgA nephropathy (50%), Henoch-Schonlein purpura (80%), and focal and segmental glomerulosclerosis (30%) being the most common (Morris 1994, p 44). Goodpastures syndrome is almost certain to recur and destroy the transplanted kidney if transplantation is not postponed for one year after circulating antiglomerular basement antibodies are no longer detectable (Allen and Chapman 1994, p 9).

2. Haemolytic Uraemic Syndrome (HUS): Transplantation should be delayed for one year after treatment of the active disease to reduce the chance of it recurring (Al-Akash and Ettenger 2001, p341). HUS has been reported to occur in up to 50% of transplanted kidneys (Miller 1991, p 6). Relapse appears to be highest when a kidney from a living related donor is used (Kendrick 2001, p 138). Recurrence has been linked to the use of cyclosporine, antithymocyte globulin and tacrolimus (Al-Akash and Ettenger 2001, p341).

3. Alport's syndrome (10%), where the glomerular basement membrane lacks the 'glomerular antigen'. After transplantation, and therefore first time exposure to glomerular antigen, patients can develop classic antiglomerular basement membrane disease. They do poorly, despite aggressive treatment similar to that used for the primary disease. Because Alport's syndrome is an inherited disorder, potential living related donors should be carefully screened to exclude asymptomatic disease (Kendrick 2001, pp 136–137).

4. Hyperoxaluria type 1 has a high rate of recurrence (33%) when renal transplant is undertaken alone. It recurs because the inborn error of metabolism that caused the initial renal failure is not affected by transplantation. It has been suggested that transplanting both kidney and liver could be an acceptable solution because both the metabolic disorder and renal failure could be solved simultaneously (Allen and Chapman 1994, p 10). Recurrence in hyperoxaluria type 11 is not as common if surgical correction of the intestinal defect is undertaken prior to transplantation (Kendrick 2001, p 138).

The above discussion is only relevant to commonly recurring diseases. For a complete review of disease recurrence, especially when the primary disease is the result of a systemic disorder refer to specialist texts.

Recipient perceptions and expectations

Transplantation is considered to be the best available treatment for end stage renal failure and is the ultimate goal of many patients. However, even those awaiting a transplant experience anxieties that they are often unwilling or unable to share. Murray and Conrad (1999) found, that while most potential recipients felt receiving a transplant would allow them to 'feel normal again', they had a number of concerns. These included fears that the transplant would fail, that they would suffer episodes of rejection, that there could be a prolonged wait to see whether the transplant would function and for how long, and the amount of medication that was required to prevent rejection. Many of the study participants felt that it was 'extremely hard to talk to their family members' about transplantation and would only discuss it if asked directly.

Most participants, (80%), attempted to avoid the subject altogether while the majority, (70%), only discussed transplant-related issues with a social worker or a nurse. When the source of the donor kidney was discussed, participants preferred to receive their transplant from either a cadaver or a living *unrelated* donor. There was very strong opposition to receiving a kidney from a family member, primarily due to the concern that the donor could later suffer renal disease and require dialysis.

2.2 Contraindications

Relative contraindications

The presence and the severity of coexisting disease impacts strongly on the outcome of transplantation and is a major factor in the decision whether transplantation is the best option for a given patient. As well as the considerations already mentioned, relative contraindications to transplantation include:

1. **Obesity:** Excessive abdominal fat can increase the technical difficulties associated with the operative procedure. Generalised obesity increases the likelihood of postoperative complications (Franklin 1998, p 388).

2. **Past history of malignancy:** Most texts discourage transplantation unless the patient has been disease-free for at least two years, for two reasons:

a)   immunosuppression can accelerate disease progression and encourage the development of metastases (Franklin 1998, p 388).

b)   it is not considered reasonable for a person with limited life expectancy undergo transplantation (Kendrick 2001, p 130).

Exceptions to the two-year wait include *in situ* lesions of the uterine cervix and basal cell carcinoma (BCC) of the skin where no waiting time is required. Routine cytology screening is recommended if uterine cancer is present. In situ lesions in melanoma, the breast, and colorectal area may not require a waiting period. A five-year wait is recommended if carcinomas of the breast and malignant melanoma have progressed beyond the in situ stage, (Kendrick 2001, p 131). These suggestions are only a guide to appropriate treatment. The type of tumour and its natural history determines individual cases and oncology consultation is recommended.

3.   **Noncompliance:** Patients who have a history of noncompliance are generally considered unsuitable as they are at high risk of organ loss if immunosuppressant drugs are not taken as required (Kendrick 2001, p 130). Because there is a degree of subjectivity in such a label, objective criteria such as attendance at outpatient appointments, ceasing substance abuse and seeking medical or psychiatric consultation when requested to do so, should be used as objective measuring criteria (Rothberg 2001, p 389).

4.   **Chronic infection:** If infective lesions are treatable with antibiotics or surgery, transplantation can be undertaken. Recurrent urinary tract infection may require unilateral or bilateral nephrectomy and patients undertaking peritoneal dialysis should be free of peritonitis for approximately six weeks (Kendrick 2001, p 130, 134, 142).

Absolute contraindications

As can be deduced from the preceding discussion, there are few absolute contraindications to transplantation. Recent malignancy and untreatable chronic infection, pulmonary and cardiovascular diseases are among the few that remain with modern management methods. Even excluding patients infected with the HIV is being reconsidered with the advent of new antiviral regimens that prolong patient survival (Kendrick 2001, p 131).

2.3 Matching the donor and recipient

Preamble

The function of the immune system is to distinguish between 'self' (cells that should be present) and 'non-self' (cells that should not be present). When cells that should be present are recognised, 'tolerance' is exhibited and the cells are free to grow and multiply in accordance with their genetic program. When foreign cells (non-self) are recognised, the immune system generates a complex set of responses that are designed to destroy the foreign cells and ensure the survival of 'self'. The purpose of this response is to prevent foreign organisms (virus, bacteria etc.), or 'altered self' (tumour cells) from multiplying and ultimately destroying the organism. The same response causes rejection of a transplanted organ. The recipient's immune system recognises the cells of the transplanted organ as 'foreign', and proceeds to destroy it.

The process of destruction commences when structures present on the foreign tissue (antigens) are recognised as not being present on self-cells ('host'). T lymphocytes (responsible for 'cell mediated immunity') and B lymphocytes (responsible for antibody production) multiply and facilitate the destruction of the foreign cells. T lymphocytes become activated to a form that is able to attach directly to foreign cells and cause this destruction ('killer' or cytotoxic T cells), while B cells provide antibody that binds to foreign cells, recruiting chemical mediators (complement) to assist with their destruction. Macrophages assist T cells to recognise a foreign antigen. With monocytes and neutrophils they are responsible for the phagocytosis that removes cellular debris once foreign tissue has been destroyed.

Histocompatibility antigens

Histocompatibility antigens are glycoproteins present on the surface of all nucleated body cells. They are often referred to as human leucocyte antigens (HLA) because they were first identified on the cell membrane of human white blood cells (leucocytes). The genes that encode (produce) these glycoproteins are called 'histocompatibility genes'. They are located on the short arm of chromosome No. 6, and are found in an area known as the 'major histocompatibility complex' (MHC). The histocompatibility antigens produced by the MHC are primarily responsible for transplant rejection when the recipient's immune system recognises the foreign antigens on donor tissue as being different, it assumes this foreign tissue to be a potential invader, and proceeds to destroy it.

There are four histocompatibility antigens: HLA A, HLA B and HLA C (the class 1 antigens) and HLA D (the class 11 antigen group). One set of these four, known as a haplotype, are inherited 'en block' from each parent giving each child's cells eight histocompatibility antigens on their cells surface membranes. Because all eight are present, they are described as 'codominant' (Hutchinson 1998, p 354).

Each HLA antigen has multiple 'alleles'. An allele is a normal variant that can be present at any gene site. A gene site is called a 'locus'. This means that the locus for HLA A will normally produce many alleles, for example 1, 2, and 3. Therefore, an individual can have a tissue type for the 'A' locus of HLA A_1, HLA A_2, HLA A $_3$, or HLA A_4 (etc.). The same applies to the other histocompatibility antigens.

Tissue typing refers to testing that identifies the eight alleles on an individual's cell membrane. Remember that because one set of four comes from each parent, every child will have two pairs of each of the four alleles. Following is an example of tissue typing for a mythical 'Ms. P':

$$A_2 \ A_{27}, \ B_{12} \ B_{17}, \ C_5 \ C_{16}, \ D_{12} \ D_{27}$$

The object of tissue typing is to match, as closely as possible, the HLA antigens of the recipient with those of the donor. Where mismatches occur, as they invariably do (with the exception of identical twins), immunosuppression is achieved with specific drugs that block the immune response and prevent destruction of the donor tissue.

Cross match

Specific cross matching between the potential recipient and the donor takes place immediately prior to transplantation. When donor lymphocytes are mixed with serum from the recipient the donor lymphocytes act as target cells for the recipient's serum (Katznelson et. al. 2001, p 51). If the donor's cells are destroyed, the result is referred to as a positive cross match. This means that the potential recipient has pre-existing 'anti-donor HLA antibodies' and any attempt at transplantation would be followed by hyperacute rejection. The types of rejection are discussed in Chapter 5.

These preformed antibodies come from three sources:

1. Pregnancy, which exposes the mother to foreign paternal HLA antigen through fetal blood.

2. Previous blood transfusion that exposed the recipient to HLA antigens on the blood donor's white cells.

3. Prior transplantation that exposed the recipient to foreign HLA antigens on the donor organ.

Cytotoxic antibodies

This test is similar to cross matching, but is not specific for a given donor. Serum is collected from potential recipients on a monthly basis and is exposed to a random panel of donor serum of known HLA specificity. This 'random panel' is supposed to represent the various HLA specificities common to the general population (Wingard 1990, p 289). If the serum of a potential recipient reacts with (destroys) the lymphocytes of 30 of the 60 donor sera to which it is exposed the potential recipient is said to have a cytotoxic antibody count of 50%. This means, that if a donor becomes available, and the recipient is considered suitable on the basis of HLA matching, the degree of mismatch (even though it is between only one of the eight alleles that *do not* match) will result in a 50% chance of hyperacute rejection.

The high chance of rejection occurs because the recipient's immune system was exposed to the offending antigen previously and has B and T memory cells already primed to respond should it appear again. Because the nonspecific cytotoxic antibody count is a guide only, the specific cross match will provide a definitive answer. However, there is often not time for a specific cross match to be performed, except in the case of living organ donation, therefore the monthly cytotoxic antibody count gives an indication of the degree of probability that the recipient will either accept, or reject, the donor organ.

Highly sensitised patients

Highly sensitised patients is a term applied to patients who have preformed anti HLA antibodies to a large percentage of known HLA antigens. These patients have an 80–90% cytotoxic antibody count, and who, because of the likelihood that they will have a positive cross match to the majority of HLA antigens on donor organs, are the least likely to receive a transplant. They have probably already received more than one transplant, and may have children to more than one partner.

Pretransplant preparation includes attempting to reduce their cytotoxic antibody count by:

1. Plasma exchange, where circulating antibodies are removed along with the discarded plasma.

2. Plasmapheresis, where separated plasma is passed through a filter that adsorbs HLA antibodies.

3. Immunoadsorption, where anti HLA antibodies are adsorbed directly onto a specifically designed adsorbent column (Wingard 1990, pp 190-191).

Treatment with immunoglobulin and cyclophosphamide has also been advocated to reduce the number of cytotoxic antibodies. To date none of these treatments has been widely accepted (Kendrick 2001, p 143).

The role of blood transfusion

In the 1960's when the role of the HLA was first recognised, it was assumed that people who had received a blood transfusion prior to transplantation would experience poorer graft survival compared with patients who had not. However, in 1972 it was noted that this was not the case. In fact, graft survival seemed longest in those patients who had received a pretransplant transfusion (Allen and Chapman 1994, p 16). By the 1980's it was accepted that nonspecific, not from a designated donor, pretransplant blood transfusion appeared to enhance graft survival. Acceptance was based on the assumption that exposing potential recipients to the foreign antigens in donated blood would induce 'immune tolerance' and enhance graft survival. In the early 1990's, immunologists again queried the 'pretransfusion effect'. It became less popular and was reserved for those patients who were considered to be at the least risk of developing cytotoxic antibodies (Allen and Chapman 1994, p 16).

Donor-specific transfusion refers to blood transfusions from a living donor known to a potential recipient. The intention is to induce immune tolerance specific to the intended donor. While donor-specific transfusions have been attempted in the past, they lost popularity with the advent of newer and more specific forms of immunosuppression. Some recent studies indicate a possible resurgence of this form of preparation, especially in children (see Chapter 4, Paediatric Renal Failure).

Immune modulation has also been successfully attempted be infusing donor-specific bone marrow where the precise mechanism of action is unknown, but is assumed to be similar to that achieved with donor-specific transfusion (Danovitch 2001, p 99).

References

In text references

Al-Akash, S., Ettenger, R., 2001, 'Kidney transplantation in children', in, *Handbook of Kidney Transplantation*, Danovitch, G., (ed.), 3rd ed., Lippincott, Williams and Wilkins, Sydney.

Allen, R., Chapman, J., 1994, *A Manual of Renal Transplantation*, Edward Arnold, Melbourne.

Briggs, J., 1994, 'The recipient of a renal transplant', in *Kidney Transplantation*, Morris, P., (ed.), 3rd ed., Saunders, Sydney.

Danovitch, G., 2001, ' Immunosuppressive medications and protocols for kidney transplantation', in), *Handbook of Kidney Transplantation*, Danovitch, G., (ed.), 3rd ed., Lippincott, Williams and Wilkins, Sydney.

Franklin, P., 1998, ' Renal transplantation', in *Renal Nursing*, Smith, T., (ed.), 2nd ed., Bailliere Tindall, Sydney.

Hutchinson, I., 1998, 'Transplant and rejection', in *Immunology*, Roitt, I., Brostoff, J., Male, D., (eds.), 5th ed., Mosby, Sydney.

Katznelson, S., Takemoto, S., Cecka, J., 2001, 'Histocompatibility testing, cross matching, and allocation of cadaveric kidney transplants', in *Handbook of Kidney Transplantation*, Danovitch, G., (ed), 3rd ed., Lippincott, Williams and Wilkins, Sydney.

Kendrick, E., 2001, 'Evaluation of the transplant recipient', in *Handbook of Kidney Transplantation*, Danovitch, G., (ed), 3rd ed., Lippincott, Williams and Wilkins, Sydney.

Miller, S., 1991, 'Medical evaluation and recipient selection', in *The Handbook of Transplant Management*, Makowka, L., (ed.), Landes, Austin.

Murphy, K., 2001, 'Psychiatric aspects of kidney transplantation', in *Handbook of Kidney Transplantation*, Danovitch, G., (ed), 3rd ed., Lippincott, Williams and Wilkins, Sydney.

Murray, L., Conrad, N., 1999, 'Perceptions of kidney transplant by persons with end stage renal disease', *ANNA Journal*, vol. 26, no. 5, pp 479–483, 500.

Rothberg, L., 2001, 'Ethical and legal issues in kidney transplantation', in *Handbook of Kidney Transplantation*, Danovitch, G., (ed), 3rd ed., Lippincott, Williams and Wilkins, Sydney.

Wingard, R, 1990, 'Immunadsorption: a novel treatment for sensitised kidney transplant candidates', *ANNA Journal*, vol. 17, no. 4, pp 288–292,328.

Recommended reading

Conrad, N., Murray, L., 1999, 'The psychosocial meaning of living related kidney organ donation: recipient and donor perspectives- a literature review', *ANNA Journal*, vol. 26, no. 5, pp 485–490.

CHAPTER THREE

Donor selection and preparation

Introduction

The first successful organ donors were the living identical twins of people with end stage renal failure. Attempts at transplantation using the kidneys of people who died following a cardiac arrest resulted in varying degrees of success. There are patients still alive today who received their transplants from donors who died as a result of a cardiac arrest, but overall, the survival rates for both organs and recipients were much lower than those of recent years.

The development of criteria for the diagnosis of 'brain death' in 1968 and its subsequent legal acceptance as an alternative way to determine whether death has occurred meant that organ donation can now be undertaken while an intact circulation maintains oxygen to tissue. Interestingly, the current worldwide shortage of organ donors has led some medical staff to reconsider the use of organs from people whose heart has stopped beating (non beating heart donors). Strict criteria apply to using such donors and acceptance of the practice is still limited.

3.1 Cadaveric (beating heart) donation

The concept of death

Historically, death has been recognised when heart and lung functions cease. Modern resuscitative techniques and life support technology have made it possible to maintain the respiratory and heart function of a person who has lost brain function and for whom there is no hope of recovery. This resulted in the recognition that the accepted definitions of 'death' needed to be expanded (Terrill and Griffiths 1997).

Death is not a single event but a process that occurs over time. As a result, nerve cells in the brain stem and medulla that control vital functions such as blood pressure, cardiac output and respiration can continue to function for a limited period of time, despite the death of cells in the remainder of the brain. Such a situation can be difficult to recognise after major trauma and might not be suspected until full resuscitative technology has been commenced. When the remaining brain cells die (brain death), the body of the brain dead person can be maintained on ventilatory and other support for several hours before the heart and lung function ceases.

The technology used to support the living can continue to be employed once brain death occurs if organ donation is a possibility. If consent for organ retrieval has not been given, life support is withdrawn, and the body is prepared for cremation or internment (Terrill and Griffiths 1997).

Death entails the irreversible loss of those essential characteristics that are necessary to the existence of a living human being. It is recommended that the definition of death should be regarded as 'irreversible loss of the capacity for consciousness, combined with irreversible loss of the capacity to breathe'. The current position in law is that there is no statutory definition of death in the United Kingdom (A Code of Practice for the Diagnosis of Brain Stem Death, 1998).

It is important to remember that a person diagnosed as being brain dead will not exhibit the skin colour alterations, coolness and absence of breathing and heart beat that are traditionally associated with death. The heart of the brain dead person still beats, their chest moves giving the appearance of breathing and they are warm to the touch. Often there are no visible signs of trauma, and the confusion and shock experienced by the family can be profound. Extreme sensitivity is required by all those associated with the care of the patient, because without the signs normally associated with death, the family can have great difficulty accepting that death has really occurred (Terrill and Griffiths 1997).

Criteria for brain death

Brain death is said to have occurred when there is irreversible cessation of all function of the brain. The diagnosis is made when there is irreversible loss of consciousness together with loss of brain stem reflexes and respiratory function, or when there is irreversible loss of blood flow through the brain. The latter is usually used when facial injury prevents brain stem reflexes from being tested. The following criteria must be confirmed prior to testing brain stem reflexes:

1. Evidence of catastrophic cerebral injury consistent with a clinical diagnosis of brain death.

2. Exclusion of conditions that can compromise the clinical assessment of brain death such as acute metabolic or endocrine disorders.

3. Absence of evidence for drug or alcohol poisoning.

4. Core body temperature $\geq 32^{\circ}$ centigrade.

(Sullivan et al. 1999, p38).

Once these criteria are met, clinical examination to exclude brain stem reflexes for facial reaction, swallowing, cough, blink, eye movement and pupillary movement is conducted. More detail can be found in Sullivan et al. in the recommended reading at the end of the chapter. If these reflexes are absent, the patient's ability to breathe without mechanical assistance is assessed as per code of practice (A Code of Practice for the Diagnosis of Brain Stem Death, 1998). Before performing the final test of the person's ability to breathe without assistance, the patient should be ventilated with 100% oxygen for 10 minutes and the $PaCO_2$ should be allowed to rise to 45 mmHg before they are disconnected from the ventilator and should be allowed to increase to 50 mmHg during the test. Once the patient is disconnected from the ventilator, and throughout the test, 100% oxygen should be administered at a rate of six litres/min. through the endotracheal tube. For the next ten minutes, or until the $PaCO_2$ rises to 50 mmHg, the patient should be observed closely for any sign of respiratory effort. At the completion of the test the patient should be reconnected to the ventilator (Franklin 1998, p 399).

If organ donation is to occur, brain death should be confirmed by two doctors, one of whom is a registered specialist, and neither of whom are in any way involved with organ donation (A Code of Practice for the Diagnosis of Brain Stem Death, 1998).

Donor criteria

The potential kidney donor can be aged up to 75 years but must have no pre-existing renal disease of significance. Brain death must have been confirmed and the donor should be maintained on a ventilator to ensure an intact circulation. No major untreated sepsis should be present and the donor must have no history of malignancy other than a primary brain tumour or minor skin lesion.

A detailed personal and past medical history should be available, and particular attention must be given to behaviour that could place the patient in a high-risk category for HIV infection. The ICU admission history should include vital signs, all medication given, time of death, urine output and laboratory data. All potential donors with known HIV and known or suspected CJD are excluded. Two relative contraindications to solid organ donation, which may be considered in life-saving situations are Hepatitis B—HbsAg and Hepatitis C—HCV antibody (Guidance on the Microbiological Safety of Human Organs, Tissues and Cells Used in Transplantation, 2000).

Causes of brain death

The 1999 ANZDATA (p 88) for the cause of donor death in Australia and New Zealand for the previous year are shown in table 5.3.1 and reflect those reported in other developed countries.

Table 5.3.1: Causes of death of kidney donors in Australia and New Zealand in 1999 (ANZDATA 2000).

Cause	Australia	New Zealand
Cerebrovascular accident	88	24
Road trauma	37	8
Other trauma	18	4
Hypoxia/anoxia	13	3
Cerebral tumour	73	0
Other	5	0
TOTAL	**164**	**39**

Similar data available in the United Kingdom can be obtained from UK Transplant.

The use of organs from donors with a cerebral malignancy is restricted to patients with a primary tumor and has only recently been accepted because of the increasing disparity between the supply and demand for organs, and the low frequency of extracranial metastases from these tumors (Chui et al.1999, p 1266). In 1997, the Council of Europe, recommended guidelines for the use of organs from donors with primary cerebral malignancy and circulated a document based on the Cincinnati Transplant Tumor Registry. Entitled 'the International Consensus Document', it advised that 'organs from donors with high-grade malignant [primary brain tumors] should not be transplanted and that donors with [primary brain tumors] of low grade, should only be considered in special circumstance' (Chui et al. 1999, p 1266).

The request for donation

Organ donation offers the only positive outcome from what is often a devastating personal loss for some families. Whatever the family's decision, their response should be accepted graciously.

Ideally, the Organ Donor Co-ordinator should be informed whenever a potential donor becomes available prior to the diagnosis of brain death. They will approach the family in a quiet, private place *after* brain death is confirmed, and after a member of medical staff, preferably a senior person who has already met the family, tells them their family member has died. It may be appropriate to have a social worker or priest present, and it is often helpful to the family if the nurse caring for the deceased person is also present as this will allow them to ask questions as needed during the ensuing hours. The subject of organ donation should not be broached until the family has accepted that the patient has died.

Organ preservation

Care of the donor: The time of death shown on the death certificate is the time at which both doctors undertaking brain death testing confirm that irreversible loss of all brain function has occurred. If the deceased person is to become an organ donor the situation is 'time critical' as the patient cannot be stabilised for a prolonged period. Once death has occurred, the care of the deceased changes from cerebral resuscitation that would be employed if recovery was an option, to that which optimises oxygen delivery to the body, and ensures good organ and tissue perfusion (Scheinkestel et al. 1995, p 51). At the time of brain stem coning, herniation of the brain stem through the medulla oblongata, there is a marked increase in circulating catecholamines that cause vasoconstriction, with subsequent ventricular failure and pulmonary oedema (Scheinkestel et al. 1995, p 52). This is usually followed by progressive hypotension and hypoperfusion that is due to the cessation of brain stem vasomotor activity (Jonas and Oduro 1997, p 124).

Numerous endocrine alterations occur and include; failure to secrete antidiuretic hormone and the subsequent development of diabetes insipidus and the risk of dehydration and hypoperfusion, reduction in thyroid hormone levels leading to anaerobic metabolism and depleted cellular energy stores, and hyperglycaemia as insulin production fails (Jonas and Oduro 1997, pp 128–129). The impaired cellular energy is thought to contribute to organ dysfunction that occurs both pre and post transplant (Power and Van Heerden 1995, p 33).

The patient becomes poikilothermic due to the loss of thermoregulation and the body temperature eventually drops to the ambient temperature. As the temperature continues to drop myocardial depression and cardiac arrhythmias occur, tissue hypoxia develops from a left shift in the oxyhaemoglobin dissociation curve, renal function begins to decline and coagulopathies develop (Jonas and Oduro 1997, pp 129–130). Electrolyte abnormalities are common, and with the exception of sodium, which tends to be elevated), are lower than normal (Powner et al. 2000, p 91).

The alterations in general homeostasis seen in the organ donor can be the result of care that was provided earlier for the patient, the processes leading to hospitalisation or to brain death itself. Fluid replacement given to support blood pressure affects water, electrolyte and acid-base status, and fluids that are lost due to diabetes insipidus affect volume status, blood pressure, tissue perfusion and cardiac output. Constant monitoring of vital signs, and of biochemical and serological values are required and therapeutic intervention titrated against the results. The 'rule of 100's and 10's' is a good working guide. Systolic blood pressure should be kept above 100 mmHg, urine output should be above 100 ml/hr, arterial PO_2 should be above 10 kPa [75 mmHg] and CVP should be above 10 mmHg (Franklin 1998, p 403).

It is beyond the scope of this text to detail the specialist care that is required if the donor organs subsequently procured and transplanted are to be in optimum condition. The interested reader is referred to the references and recommended reading for the chapter.

Care of the organs: Operative details vary between units, but the principles of generous exposure, organ mobilisation and placement of cannulae for later perfusion and cooling are common to them all. If the patient is a multiorgan donor, the thoracic organs are removed first, followed by the liver and pancreas and finally by the kidneys. Ventilation is discontinued when the aorta is cross clamped, and organ perfusion and 'blood washout' commences at this time.

When the blood supply ceases at the time of cross clamping, the lack of oxygen to tissues causes cellular ischaemia. Cooling the organs by using both cooled perfusion fluid and packing in an ice slush reduces cellular metabolism and decreases the possibility of damage from 'warm ischaemic time—the time between suspension of the circulation and cooling of the organs (Franklin 1998, p 408). Because ventilation and blood supply are maintained until the perfusion equipment is in place, warm ischaemic time can now be kept to a minimum of a few minutes. Cold ischaemic time generally refers to the time between the beginning of cooling during organ retrieval and rewarming that occurs when are completed. Some units refer to 'cold ischaemic time' as the period of cold storage or machine perfusion, and to 'rewarm time' as the time between removal from cold storage and the release of the vascular clamps (Gritsch et al. 2001, p 127). The perfusion solution is similar in content to intracellular fluid and helps to stabilise the cell membrane and reduce intracellular swelling.

Most cadaver donors receive large doses of corticosteroids in an attempt to deplete circulating lymphocytes (Gritsch et al. 2001, p 127). Mannitol can be given to promote diuresis as well as drugs to prevent clotting and maintain vascular tone. In Australia and the UK many centres will give methylprednisolone (1 gm) and broad-spectrum antibiotics at the start of the procedure. Heparin is given prior to placement of the perfusion cannulae and chlorpromazine is given immediately prior to circulatory arrest to assist renal blood flow following implantation. However, this process may vary from centre to centre and is dependent on local policy.

After the organs are removed and examined to exclude surgical trauma and anatomical abnormality, the kidneys are either flushed with a preserving fluid and stored on ice at approximately 4° centigrade, or they are maintained by a perfusion device that pumps cold colloid solution continuously through the renal artery. The kidneys are maintained in a sterile environment and transported on ice to the recipient hospital. At the time of organ retrieval a specimen of splenic and lymph node tissue is also removed for retrospective cross matching between donor and recipient(s).

Organ allocation

In Australia, organs are allocated and distributed in accordance with data supplied by a computer-based system known as the National Kidney Matching Scheme and staff from the tissue laboratory and donor co-ordinators, are responsible for operating the system in each state (Australian National Organ Allocations Protocol 1999, p 28). Kidneys are allocated in accordance with blood group and 'a computer calculated score based primarily on the degree of matching at the HLA B and DR loci, and secondarily on such factors as A locus matching, waiting time, and degree of sensitisation' (National Guidelines for Organ and Tissue Donation 1999, p 46) The most closely matched recipients with a negative cross match are eligible for transplantation. In the United Kingdom, UK Transplant manage the allocation of all human organs similar to that of Australia.

3.2 Living Donors

The related donor

The first successful organ transplants were from the identical twins of people with end stage renal failure. Because these siblings were genetically identical, no immunosuppression was required. As knowledge of the immune system increased and methods of suppressing it were developed, the use of living related donors was extended to include first-degree relatives—parents, children or siblings, who were matched for at least one haplotype. The advent of more selective immunosuppressive therapies and the continuing lack of donor organs has encouraged the use of relatives who do not share a common haplotype, and even those who are biologically unrelated.

The fact that organs transplanted from donors who are not matched at either haplotype do as well as, or better than, six antigen matched cadaveric transplants, suggests that the excellent condition of the kidney at the time of transplantation has a major effect on graft survival (Gritsch 2001, pp 111–112). In Australia during 1999, 37% of all transplants performed were from living donors, of these 26% were from unrelated donors, with 77% being from spouses (ANZDATA 2000, p75). In England living related kidney donors increased by 7%—286 in 2000 to 307 in 2001 (UK Transplant Statistics, 2001).

The unrelated donor

Most transplant units now accept what are commonly known as 'emotionally related donors'. This term is applied to people such as spouses, close friends, and stepchildren who are not biologically related to the recipient, but who wish to donate a kidney Some centres accept 'altruistic donors', people who have no relationship with the recipient, but who feel that they are in a position to help another human being to achieve optimum health. Within the United Kingdom, ULTRA (The Unrelated Live Transplant Regulatory Authority) approve all transplant operations involving a living donor who is not a close blood relative of the recipient.

The potential benefits for the recipient of receiving a kidney from a living donor need to be weighed against the possible harms that may occur to the donor. Most transplant units have rigorous acceptance criteria for live donor transplants that includes evaluation of the physical and emotional health of the donor and their reasons for wishing to donate.

Potential benefits for the recipient include improved short and long term results, more consistent early functioning, avoidance of prolonged waiting time, convenient timing of the surgery and less aggressive immunosuppression. Potential harms for the donor include psychological stress, the risks associated with invasive physical evaluation and surgery, long term morbidity (mild hypertension and proteinuria), and renal impairment due to unrecognised disease (Gritsch 2001, p 112).

Some texts claim emotional benefits for the donor, and while this may be true for successful transplants, rejection of the kidney, especially shortly after surgery, or severe illness in the recipient can have profound and long lasting effects on the donor. Similarly, the recipient can experience guilt or anger if the kidney is rejected, or if they are unwell following surgery. The emotional consequences of live organ donation are extremely complex and specialist nephrology and psychiatric texts are available that address this subject in detail.

Buying and selling of organs for transplantation is an issue that also involves living unrelated donors and is surrounded by controversy. The first recorded instance of organ purchase was in 1971 when a potential kidney recipient introduced his 'cousin' as a living related donor. It transpired that the donor was actually an unrelated paid stranger (Rothenberg 2001, p 383). This case occurred in India where buying and selling kidneys is accepted practice and where advertisements for both purchase and sale are common. There is also evidence to suggest that wealthy people from other countries have travelled to India and other underdeveloped countries to purchase kidneys. The illicit nature of these practices means that care is often substandard and access to post transplant care, including immunosuppression, is lacking (Rothenberg 2001, p 384, Salahudeen et al., 1990 pp725–727).

Western nations have condemned these practices and Western doctors who participated in transplant procedures using purchased organs have been disciplined

(Rothenberg 2001, p 384). There are many arguments for, and against, buying and selling organs, most of which centre around the right of a person to do what they wish with their body and its parts, versus the exploitation of needy people in difficult financial or social circumstances.

A somewhat modified method of increasing donor supply is known as 'rewarded gifting'. Proponents of such a system suggest that the living organ donor, or the family of deceased organ donors, be rewarded with schemes that provide indirect financial assistance such as reduced health insurance fees, income tax rebates, or assistance with the costs associated with burial (Rothenberg 2001, p 384).

Live donor nephrectomy

Most kidneys are removed from living donors through a flank incision, although the use of laparoscopic surgery is becoming increasingly popular. After the kidney is removed it is placed on ice slush and flushed with heparinised preservation fluid. The recipient is transported to the operating suite a short time after the donor and prepared for surgery in an adjacent theatre. The recipient surgery is planned so that there is minimal cold ischaemic time, and after inspection of the donor kidney to exclude surgical trauma and previously unrecognised disease, it is taken to the adjacent theatre and placed into the recipient.

3.3 Other options

The cadaveric (non heart beating) donor

In an attempt to increase the number of organs available for transplantation, some units are currently considering the use of organs from deceased, non beating heart donors (Leishman and Varga 2000, p 77). Organs are procured from these donors in either a 'controlled' or an 'uncontrolled' setting. A controlled setting is one in which the family has decided to discontinue life support, and where cardiac arrest is expected to follow shortly after its discontinuation. Uncontrolled settings are those where cardiac arrest is not expected, and therefore where no provision for organ retrieval has been made. Donors in this category have been divided into four subsections based on the Maastricht Categories (Koostra 1995 p 2965). These are:

1. Dead on arrival.

2. Unsuccessful resuscitation.

3. Awaiting cardiac arrest.

4. Cardiac arrest while brain dead.

Because professional and community concerns around the use of non heart beating donors can reasonably be anticipated, it is imperative that guidelines based on sound legal and ethical principles underpin the retrieval policies of any unit considering the use of such donors.

References

In text references

ANZDATA Registry Report, 2000, 'Australia and New Zealand Dialysis and Transplant Registry, Adelaide, South Australia.

Australian National Organ Allocation Protocols, 1999, Overview of 1999 changes, TSANZ.

Australian and New Zealand Intensive Care Society, 1993. 'Guidelines on brain death and organ donation' a report to the ANZICS Working Party on Brain Death and Organ Donation.

Chui, A., Herbertt, K., Wang, L., Kyd, G., Hodgeman, G., Verran, D., DeLeon, C., Sheil, A., 1999, 'Risk of tumour transmission in transplantation from donors with primary brain tumours', *Transplant Proceedings*, vol. 31, pp 1266–1277.

DoH (1998), A Code of Practice for the Diagnosis of Brain Stem Death. Department of Health, London.

DoH (2000), Advisory Committee MSBT. *Guidance on the Microbiological Safety of Human Organs, Tissues and Cells Used in Transplantation*. Department of Health, London.

Franklin, P., 1998, 'Renal transplantation', in *Renal Nursing*, Smith, T., (ed.), 2nd ed., Bailliere Tindall, Sydney.

Gritsch, H., Rosenthal, J., Danovitch, G., 2001, 'Living and cadaveric organ donation', in *Handbook of Kidney Transplantation*, Danovitch, G., (ed) 3rd ed., Lippincott, Williams and Wilkins, Sydney.

Jonas, M., Oduro, A., 1997, 'Management of the multi-organ donor', in.), *The Multi-Organ Donor*, Higgins, R., Sanchez, J., Lorber, M., Baldwin, J., (eds.) Blackwell Science, Melbourne.

Koostra, G., 1995, 'Statement on non-heart beating donor programs', Transplant Proceedings, vol. 27, pp 2965–2970.

Leishman, R., Varga, C., 2000, 'Maximising liver transplantation from non-heart beating donors', *Progress in Transplantation*, vol. 10, no. 2, pp77–80.

National Guidelines for Organ and Tissue Donation, 1999, 'The role of tissue typing in transplantation, HLA typing, screening and cross-matching', Australasian Transplant Co-ordinators Association, Inc., Sydney.

National Operating Theatre Guidelines for Organ and Tissue Donation, 1999, 'Outline of operative procedures', Australasian Transplant Co-ordinators Association, Inc., Sydney.

Power, B., Van Heerden, P., 1995, 'The physiological changes associated with brain death-current concepts and implications for the treatment of the brain dead organ donor', *Anaesthesia and Intensive Care*, vol.23, no. 1, pp 26–36.

Powner, D., Kellum, J., Darby, J., 2000, 'Abnormalities of fluids, electrolytes, and metabolism of organ donors', *Progress in Transplantation*, vol. 10, no. 2, pp 88–94.

Rothenberg, L., 200, 'Ethical and legal issues in kidney transplantation' in *Handbook of Kidney transplantation,* in Danovitch, G., (ed), 3rd ed., Lippincott, Williams and Wilkins, Sydney.

Salahudeen, A., Woods, H., Pingle, A., Nur-El-Huda Suleyman, M., Shakuntala, K., Nandakumar, M., Yahya, T., Daar, A., 1990, 'High mortality rate among recipients of bought living unrelated kidneys', *The Lancet*, vol. 336, pp725–728.

Scheinkestel, C., Tuxen, D., Cooper, D., Butt, W., 1995, 'Medical management of the (potential) organ donor', *Anaesthesia and Intensive Care*, vol. 23, no. 1, pp 51–59.

Statement and Guidelines on Brain Death and Organ Donation, 1993, 'Statement and guidelines on the certification of brain death', Australian and New Zealand Intensive Care Society.

Sullivan, J., Seem, D., Chabalewski, F., 1999, 'Determining brain death', *Critical Care Nurse*, vol. 19, no. 2, pp 37–46.

Terrill, B., Griffiths, M., 1997, 'Discussion paper one: ethical and clinical implications of brain death', Patient Care Ethics Committee Newsletter, Austin and Repatriation Medical Centre, Melbourne.

www.doh.gov.uk/ultra

www.uktransplant.org

Recommended reading

Sullivan, J., Seem, D., Chabalewski, F., 1999, 'Determining brain death', *Critical Care Nurse*, vol. 19, no. 2, pp 37–46.

Pallis, C., 1995, 'Further thoughts on brainstem death', *Anaesthesia and Intensive Care*, vol. 23, no. 1, pp 20–23.

Truog, R., 1997, 'Is it time to abandon brain death?', Hastings Center Report, vol. 27, no. 1, pp 29–37.

Kerridge, I., Lowe, M., McPhee, J., Saul, P., Williams, D., 1999, 'Death, dying and donation: organ transplantation and the diagnosis of brain death', The Australian Institute of Health, Law and Ethics, Issues paper no.10, pp1–8.

CHAPTER FOUR

The perioperative period

Introduction

Only a quarter of renal transplant recipients have an uncomplicated course. Ideally, they would not have preformed antibodies to histocompatibility antigens (HLA), and would be free of medical problems other than end stage renal disease. The donor kidney would come from 'a two haplotype matched sibling or otherwise, a left sided, HLA compatible, cadaver kidney retrieved from a haemodynamically stable, young, beating heart donor at the recipient's own hospital' (Allen and Chapman 1994, p 110). The surgical procedure would follow shortly after the cadaver donor procedure and urine would start flowing within minutes of releasing the vascular clamps towards the conclusion of the recipient surgery. Maintenance immunosuppression would minimise episodes of acute rejection and side effects would be negligible.

So why is transplantation still viewed as a challenge?

> *A quarter of the recipients will have no primary … function, will require … temporary dialysis and expect a one year graft survival of 10 to 20% less than that achieved by patients who do have primary renal function. At least 60% … will have at least one episode of acute rejection …, and about 5% will have technical complications requiring … surgical intervention*

(Allen and Chapman 1994, p 111).

The success or failure of the transplantation process often rests with the attention to detail that occurs during the perioperative period.

4.1 The immediate preoperative period

From initial contact to hospital

Most potential transplant recipients carry a paging device so they can be contacted at any time or place should a suitable donor become available. If, for any reason, they are not contactable using a paging device, most will make alternative arrangements so that the possibility of receiving a transplant is not missed.

Patients report mixed feelings when they receive 'the telephone call'. Many report anticipation and excitement at the possibility of a life without dialysis, fear that the operative procedure might not go well or that the transplant will fail, and sadness that they were given this chance through the death of another human being. Some transplant units contact two patients and ask both of them to come to the hospital to be prepared as the eventual recipient. This is done so that in the event of a negative cross match between the donor and the first potential recipient the cold ischaemic time is not unnecessarily prolonged by the need to contact a second patient. Although medically efficient, this practice inevitably means that one person goes home without a transplant. The experience of 'being second in line' was explored in a study by Sloan and Gittings (1999), and is listed as recommended reading at the end of the chapter.

After preliminary questions about their immediate state of health and checking that there are no signs of infection or general illnesses, patients are asked to fast and come into the hospital where a routine nursing assessment and admission is completed. Urinalysis is performed with bacterial analysis if possible. Blood samples are taken for serum biochemical and serological analysis and the final cross matching. Skin, nose and throat swabs are taken to exclude infection and most units also swab the exit sites of peritoneal and subclavian catheters.

Preoperative dialysis may be required, especially if the patient is markedly volume expanded or hyperkalaemic. If haemodialysis is undertaken, minimal heparin should be used and, if peritoneal dialysis is used, the peritoneal cavity should be drained and the catheter capped after the final exchange. Immunosuppressive therapy is commenced prior to theatre if it is part of the transplant unit's policy.

The final surgical preparation and preoperative check list is the same as that used for any patient preparing for major surgery. If drugs for use during surgery are to accompany the patient to the theatre they should also be checked at this time.

4.2 The intraoperative period

Anaesthesia

Transplantation is usually treated as an emergency procedure because most patients have either eaten or received oral cyclosporine. The hyperemetic state often induced by uraemia and dialysis promotes increased secretion of gastric juices, peptic ulceration and gastric atony, resulting in the need for either 'rapid sequence induction of anaesthesia with preoxygenation and cricoid pressure or an awake intubation' (Freeman and Wels 1991, pp 153–154). Succinylcholine chloride as a muscle relaxant should be avoided during intubation due to its potassium elevating effects and the reduction in protein binding sites that occurs with uraemia means that lower doses of the chosen induction agent are usually required.

Maintenance anaesthesia is best achieved with an inhalation agent such as isoflurane and nitrous oxide because both of these agents are excreted via the lungs. Narcotics should be administered with care because prolonged depression of the central nervous and respiratory systems can occur (Freeman and Wels 1991, p154). Peripheral nerve stimulators should be used to monitor neuromuscular blockade. Although regional and spinal anaesthesia have both been used successfully during renal transplantation, it is more common to use general anaesthesia.

Transplantation technique

The most common approach is via an oblique incision from the symphysis pubis to the midline, 'curving in a lateral superior direction to the iliac crest' (Gritsch and Rosenthal 2001, p 147). The incision can be easily extended upwards towards the rib, or downwards to the flank, if necessary. There are three different approaches to the placement of the kidney:

1. The location is on the right side of the recipient, irrespective of the side of origin in the donor. This approach is chosen because of the ease of access to the iliac vein compared to left sided placement.

2. The location is contralateral to the kidney's position in the donor (a right donor kidney is placed in the left side of the recipient, and vice versa). This approach is preferred when the hypogastric artery is used for the arterial anastomosis. It also locates the renal pelvis anteriorly, facilitating access if ureteral repair is needed.

3. The location is ipsilateral to the position in the donor (a right sided donor kidney is placed in the right side of the recipient, and vice versa). This approach is chosen when the external iliac artery is to be used for the arterial anastomosis.

These placement choices refer to first transplants. Second transplants are usually placed on the side opposite to the first. If third or fourth transplants are undertaken, the choice of location depends on factors such as the presence of adhesions and the availability of vessels suitable for anastomosis (Gritsch and Rosenthal 2001, p 147).

The renal artery can be anastomosed to the external iliac artery (most frequently chosen in adults), the hypogastric artery, the common iliac artery, or the aorta in children. In cadaveric donation, a patch of aorta, a 'Carrel' patch is taken with the donor artery(s) attached and is anastomosed intact. This is not possible in living-related donation and the donor artery(s) are anastomosed directly to the recipient vessels. The donor renal vein is anastomosed to the recipient external iliac vein, or the vena cava in children.

The donor ureter is preferentially placed into the recipient bladder using a technique that prevents post transplant reflux. However, it can also be placed into the ipsilateral ureter, or a previously constructed ileal or colonic conduit. Some surgeons place an indwelling stent as an initial support for the ureteric anastomosis and remove it after approximately six weeks.

Drug and fluid management

Adequate perfusion is vital during the operative procedure, and the patient should be kept slightly volume expanded if cardiac status is stable, to allow the newly transplanted kidney to function properly. Prior to release of the vascular clamps up to 1 gm of methylprednisolone is given together with diuretics such as mannitol and frusemide. Verapamil can also be given directly into the renal artery but great care is required in patients taking beta blocking agents because complete heart block can occur. Verapamil is given to reduce capillary spasm and increase renal blood flow (Gritsch and Rosenthal 2001, p 150).

4.3   The immediate post operative period

Intensive care

It is not usual for patients to require intensive care, unless their condition prior to surgery was poor, or their intraoperative course was stormy. However, many prefer that the recipients of dual organs (heart/kidney, liver/kidney and pancreas/kidney) spend the first twenty four to forty eight hours after theatre in the intensive care, or specialist transplant unit setting. Apart from the immediate access to respiratory and cardiac support technology available in intensive care units, one-to-one nursing ensures that the recipient does not have to compete with the needs of other patients during this critical period.

The renal ward

The majority of patients return to a specialist setting, and the psychological advantages of a familiar staff and environment. Systemic or regional analgesia will be required and is often delivered by the patient in predetermined amounts. Care should be taken to ensure that the effects of intraoperative narcotic or neuromuscular blockade do not persist and cause hypoventilation. Hypertension and tachycardia are common, and should be treated with an antihypertensive agent after excluding pain, hypoxaemia, CO_2 retention, and clot retention in the bladder (Freeman and Wels 1991, p 156). Early postoperative bleeding should be expected in any patient who experiences a rapid decrease in haemocrit, and whose blood pressure does not respond to saline infusion (Amend et. al. 2001, p 168).

Most patients return from theatre with an indwelling urinary catheter to allow urine output to be measured precisely over very short periods of time, often less than one hour. They also have a drain tube(s) draining the perirenal bed, peripheral venous access for analgesia (often patient-controlled), blood taking and drug administration, central venous access that is also used for drug administration and estimation of central venous pressure. 'Aggressive' hydration is required in the immediate postoperative period, with central venous pressure usually kept at 10 cms H_2O [7.4 mm Hg] and up to 15 cms H_2O [11 mm Hg] if urine production is poor, and cardiac status is stable (Allen and Chapman 1994, p 114).

As with all perioperative management, individual patient physiology and unit protocols dictate the precise parameters. As a general principle, the less invasive the monitoring devices the better. Renal transplant recipients are immunosuppressed prior to surgery because of their illness, and more so after surgery due to immunosuppressive drugs required to reduce the possibility of rejecting the kidney. Catheters, drain tubes, and intravenous access should all be removed as soon as possible. Where possible, the patient should be received into a single room with private bathroom facilities. Reverse barrier nursing is no longer considered necessary by most units, but the prevention of cross infection remains paramount.

Three common patterns of graft function are usual. The kidney either functions well with good clearances of water and solute, functions adequately for water removal but solute clearance is inadequate, or there is a period of oliguria or anuria, usually requiring dialysis, prior to diuresis and normal function. Cardiac preload should be monitored and maintained within the guidelines for each unit. Dopamine and/or a diuretic may be administered if cardiac preload is adequate (Freeman and Wels 1991, p 157).

Immunosuppressive therapy is continued in accordance with the protocol of the individual unit. A discussion of the type, and dose, of the drugs used, their mode of action, and their side effects are beyond the scope of this text. As a brief summary, most protocols include the use of the calcineurin inhibitors (cyclosporine or tacrolimus) often commenced in the immediate preoperative period, steroids (prednisolone) usually commenced intraoperatively, adjunctive agents such as azathioprine or mycophenolate mofetil (antimetabolites), and calcium channel blockers (diltiazim and verapamil). The latter two drugs do not provide immunosuppression themselves, but potentiate the action of the calcineurin inhibitors and allow lower doses to be used while achieving the same degree of immunosupression (Danovitch 2001, pp 101-105). Antilymphocyte preparations (ATGAM and OKT$_3$), and the more recently developed chimeric monoclonal antibodies (basiliximab [Simulect] and daclizumab [Zenapax]), may also be included, but are not usually introduced as first line therapy.

References

In text references

Allen, R., Chapman, J., 1994, *A Manual of Renal Transplantation*, Edward Arnold, Melbourne.

Amend, W., Vincenti, F., Tomlanovich, S., 2001, 'The first two post-transplant months' in *Handbook of Kidney Transplantation*, Danovitch, G., (ed.), 3rd ed., Lippincott, Williams and Wilkins, Sydney.

Danovitch, G., 2001, ' Immunosuppressive medications and protocols for kidney transplantation', in *Handbook of Kidney Transplantation*, Danovitch, G., (ed.), 3rd ed., Lippincott, Williams and Wilkins, Sydney.

Freeman, J., Wels, J., 1991, 'Anaesthesia for organ transplantation', in *The Handbook of Transplant Management*, Makowka, L., (ed.), Landes, Austin.

Gritsch, H., Rosenthal, J., 2001, 'The transplantation operation and its surgical complications', in *Handbook of Kidney Transplantation*, Danovitch, G., (ed.), 3rd ed., Lippincott, Williams and Wilkins, Sydney.

Sloan, R., Gittings, J., 1999, 'Hearing the silence of patients who did not receive an anticipated organ transplant: "being second in line", *ANNA Journal*, vol.26, no. 1, pp 375–379, 448.

UK Transplant Activity (2001). Website: www.uktransplant.org.uk/statistics

Recommended reading

Danovitch, G., 2001, ' Immunosuppressive medications and protocols for kidney transplantation', in *Handbook of Kidney Transplantation*, Danovitch, G., (ed), 3rd ed., Lippincott, Williams and Wilkins, Sydney.

Complications of transplantation

Introduction

The success of the early postoperative period is largely dependent on the patient's state of health prior to surgery, especially cardiovascular and nutritional status, and to the effects of antirejection therapy on both the kidney and the patient. While these factors remain important throughout the life of the transplant, the most significant risk to long term patient survival stems from cardiovascular disease, malignancy and infection. Cardiovascular death can reflect the results of prolonged uraemia and the need for renal replacement therapy pretransplant. Malignancy and infection relate to the effects of long term immunosuppression. As knowledge of the immune system increases, hopefully these problems will decline.

5.1 Primary lack of function

As suggested by Allen and Chapman (1994, p 128), the situations outlined in this section refer to a lack of function that occurs during the first post transplant week, and which requires dialysis in a patient who was previously dialysis dependant. There is some obvious overlap between some of the conditions causing 'primary' dysfunction and 'early' dysfunction.

Hyperacute rejection

Hyperacute rejection occurs when the recipient has preformed antibodies to donor histocompatibility antigens. It is rarely seen now that results of the final lymphocyte cross match can be made available prior to transplantation. When hyperacute rejection does occur, it is often apparent immediately the vascular clamps are released and the donor kidney becomes swollen, flaccid, and develops a patchy blue discoloration instead of the expected even pink colour, accompanied by firm, pulsatile blood flow. There is no accepted treatment for hyperacute rejection and the kidney usually has to be removed. It can be removed prior to closure of the abdominal wound if the condition is recognised in the operating theatre. If it is not apparent until some hours after surgery additional surgery is necessary (Neumann 1997, p 521).

Limited success has been reported using plasma-exchange (Allen and Chapman 1994, p 141). Treatment using immunoadsorbent columns to remove preformed antibodies is said to be successful if it is undertaken *prior* to transplantation (Wingard 1990). Hyperacute rejection has also been described when the blood groups of donor and recipient are incompatible (Franklin 1998, p 429).

Accelerated rejection occurs, some one to four days after transplantation, and often follows apparently good initial function. The graft is tender and the patient febrile and urine output ceases abruptly. Although not due to preformed antibodies, and despite a negative cross match, accelerated rejection is thought to be due to previously sensitised B and T cells. Treatment is with high dose steroids, but is often unsuccessful (Allen and Chapman 1994, p 141).

Acute tubular necrosis

The majority of patients with nonfunctioning transplants received donor kidneys damaged by the ischaemia that follows imperfect preservation, prolonged warm or cold ischaemic time, donor hypotension, prolonged vascular anastomosis or recipient hypoperfusion (Allen and Chapman 1994, p 136). If urine output does not commence within a few hours of transplantation, despite adequate hydration, acute tubular necrosis (ATN) can be diagnosed with reasonable certainty. One of the management difficulties with a delay in graft function that persists for several days, is determining whether the cause is really due to ATN, in which case the immunosuppressive regime usually remains unchanged, to early rejection, in which case immunosuppressive therapy may be increased, or to the nephrotoxic side effects of some immunosuppressive agents in which case the dose would be decreased. Ultrasonography and renal biopsy best determine which of these three possibilities is the cause.

Vascular complications

Arterial occlusion, venous occlusion and graft rupture are the primary vascular causes for lack of early function. Arterial occlusion is uncommon, and unless recognised and treated during surgery, its effects are rarely reversible. The usual causes are hyperacute rejection, renal artery spasm, and malrotation of either of the vascular anastomoses (Allen and Chapman 1994, p 135). Venous thrombosis is also uncommon, and tends to be associated with rupture of the kidney. Graft salvage is possible if the situation is recognised early, and if normal venous return is established. This return to normal function usually follows a short period of ATN (Allen and Chapman 1994, p 154).

Graft rupture is the most rare of the vascular complications, but can be the most devastating, often placing the patient's life at risk. It was previously seen following ATN in non beating heart donors, and occurred typically along the convex border; a fact that prompted many surgeons to perform a prophylactic donor kidney capsulotomy at the time of transplantation. The most common cause of graft rupture since the use of beating heart donors is renal vein thrombosis, and as mentioned before, the kidney may be salvaged after successful renal vein thrombectomy.

5.2 Early dysfunction

Acute rejection

Acute rejection is by far the most common form of rejection. Although it can occur at any time, it occurs most frequent during the first three transplant months. It is usually the result of a cell-mediated response involving T cells and is treated with high dose steroids. Most patients respond to this treatment. Those who do not respond are treated with an antilymphocyte preparation such as OKT3 (Shapiro and Simmons 1991, pp177-178). Less frequently, acute rejection is antibody-mediated, resulting in a necrotising arteritis that responds poorly to treatment (Nast and Cohen 2001, pp 296–297).

Urinary complications

Urinary leaks typically become apparent within the first few postoperative days, or follow the onset of diuresis, if function has been delayed. They occur anywhere between the renal calyx and the bladder and can be due to either technical error, as with failure to obtain a watertight seal at the point of anastomosis, or to necrosis and sloughing of the ureter if the donor blood supply was compromised during retrieval (Gritsch and Rosenthal 2001, p 156). Leaks due to technical errors, and obstruction due to kinking or overly tight suturing are usually apparent earlier than those due to ureteral sloughing (Allen and Chapman 1994, p141). Kinks and obstruction can usually be reversed, but avascular necrosis of the transplanted urinary system, which can present as late as six months after the transplant may require nephrectomy.

Apparent primary or early nonfunction can be due to catheter blockage by a blood clot and should be excluded by bladder washout. Occasionally a large clot will require removal via cystoscopy.

Acute renal failure

Acute renal failure is usually reversible if the cause is recognised and treated early. It follows the same classification as that for the nontransplant recipient (Allen and Chapman 1994, p 152). Prerenal failure is a consequence of vascular volume depletion (hypo-perfusion, blood loss or septicaemia), cardiac failure, and either stenosis or occlusion of the renal artery. ATN follows either ischaemic damage during retrieval or preservation, and nephrotoxicity due to immunosuppressive, radiodiagnostic, or anti microbial agents. Postrenal failure occurs due to obstruction at any point along the collecting system. Management principles include the maintenance of adequate fluid volume, which depends on early recognition of volume deficits, prevention and treatment of infection, and avoiding nephrotoxic substances. The latter two principles are not always easy to adhere to because the aminoglycoside antimicrobial agents, and immunosuppressive drugs such as cyclosporine, are all nephrotoxic at higher doses.

5.3 Late dysfunction

Chronic rejection

Chronic rejection refers to the slow, progressive decline in function that is treatment resistant, and that follows tubular alterations consistent with ischaemic injury, which occur over a period of months to years (Neumann 1997, p 522, Allen and Chapman 1994, pp 170–171). In many ways, the course of chronic rejection parallels that of chronic renal failure and may not become clinically apparent until the glomerular filtration rate falls below 25% of normal (20–25 ml/min.). Renal function is progressively unable to support homeostasis and eventually dialysis is required for survival. Prevention of graft loss is not simple. At best it can be delayed by the rigorous treatment of acute rejection, prevention of arterial damage caused by occlusion and intimal thickening, and avoiding the damage caused by hypertension (Allen and Chapman 1994, pp 174).

Other causes for late dysfunction

Causes for late loss of function include the recurrence of primary renal disease, chronic cyclosporine toxicity requiring a reduction in dose and therefore incurring the risk of acute rejection, renal artery stenosis, stenosis of the transplant ureter, and transplant vesicoureteric reflux (Allen and Chapman 1994, pp 168–192).

5.4 Infection

Opportunistic Infection

The term 'opportunistic infection' is used to describe infection that occurs due to an organism normally present in either the body or the environment of the host that does not cause problems as long as the person's immune system is intact. Micro-organisms previously considered harmless to humans often become pathogenic with the advent of medical technologies that can sustain life in patients who would otherwise die (Pritchard 1989, p 36).

General principles

Vaccination, immunoglobulin, and antibiotics are the main prophylactic treatment used to prevent infection in immunosuppressed patients. Reverse barrier nursing is seldom used in modern transplant practice, but the principles for prevention of cross infection still apply and should be strictly adhered to. In parts of the world where tuberculosis remains endemic, prophylactic treatment with isoniazid is commenced at the same time as immunosuppression. Pneumocystis carinii, a protozoan infection known to cause life threatening pneumonia in immunosuppressed patients, is now able to be effectively eliminated with low dose co-trimoxazole during the first six post transplant months (Allen and Chapman 1994, pp 219–220). Antifungal agents in lozenge form are used routinely to prevent oral thrush and acyclovir is used prophylactically to reduce the likelihood of oral infection with the herpes simplex virus. Basic nursing care goes a long way towards preventing oral infections. Mouth rinses, gentle tooth brushing and the application of gels to inflamed or cracked mucous membranes are the mainstay of treatment (Campton 1991, p 40).

Opportunistic organisms

Opportunistic infection is possible with many organisms. Only those most commonly encountered are reviewed in this section.

Viral infection: Infection with the cytomegalovirus (CMV) is common during childhood and usually passes without causing major illness and leaves the child with antibodies to the disease. However, infection in the immunocompromised patient can be life threatening (Lott 1995, p 599). Four modes of presentation have been identified:

1. A recipient who has not been exposed to the virus as a child can develop primary disease from an infected donor kidney or from a blood transfusion with blood from an infected donor.

2. A recipient who was exposed to CMV as a child can have the disease process reactivated as a result of the immunosuppressive regimen that accompanies transplantation.

3. The CMV-positive patient can develop what is called CMV 'super-infection', which is infection that occurs during antimicrobial treatment for another condition, where the normal flora are altered and opportunistic organisms are favoured.

4. Reinfection with a strain of donor CMV different from that which caused the initial infection in the recipient to which the recipient demonstrates antibodies (Allen and Chapman 1994, p 221).

Both prevention and prophylaxis are attempted. Where possible, a seronegative donor is matched with a seronegative recipient. Where this is not possible, CMV immunoglobulin, or antiviral agents such as acyclovir or ganciclovir are usually be used (Lott 1995, p 601).

The presence of both Hepatitis B and C in the recipient impacts on the decision to transplant, patients who have evidence of either disease do less well in both the long and short term than those who do not. Liver biopsy for patients with either disease is recommended. Transplantation can go ahead if the disease is only minimal and it is recommended that antiviral drug therapy be used. Transplantation is not recommended for patients with evidence of active disease (Fabrizi and Martin 2001, pp 263–270). All donors are now screened for evidence of both diseases, and, with the dearth of donor organs, some units consider it reasonable to transplant kidneys from donors positive to either Hepatitis B or C into recipients who are also positive to either of these diseases, but the practice remains controversial (Neyhart 1995, p589). Other viruses that cause difficulties include the Epstein-Barr, herpes simplex and varicella zoster viruses. Transmission of papillomavirus and polyomaviruses also occurs, but is rare.

Bacterial infection: Gram-positive bacteria are a common cause of septicaemia, wound and line infection in the postoperative period, with methicillin-resistant staphylococcus aureus (MRSA) and clostridium difficile (causing diarrhoea) being frequent offenders. Gram-negative bacteria such as (Eschericia, Klebsiella, Proteus), Legionella pneumophilia, mycobacteria (tuberculosis) and psittacosis cause other infection.

Fungal infection: Although reported as occurring less frequently in renal transplant recipients than in recipients of other solid organ transplants, the mortality rate from fungal infection is high. Most infections are the result of either nosocomial or environmental organisms and include candida, aspergillus, zycomycosis and cryptococcus. Diagnosis is often difficult causing delayed treatment. Initial prophylaxis against candidiasis, as already mentioned, is common. Some patients are placed on long term prophylaxis if they are at risk of the less common and frequently fatal forms of fungal infection (Kubac et al. 2001, p 243–249).

5.5 Long term complications

Transplantation is a treatment, not a cure

This phrase should be remembered. Whilst successful transplantation provides many recipients with years of dialysis-free time, for most it does not last forever. The long term effects of continued immunosuppression are responsible for the majority of side effects, and for some patients they are the limiting factor in the life of their transplant.

Cardiovascular disease is a leading cause of death after transplantation. It tends to be associated with the degree of cardiac damage that was present prior to transplantation.

Diseases that are directly attributable to the effects of immunosuppression are:

1. Cataracts, which are associated with long term steroid use and occur in up to 40% of patients (Allen and Chapman 1994, p 248).

2. Ischaemic necrosis, particularly of the femoral head, is associated with long term steroid use. Leaks due to technical errors and obstruction due to kinking or over tight suturing are usually apparent earlier than those due to ureteral sloughing, which are not usually apparent until four or five days after the transplant (Allen and Chapman 1994 p 141). Kinks and obstruction can usually be reversed, but necrosis of the transplanted urinary system that can present as late as six months after the transplant may require nephrectomy.

3. Hepatic disease, which was not previously recognised as causing problems, has become apparent with the longer survival of patients using hepatotoxic drugs.

4. Malignancy, due to the presence of oncogenic viruses, and to the oncogenic effects of generalised long term immunosuppression is of particular concern. The common cancers are squamous cell carcinoma of the skin, vulva, and uterine cervix, lymphoproliferative disorders, Kaposi's sarcoma, and leukaemia, all of which are associated with the long term suppression of immunosurveillance, and which are as yet unavoidable in suppression of the immune response.

References

In text references

Allen, R., Chapman, J., 1994, *A Manual of Renal Transplantation*, Edward Arnold, Melbourne.

ANZDATA registry Report 2000. 'Australia and New Zealand Dialysis and Transplant Registry' Adelaide, South Australia.

Campton, C., 1991, 'Oral care for the renal transplant patient', *ANNA Journal*, vol. 18, no., 1, pp 39–41.

Fabrizi, F., Martin, P., 'Hepatitis in kidney transplantation', in *Handbook of Kidney Transplantation*, Danovitch, G., (ed.), 3rd ed., Lippincott, Williams and Wilkins, Sydney.

Franklin, P., 1998, 'Renal transplantation', in *Renal Nursing*, Smith, T., (ed.) 2nd ed., Bailliere Tindall, Sydney.

Gritsch, H., Rosenthal, J., 2001, 'The transplant operation and its surgical complications' in *Handbook of Kidney Transplantation, Danovitch*, G., (ed.) 3rd ed., Lippincott, Williams and Wilkins, Sydney.

Smith, T., (ed.), Kubak, B., Pegues, D., Holt, C., 2001, 'Infectious complications of kidney transplantation and their management, in *Handbook of Kidney Transplantation*, Danovitch, G., (ed), 3rd ed., Lippincott, Williams and Wilkins, Sydney.

Lott, S., 1995, 'Cytomegalovirus prophylaxis in kidney transplantation recipients', *ANNA Journal*, vol. 22, no. 6, pp 599–602.

Nast, C., Cohen, A., 2001, 'Pathology of kidney transplantation', in *Handbook of Kidney Transplantation*, Danovitch, G., (ed), 3rd ed., Lippincott, Williams and Wilkins, Sydney.

Neumann, M., 1997, 'Evaluation of the paediatric renal transplant recipient', *ANNA Journal*, vol. 25, no. 5, pp 515–523, 538.

Neyhart, C., 1995, 'Hepatitis C virus and its impact on transplantation' *ANNA Journal*, vol. 22, no. 6, pp 587–589.

Pritchard, R., 1989, 'The immunocompromised patient: new opportunities for fungi', *Today's Life Science,* September, pp 36–37, 39–41, 44–45.

Shapiro, R., Simmons, R., 1991, 'Kidney transplantation' in *The Handbook of Transplant Management*, Makowka, L., (ed.), Landes, Austin.

Wingard, R., 1990, 'Immunoadsorption: a novel treatment for sensitised kidney transplant candidates, *ANNA Journal*, vol. 17, no. 4, pp 288–292, 328.

Recommended reading

Schlatter, S., McNatt, G., 1995, 'Risk of community infections in transplant patients: a literature review', *ANNA Journal*, vol. 22, no. 6, pp 590–595, 630.

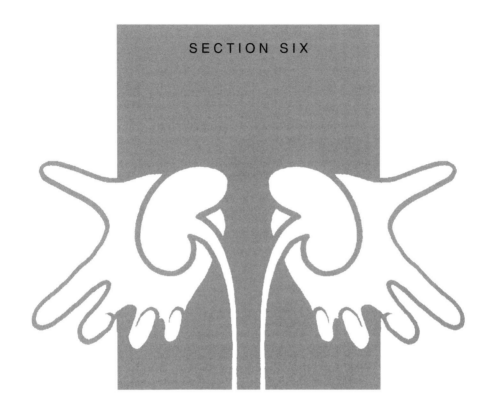

SECTION SIX

Renal function in the child

Introduction

The successful management of children with renal failure can only be achieved if the practitioner has a thorough understanding of the development of normal renal function and the alterations that occur to metabolic balance during childhood. The kidney in the newborn is immature, buffering capacity is reduced and the ability to conserve and excrete sodium is limited. Even when quite severe renal disease is present, serum biochemistry can be normal at birth because the mother maintains fetal homeostasis. When a severely affected infant is born, especially when multiple defects are present, the ethical and moral implications of attempting renal replacement therapy can be considerable. A thorough working knowledge of the expected prognosis is required prior to commencing treatment because the mortality rate for both acute and chronic renal failure in infants remains high.

1.1 The development of renal function

Development of renal function

The kidney begins to develop in the fifth week of intrauterine life and is not complete until between twelve and eighteen months after birth. Urine production commences at approximately ten weeks of intrauterine life and increases to about 28 ml/hour immediately prior to birth. Fetal urine is the major component of amniotic fluid and significant reduction in the amount of amniotic fluid (oligohydramnios) is usually associated with renal disease in the baby. Prior to birth, the fetus does not require intact renal function because the mother provides homeostasis. It is therefore possible for a child with bilateral renal agenesis (congenital absence of both kidneys) to survive for several days after birth (Roy 1994, p 411–412).

At birth, the kidney contains only 17% of its cellular components. Postnatal cell division is complete by six months and subsequent growth is due to increased cell size. Although nephron formation is completed prior to birth, the superficial cortical nephrons are not functionally mature (Donckerwolcke 1996, p 863) and the juxta medullary nephrons are responsible for the bulk of the glomerular filtrate. Glomerular filtration rate increases from the 28 ml/hr immediately prior to birth, to 48 ml/hr by one month and 80 ml/hr by six months (Donckerwolcke et. al. 1996, p 863). At birth, the serum creatinine reflects maternal renal function but falls progressively from day five to between 25 and 50 mmol where it remains until approximately two years of age. Thereafter it rises progressively to reflect adult levels by adolescence (Wolfish 1998, p97).

A discussion of congenital problems identifiable at birth is beyond the scope of this text but the interested reader is referred to specialist texts or those texts that contain specific sections on paediatric renal disease.

Metabolic and fluid balance

According to Donckerwolcke et al. (1996, p 864) 'the requirement for water is directly proportional to energy expenditure'. This means that, with a normal basal metabolic rate, the requirement for water is 1000 ml/m^2 of body surface area. Conditions such as hospitalisation increases these requirements by 50%, and each 1^0 increase in body temperature above 37^0 results in a further increase of 12%. In infants and to a lesser degree, older children, the ratio of surface area to weight is increased, resulting in a higher energy requirement and an increase in water requirements up to five times higher than that of an adult (Donckerwolcke et al. 1996, p 864). As a consequence, serious acid-base and electrolyte abnormalities can occur suddenly in an infant with renal failure.

The small child is unable to make known its need for fluid when volume is depleted, or when serum sodium is elevated.

1.2 Causes of renal failure

Acute renal failure

Acute renal failure is more common in the neonatal period than at any other time during childhood. This is because the low glomerular filtration rate, designed (presumably) to prevent over perfusion and subsequent salt and water loss, combined with the normal low glomerular blood flow and high renal vascular resistance, leaves minimal functional renal reserve (Donckerwolcke et al. 1996, p 864). This means that minor assaults to renal blood flow often result in an acute renal failure that would be compensated for by the mature kidney.

Acute renal failure in the newborn is frequently caused by prerenal conditions that respond well to normalising the blood volume. Treatment needs to be tailored to the cause and varies widely depending on the expected quality of life for the infant. For example, it would be inappropriate to commence treatment of an infant with bilateral renal agenesis because the condition is incompatible with life and the child could not be maintained on dialytic therapy until it achieved a suitable weight for transplantation. Causes of acute renal failure in the newborn are classified in the same way as in the adult, but the causes differ, and include:

1. **Prerenal:** Hypotension and hypovolaemia (septic shock, maternal antepartum haemorrhage and twin-to-twin transfusion), congestive cardiac failure, hypoxia, asphyxia and dehydration.

2. **Intrinsic renal:** Congenital abnormalities, acute tubular necrosis, vascular disease and inflammation (pyelonephritis, toxoplasmosis and syphilis).

3. **Postrenal:** Congenital abnormalities (posterior urethral valves, neurogenic bladder), and tumours (nephroblastoma and mesoblastic nephroma).

(Wolfish 1998, p 99).

The most common cause of ARF in the older child is haemolytic uraemic syndrome (Hicklin and De Sousa 1998, p 366). Injury, especially burns, and glomerulonephritis are two other common causes.

Chronic renal failure

Chronic renal failure (CRF) in childhood is associated with most of the problems seen in adults and many more. Although the use of rHuEPO and the introduction of growth hormone have improved the physical growth of children with renal disease, short stature and its accompanying psychosocial problems, especially with older children, remains an issue. Excellent dialysis and early transplantation are primary goals, as is the normalisation of pH and calcium/phosphate balance.

Psychosocial problems are often aggravated by the time required for treatment, which in turn prevents normal schooling and social activity. Frequent illness and hospitalisation are two other primary problems that require major adjustment by both the parents and the child.

Major moral and ethical dilemmas arise when determining whether dialysis should be offered to a child with end stage renal failure, and can only be decided on an individual basis. Questions relating to the possibility of independent existence and quality of life arise as they do for adults, especially in children with multiple handicaps.

Aetiology of end stage renal failure (major causes only)

1. Glomerulonephritis, commonly focal sclerosing and membranoproliferative types.

2. Congenital or hereditary disease.

3. Reflux nephropathy.

4. Obstructive nephropathy.

5. Collagen disease.

6. Interstitial nephritis.

7. Cystic disease.

8. Hypertension.

(Wassner1997, p 1317).

The use of renal replacement therapies to treat both acute and chronic renal failure during infancy and childhood are addressed in the following chapters.

References

In text references

Donckerwolcke, R., Broyer, M., Chantler, C., Rizzoni, G, 1996, 'Renal replacement therapy in children' in *Replacement of Renal Function by Dialysis,* Jacobs, C., Kjellstrand, C., Koch, K., (eds.), 4th ed., Kluwer Academic Publishers, Boston.

Hicklin, M., De Sousa, M., 1998, 'Children with renal problems', in *Renal Nursing*, Smith, T., (ed.), 2nd ed., Bailliere Tindall, Sydney.

Roy, L., 'Paediatric nephrology' in *Textbook of Renal Disease*, Whitworth, J., Lawrence, J., (eds.), 2nd ed., Churchill Livingstone, Melbourne.

Wassner, S., 1997, 'Conservative management of chronic renal insufficiency', in *Paediatric Nephrology*, Holliday, M., Martin-Barrett, T., Ellis, E., (eds.), 3rd ed., William and Wilkins, Sydney.

Wolfish, N., 1998, 'Paediatric nephrology', in *Caring for the renal patient*, Levine, D (ed.), 3rd ed., Saunders, Sydney.

Extracorporeal management

Introduction

Historically, paediatric haemodialysis refers to extracorporeal renal replacement therapy in children under the age of 15 years. The group classified as 'adolescent' is generally accepted as being between 15 and 19 years, and these patients with end stage renal failure often continue to dialyse in the paediatric units to which they have become accustomed. Many children have attained their adult height and weight as they near the end of adolescence, and can be dialysed using the same software and treatment parameters as adults.

However, neonates, infants and smaller children have special requirements. It is towards this group that this chapter is directed. Children undergoing extracorporeal renal replacement therapy require dialysers and blood lines that limit the amount of extracorporeal blood volume. Clearances for both metabolic waste products and body fluid need to be calculated according to body weight. Paediatric renal replacement therapy is a specialty of its own. This chapter seeks to introduce the reader to the principles involved in paediatric renal care and provide nurses who wish to practice in this area with an overview of the treatment parameters.

2.1 Haemodialysis

Beginning principles

Paediatric dialysis programs involve children of all ages from neonates who weigh less than 1kg, to mature adolescents. Caring for children with end stage renal failure, especially those for whom dialysis has been suggested, requires a nurse who possesses special skills from both the paediatric and dialysis arenas of nursing. There are many aspects of renal nursing that are similar in adults and children but it should be remembered that a child is not a small adult. The treatment requirements of a child include many unique differences in relation to:

1. renal replacement therapies

2. growth and development

3. psychosocial demands.

The optimal treatment of a child with end stage renal failure is a successful renal transplant (Allen and Chapman 1994, p 254) because this enables all the functions of the kidney to be replaced rather than the temporary restoration of fluid and electrolyte balance by haemodialysis. Unfortunately many children cannot receive a renal transplant before uraemic symptoms appear and require a period of time on some form of renal replacement therapy.

The goal of the paediatric renal dialysis program is to maximise the biochemical and psychosocial management of the child. One of the challenges in paediatric dialysis is to maintain a patent and infection-free vascular access that functions as a 'lifeline' for the child (Taylor 1996, p 486). Special consideration should be given to the choice of dialyser, lines and blood flow rate. These are selected according to the body surface area and weight of the child (Stewart et al. 1988, p 163–165).

The indications for dialysis in children with acute renal failure do not differ markedly for those in adults and include hyperkalaemia, intractable acidosis, symptomatic volume expansion, severe azotaemia, symptomatic uraemia, symptomatic metabolic disturbance, the requirement for fluid removal to optimise nutrition, transfusion or medication administration (Donckerwolcke et al. 1996, p 864). Dialysis is usually commenced when the glomerular filtration rate falls to 20ml/min/1.73m^2 in end stage renal disease.

The dialysis prescription

Technically, paediatric haemodialysis is similar to adult dialysis. The choice of dialyser, extracorporeal circuit volume and blood flow rates require specific consideration prior to commencing a child on haemodialysis According to Donckerwolcke et al. (1996, p 104–105) these considerations can be divided into two primary groups.

1.   The extracorporeal circuit

a)   Extracorporeal circuit volume

The amount of blood occupied by the bloodlines and dialyser should not exceed 10% of the patient's total blood volume. If the child is severely anaemic (Hb <5–6g/dL), the extracorporeal circuit volume should not exceed 7 %. The total blood volume can be determined by multiplying the child's weight by 80mls.

The circuit is usually primed using isotonic saline if the child is normovolaemic, or hypervolaemic but without symptoms (Gruskin et al. 1992, p 835). If the child is hypovolaemic and symptomatic, or has hypoalbuminaemia, standard conc albumin can be used to prime the lines and dialyser. Whole blood can also be used in anaemic children or when dialysis is necessary but appropriately downsized extracorporeal equipment is not available (Gruskin et al. 1992, p 835).

b)   Blood lines and dialysers

The surface area of the dialyser selected should not exceed the surface area of the child and is determined by patient's body surface area (BSA).

BSA can be determined by:

i)   multiplying the child's height by its weight

ii)   dividing the result by 3600

iii) determining the square root of the result.

Mathematically this is expressed as:

SA (m^2) = $\sqrt{}$ ([Ht in cms x Wt in kgs] ÷ 3600).

This conversion is known as the Mostellar equation (Kemp and McDowell 1997). The body surface area can also be determined by plotting the height and weight of the child on a nomogram (Kemp and McDowell 1997).

c)   Blood flow rate, which is determined by the child's size, blood volume, blood pressure and tolerance for dialysis

Blood flow rate (ml/min) should not exceed 2.5 x weight (kg) + 100.

2. Treatment parameters

a) Fluid replacement for hypotension should not exceed a maximum of 10ml/kg body weight and may be given in divided doses.

b) Ultrafiltration should not exceed 5% of total body weight for each dialysis session (Nevins and Mauer 1993, p 349–353). Neonates may be best managed when dialysed on scales accurate to +/- 5.0gms (Fine and Tejani 1994, p 561).

c) Clearance rates for urea should not exceed 3 mls/min/kg body weight, with 1.5 to 2 ml/min/kg body weight suggested for extremely uraemic children (Fine and Tejani 1994, p 561). If the calculation gives a blood flow rate slow enough to incur the risk of clotting, it may be more appropriate to reduce the hours of treatment and increase the blood flow rate, to ensure that overall clearance remains at the recommended level. Failure to do so predisposes the child to the possibility of disequilibrium.

The Gambro Mini Minor, Gambro Minor (parallel plate dialysers), and the Baxter CF 1211 L (a hollow fibre dialyser) are two types of dialysers suitable for use with infants and small children (Mendley et al. 2001, p 564). Hypothermia is a real concern when using isolated ultrafiltration on a child—loss of heat to the environment can occur quite quickly. Core body temperature should be monitored continuously (Fine and Tejani 1994, p 563).

2.2 Vascular access

Some differences between children and adults

It is well recognised that there are special problems in performing haemodialysis in the paediatric population. Adequate vascular access and proper choice of dialysers are particular problems. Paediatric nephrologists, surgeons and nephrology nurses all find it challenging to maintain reliable, long term vascular access in children.

The principles of obtaining and maintaining suitable vascular access in children do not differ markedly from those that apply to adults. Smaller catheters and cannulation needles with a shorter length and reduced bore size are available to assist with complying with these principles. Most of the difficulties occur because of the small size of the vessels involved.

Temporary vascular access: Central venous catheters can be percutaneously inserted into either the superior vena cava, recommended for short term dialysis or the inferior vena cava if the child is sedentary or confined to bed. The subclavian vein approach is preferred for easier catheter management and also the catheter can be anchored to the chest wall (Sherman 1993, p 345). These vessels are recommended because they are the only ones that provide adequate blood flow rates. In the former, the approach is usually via the subclavian or internal jugular vein, and in the latter it is usually via the femoral vein (Sherman 1993, p346). If the umbilical vein is still patent in neonates it can be used to access the inferior vena cava (Mendley et al. 2001, p 573).

Double lumen catheters are commonly used to achieve adequate dialysis. Sizes vary from 10Fr for infants and small children to 12Fr for bigger children and adolescents. The catheters are placed under general anaesthesia and radiological guidance to achieve safe and reliable catheter placement. Placement of the tip is critical to achieve adequate flows (Sherman 1993, p 346).

Permanent vascular access: Vascular access in infants and small children with end stage renal disease has to be created by a surgeon with 'great judgment and a refined technique' (Sherman 1993, p 346). The types of vascular access for children include an arteriovenous fistula, bridging an artery and vein with a synthetic graft, or a long term indwelling catheter especially for children weighing less than 25 kg. The small size of the blood vessels can make creating a natural arteriovenous fistula difficult. The patient's size, age and the expertise of the surgeon influence the choice between these two techniques.

Microsurgical techniques have been used very successfully to create arteriovenous fistulae using the distal radial artery and the cephalic vein. However, long maturation periods of 6–8 weeks are required for the fistula to develop sufficiently. Bridge grafts are usually located in the upper arm of children weighing < 25 kg and in the forearm of children weighing > 25 kg. The advantages of upper arm grafts include higher flow rates, patent access for a longer period of time, and free forearm movement during dialysis. Both native and graft fistulae provide good blood flow rates in most cases, but graft fistulae have a higher incidence of stenosis and thrombosis than native vessels and the frequently require surgical correction (Alexander et al. 1999, p 522).

Other disadvantages of native and graft fistulae are similar to those seen in adult patients and include high infection rates, the risk of venous hypertension and the development of arterial steal syndromes (Sherman 1993, p 345–347). The placement of graft fistulae in the lower limb has the advantage of allowing freedom of movement during dialysis but is often avoided because of the risk of limb oedema and hypertrophy (Mendley et al., p 573).

2.3 Anticoagulation

For haemodialysis

'The standard anticoagulation used in paediatric haemodialysis is heparin, which binds to and converts antithrombin 111 to a rapid inhibitor of thrombin' (Geary 1993, p 357–359). Because of the potential bleeding problems that can arise with anticoagulation it is preferable to use minimal heparin in children. The Activated Clotting Time (ACT) is commonly used to determine the heparin dose required. Once the baseline ACT is established, the initial heparin dose will vary according to the child's weight. Gruskin et al. (1992, p 842) suggest that the initial loading dose should be 50 IU/kg body weight, followed by either an hourly infusion of 50 IU/kg body weight, or a second bolus of 25 IU/ kg after 2 hours.

Lower doses may be required for children weighing < 15kg, those who have recently undergone surgery or who have bleeding problems. The ACT is measured at regular intervals, initially every two minutes, and the heparin dose is titrated to maintain the ACT at 150% of the baseline averaged for the time of treatment. This will achieve the desired anticoagulant effect in the extracorporeal circuit with minimal systemic heparinisation of the child. The total dose for a three-hour dialysis treatment should be less than 100 IU/kg (Geary 1993, p 357–359). Low dose heparin with the ACT kept to an average of 125% above the base line can be used if the potential for bleeding is high (Fine and Tejani 1994, p 564). The lower blood flow rates used with children mean that clotting is a major problem (Geary 1993, p 357–359), and can limit the use of low dose protocols.

Heparin-free dialysis is of limited value in children, especially neonates and small babies because the fluid used to keep the dialyser patent may necessitate an ultrafiltration rate that exceeds safe limits. Regional heparin can also be used, however the side effects of anaphylaxis and rebound heparinisation are common (Gruskin et al. 1992, p 842). Antiplatelet drugs, regional citrate anticoagulation and prostacyclin have been used with varying degrees of success (Gruskin et al. 1992, p 842).

For haemofiltration

As for haemodialysis, heparin remains the most frequently used anticoagulant, however the, routine use of anticoagulation with continuous therapies has recently been questioned (Smoyer et al., 1995, p 640). Smoyer et al. suggest that improvements to the biocompatibility of blood lines, dialysers and membranes encourage attempts to use treatments that are free from anticoagulation and that this therapy offers special benefits for children 'who are coagulopathic due to sepsis or disseminated intravascular coagulation' (Smoyer et al. 1995, p 640).

2.4 Complications

Physiological complications of haemodialysis

Although the complications of haemodialysis in children and adults are similar in some areas, there are some specific differences in children. Close monitoring of vital signs is central to the care of the child during the haemodialysis procedure. Paediatric patients are more prone to cardiovascular instability due to their small blood volume. Excessive weight loss is a real threat and can lead to hypotension. The risk of hypothermia is also very high especially in the infant. (Stewart et al. 1988, p 160–164).

The dialysis disequilibrium syndrome is a common and potentially serious cause of acute illness in children undergoing haemodialysis. It is reported as being more common in children than in adults (Mendley et al. 2001, p 563) and it occurs less frequently in children undergoing peritoneal dialysis. In 1984 Polinski (p 324) stated that dialysis disequilibrium 'occurs in a third of paediatric patients … an incidence four times that reported in adults'. Although this reference is dated, it serves as a reminder of the differences between dialysing adults and dialysing children. More recent research comparing the two groups does not appear to have been undertaken. The initial clinical features include irritability, restlessness, lethargy, nausea, vomiting and headache. If these symptoms are not recognised early, visual disturbances, confusion, muscle twitching, hypertension and myoclonic asterixis can develop.

If treatment is not provided immediately life threatening complications such as convulsions, coma and cardiac arrhythmias can occur (Gruskin et al., 1992, p 851–852). Disequilibrium tends to develop towards the end of dialysis but can begin anytime within 24 hours after dialysis finishes. The cause appears to be rapid correction of uraemia and could be attributed to the use of dialysers with higher surface areas compared to the child's surface area and/or high blood flow rates that could result in higher urea clearances. According to Gruskin al. (1992, p 852) the onset of dialysis disequilibrium can be avoided by performing shorter treatments using lower blood flow rates, with urea clearances of 1–1.5ml/minute/kg and by infusing 1gm/kg body weight of Mannitol 25% over the course of the treatment. The treatments should also be performed on a daily basis with the time increased slowly over days.

Other complications, such as the risk of hypotension and seizures especially as a consequence of the development of the disequilibrium syndrome are similar to adults.

2.5 Haemofiltration

Slow continuous therapies

Slow continuous therapies are used for critically ill paediatric patients where neither haemodialysis nor peritoneal dialysis can provide optimal management. The slow therapies provide safe, effective and gentle means of solute clearance and fluid removal. The types of modalities, excluding the automated therapies, are the same as those used for adults. At the time of writing, automated therapies are not commonly used with children. Indications for slow continuous therapies include:

- Fluid overload in the presence of acute renal failure.

- The need for fluid removal to allow for intravenous infusions eg. medications.

- Total parenteral nutrition.

Continuous haemofiltration is better tolerated than haemodialysis especially in the smaller population. Furthermore, a larger fluid removal can be achieved over a 24-hour period (Lieberman 1992, p 373).

Research survey: Seven paediatric renal units in Australia were surveyed in 1999 to assess dialytic management of acute renal failure in neonates and children weighing less than 10 kg (Jeyakumar 1998). The purpose of the survey was to:

1. Determine the treatment modalities that were offered.

2. Identify personnel performing the treatment.

3. Determine the frequency of treatment that was used.

4. Classify problems that were encountered.

The findings revealed that paediatric nephrology nurses in three units were involved with providing back up support and education to nurses in neonatal intensive care units and paediatric intensive care units. The remaining four units offered slow continuous therapies in consultation with the paediatric nephrologist. Average numbers of neonates and children treated per unit ranged from 1 to 3 per annum. The problems encountered included difficulties with access, technical/mechanical problems and shortage of competent staff. Treatment modalities offered included CVVH and CVVHD. CAVH and CAVHD have not been used in Australia for several years, although they remain options in other countries.

References

In text references

Alexander, S., Harmon, W., Jabs, K., Warady, B., 1999, Chronic dialysis in children, in Henrich, W., (ed.), *Principles and Practice of Dialysis,* (2nd ed.), Williams and Wilkins, Maryland.

Allen, R., and Chapman, J., 1994, 'Paediatric renal transplantation', in *A Manual of Renal Transplantation*, Arnold, E., (ed.), Edward Arnold, Melbourne.

Donckerwolcke, R., Broyer, M., Chantler, C., Rizzoni, G, 1996, 'Renal replacement therapy in children' in *Replacement of Renal Function by Dialysis,* Jacobs, C., Kjellstrand, C., Koch, K., (eds.), 4th ed., Kluwer Academic Publishers.

Donckerwolcke, R., Bunchman, T., 'Haemodialysis in infants and small children', *Paediatric Nephrology*, vol. 8, pp 103–105.

Fine, R., Tejani, A., 1994, 'Dialysis in infants and children', in *Handbook of Dialysis*, Daugirdas, J., Ing, T. (eds.), 2nd ed., Little, Brown and Co. Boston.

Geary, D., 1993, 'Paediatric Dialysis', in *Dialysis Therapy*, Nissenson, A., Fine, R., (eds.), 2nd ed., Hanley & Belfus Inc. Philadelphia.

Gruskin, A., Baluarte, H., Dabbagh, S., 1992. 'Haemodialysis and peritoneal dialysis, in *Paediatric Kidney Disease*, Edelmann, C., (ed) 2nd ed., Little Brown and Co., Boston.

Jeyakumar, Y., 1998, 'Neonatal dialysis: the nursing approach', Unpublished Survey, Paediatric Dialysis Unit, Monash Medical Centre, Clayton, Victoria.

Kemp, C., McDowell, J., 1997 (chief eds.), *Paediatric Pharmacopoeia,* 12th ed., Royal Children's Hospital, Victoria.

Lieberman, K., 1993, 'Continuous Arteriovenous Renal Replacement in Children' in *Dialysis Therapy,* Nissenson, A., Fine, R., (eds.), 2nd ed., Hanley and Belfus Inc. Philadelphia.

Mendley, S., Fine, R., Tejani, A., 2001, 'Dialysis in infants and children' in *Handbook of Dialysis,* Daugirdas, J., Blake, P., Ing, T., (eds.), 3rd ed.,, Lippincott Williams and Wilkins, Philadelphia.

Nevins, T., Mauer, S., 1993. 'Infant Hemodialysis', in *Dialysis Therapy*, Nissenson, A., Fine, R., (eds.), 2nd ed., Hanley & Belfus Inc., Philadelphia.

Polinsky, M., 1984, 'Neurologic Complications of ESRD, Dialysis and Transplantation', in *End Stage Renal Disease in Children*, Fine, R., Gruskin, A., (eds.), W. B. Saunders Company, Philadelphia.

Sherman, N., (1993). 'Paediatric Dialysis', in *Dialysis Therapy*, Nissenson, A., Fine, R., (eds.), 2nd ed., Hanley & Belfus Inc.Philadelphia.

Smoyer, W., Sherbotie, J., Gardner, J., Bunchman, T., 1995, 'A practical approach to continuous hemofiltration in infants and children', *Dialysis and Transplantation*, vol. 24, no. 11, pp 633–640.

Stewart, C., Katz, S., Kaskel, F., 1988, 'Unique Aspects of the Care of Pediatric Dialysis Patients', *Seminars in Dialysis*, vol.7, no 3, pp 160–168.

Recommended reading

Bunchman, T., Donckerwolcke, R., 1994, 'Continuous arterial-venous diahemofiltration and continuous veno-venous diahemofiltration in infants and children, *Pediatric Nephrology*, vol. 8, pp 96–102.

Donckerwolcke, R., Bunchman, T., 'Haemodialysis in infants and small children', *Paediatric Nephrology*, vol. 8, pp 103–105.

FDA Alert, 2000, (editorial), FDA issues warning on use of triCitrasol as a dialysis catheter anti-coagulant, *Dialysis and Transplantation*, June, p 310.

McDonald, D., Martin, R., 1995, 'Use of sodium citrate anticoagulation in a pediatric continuous venovenous hemodialysis patient', *ANNA Journal*, vol.22, June, no. 3, pp 327–328.

Taylor, J., 1996, 'End Stage Renal Disease in Children: Diagnosis, Management, and Interventions', *Paediatric Nursing*, vol. 22, no 6, pp 481–489.

CHAPTER THREE

Paediatric peritoneal dialysis

Introduction

It is generally accepted that young patients are usually best treated with peritoneal dialysis rather than haemodialysis and that CCPD is preferable to CAPD. However, the use of peritoneal dialysis as a renal replacement therapy in children differs in a number of aspects from its use in adults. As with paediatric haemodialysis, the body surface area of the child as well as the peritoneal surface area, are key components to successful dialysis. Paediatric renal replacement therapy is a specialty of its own and this chapter introduces the reader to the principles involved and provides an overview of the treatment parameters.

3.1 The paediatric peritoneal membrane

A brief history of paediatric peritoneal dialysis

Alexander (1996, pp 1339–1340) reported that using a peritoneal membrane to treat severe illness in children dates back approximately 75 years when intraperitoneal injections of fluid were used to rehydrate severely dehydrated children. The earliest reported use of the peritoneal membrane to replace renal function can be found in 1948 (Bloxsum & Powell pp 52–57) and in 1949 (Swan & Gordon pp 586–595). The technique used appears to be similar to the continuous lavage that was described in the introduction to Chapter 1 of this book.

These first treatments were performed using metal cannulae and the initial enthusiasm for the treatment appears to have waned shortly after these cases were reported. Flexible cannulae became available during the 1950's and the successful use of IPD to treat infants with acute renal failure was first reported in 1961. This was followed by worldwide reports of the efficacy of IPD to treat children with acute

343

renal failure. However, little was available to treat those with end stage renal disease because each treatment required the insertion of a new catheter. The development of a catheter suitable for long term use in 1960's and the subsequent availability of an automated dialysate delivery system made peritoneal dialysis a realistic treatment option for children with end stage renal failure.

The treatment remained unpopular with paediatric nephrologists however, possibly because it retained many of the 'most undesirable features of chronic hemodialysis' (Alexander 1996, p 1340). These included dietary and fluid restrictions, immobility during treatment and complex machinery that required extensive supervision.

In 1976 Popovich et al. described a treatment modification that enabled 'continuous therapy', now known as CAPD, which is perhaps the peritoneal dialysis equivalent of the Schribner shunt for haemodialysis. Treatment at home was now available to the child with end stage renal failure. The first treatment of a child at home occurred in 1978. Since that time CAPD and its various modifications has become the most frequently used treatment for renal replacement therapy in children.

Anatomy and physiology

The construction of the visceral and parietal layers of the peritoneal membrane, the blood supply to, and the lymphatic drainage from, each of these layers is largely the same as adults. The major difference between the peritoneal membrane of the child and the adult is its size. The difference in size is a one of the principle reasons that peritoneal dialysis is the preferred treatment in children. It is generally accepted that the peritoneal membrane of the child is functionally different from that of the adult and that normal growth and development results in alterations to the transport characteristics of the peritoneal membrane (Alexander et al. 1999, p 509).

Early studies indicated that, when scaled for body size, the infant peritoneal membrane is almost twice that of the adult (Alexander 1996, p 1341). However, subsequent studies have failed to demonstrate that this is the case or to confirm clinically relevant improvement in solute and/or water transport. The only exception is protein, where losses have been demonstrated to be greater in the child than in the adult. Recent data seems to suggest that, when properly adjusted for body size, the function of the child's peritoneal membrane is comparable to that of an adult. However, the relative paucity of studies in children suggests the need for further research in the area (Alexander 1996,p 1341).

3.2 Peritoneal access

Why peritoneal dialysis?

The difficulties in finding vascular access and maintaining adequate blood flow for haemodialysis makes peritoneal dialysis an obvious choice for the paediatric population. The success of peritoneal dialysis in children depends greatly on the technique of catheter placement and the level of expertise of the surgeon. Special considerations are required with regards to the type and size of the catheter (Tank et al. 1993, p 359).

Catheters for acute renal failure

A reliable catheter is the foundation of successful peritoneal dialysis. A variety of temporary catheters are available and have been used successfully in the paediatric population. The catheters available for acute dialysis include Trocath paediatric catheter with stylet, Cook paediatric catheter and Tenckhoff paediatric single-cuff straight and curled catheters. Although the choice of a temporary catheter depends largely on the paediatric nephrologist, the most commonly used is the Trocath, which has been renowned for its excellent flow characteristics and fewer complications (Debeukelaer et al. 1999 p 535).

The temporary catheter can be placed quickly and easily by the paediatric nephrologist under local anaesthetic, although sedation is also often used. This eliminates the risks and delays associated with an anaesthetic and a surgical procedure. The common disadvantage of the percutaneous catheter is poor catheter function due to the omentum enveloping and blocking the catheter (Alexander 1996, p 1343). The technique for insertion is the same as that used with adults and the catheter size is determined by the size of the child. If a Trocath or similar style of catheter is used, care must be taken to ensure that the tape used to secure the catheter supports it in the correct position and does not drag on the exit site.

Catheters for end stage renal failure

Peritoneal dialysis catheters are readily available in various configurations. Straight, curled and swan neck Tenckhoff catheters come with either one or two dacron cuffs that are can be customised to suit the child. Tenckhoff catheters come in three different sizes to cater for the neonate weighing less than 3kg, infants weighing between three and 10kg and children weighing more than 10kg. Controversy still surrounds the selection of single or double cuffed catheters. Early experience with double cuffed catheters reported an associated extrusion of the superficial cuff and the subsequent development of exit site and tunnel infections. The high rate of extrusion was most probably related to the thin abdominal wall and lack of subcutaneous fat seen in most infants and small children.

However, more recent data suggests that the rate of peritonitis is equally high using single cuff catheters (Alexander et al. 1999, p 518). According to Fine and Tejani (1994 p 556) single cuffed catheters are preferred because they are easier to insert and remove, especially in children with minimal subcutaneous tissue. The most recent study, the North American Paediatric Renal Transplant Cooperative Study, suggests a reduction in peritonitis rates if double cuffed catheters are used (Mendley et al. 2001, p569). The only catheter that should be avoided in children is the column-disk catheter because it carries the risk of entrapping the bowel between the columns of the device.

In 1991, in an attempt to reduce exit site infections, Twardowski et al. designed and implanted the first Swan Neck Presternal Catheter in an adult. Two months later Warchol et al. introduced the presternal catheter in children. This catheter consists of a 'Coilcath' catheter as the abdominal portion and a presternal tube joined by a titanium connector in the subcutaneous space of the epigastrium. The exit site is located on the chest wall at the level of the second or third rib. The main indications for using the Swan Neck Presternal Catheter include obesity, the presence of ureterostomies, urinary incontinence and previous multiple exit site infections. The disadvantages include local trauma associated with the long subcutaneous tunnel, and disconnection of the two parts of the catheter. Although this style of catheter reduces the risk of exit site infections, the location of the exit site poses a problem. Therefore, this catheter is usually reserved for cases where it is specially indicated (Warchol et al.1999, p18—187).

While catheters designed for use in end stage renal disease are inserted under general anaesthetic by a surgeon, and many acute catheters are inserted under local anaesthetic by a nephrologist, both procedures are often undertaken in the presence of a renal nurse who initiates the dialysis procedure. Technical considerations include sealing the peritoneum around the catheter with a purse string suture that is also affixed to the deep cuff to prevent leaking. A second purse string suture is used to seal the posterior rectus sheath and is fixed to the upper part of the cuff to prevent leakage and displacement of the catheter. Partial omentectomy is often performed to prevent blockage of the catheter by the omentum (Mendley et al. 200, p 569). It is usual to stitch the catheter tip to the bladder dome for boys and into the Pouch of Douglas for girls. As with adults, caudal placement of the exit site is preferred because it is associated with fewer episodes of peritonitis (Alexander et al. 1999, p 518).

3.3 Treatment modalities

Which therapy is best suited to the child?

It is well documented that the preferred method of dialysis in the paediatric population with end stage renal failure is peritoneal dialysis because of the ease of obtaining peritoneal access and the relative ease with which the procedure can be performed. The two modalities offered are Continuous Ambulatory Peritoneal Dialysis (CAPD), and Continuous Cycling Peritoneal Dialysis (CCPD). For infants, and children up to 11years, CCPD is often the preferred method for a number of reasons:

• There are fewer connection breaks reducing the likelihood of peritonitis.

• Therapy is undertaken at night while the child is asleep.

• Working parents, or parents who have other children requiring attention during the day, are able to attend to these activities.

• An automated machine that can be programmed to deliver the desired exchanges with precision is used.

• Daytime freedom allows for enhanced oral nutritional intake and freedom to attend school without interruptions.

The wishes of adolescents 12 years and older need to be considered, because their co-operation is important for the treatment to succeed. Both modalities are offered, because older children are usually capable of performing the procedure unassisted. Both CAPD and CCPD give these children independence and facilitate optimal school attendance. The reluctance to undergo peer scrutiny while doing a bag exchange at school often influences the choice of modality in this group. Peritoneal dialysis is also preferred for the treatment of children with acute renal failure, although continuous haemofiltration may be required for those who are haemodynamically unstable or who do not have an intact peritoneum (Alexander 1996, p1343).

The dialysis prescription

The dialysis prescription is similar to that of the adult patient with the exception of the volume per exchange. In an acute situation where the child requires dialysis as soon as the catheter is inserted, dialysis is initiated with very small volumes,

15–25ml/kg/exchange. The volumes per exchange are increased gradually to a maximum of 35–50ml/kg/exchange. The exchange is only increased when dialysate leak has been excluded. During the immediate post operative period it is very important to keep the child quiet and comfortable, because crying and moving around can increase the intra-abdominal pressure increasing the risk of leakage around the exit site (Holloway 1993, p 362–363).

Assessment of adequacy

K^t/V and creatinine clearance should be used to monitor dialysis therapy in children as it is in adults, and both should be recorded until such time as it becomes apparent which one is the most useful guide in paediatric patients. Until specific data becomes available for children, 'adult guidelines and targets should be considered acceptable minimum levels of therapy in children' (Alexander et al. 1997, p S26).

Although residual renal function persists for a time in children, it eventually ceases as it does in adults. If a child is too young to collect a timed urine sample, the dialysis prescription should be designed as though there was no urinary output rather than catheterise the child. When using a peritoneal equilibration test, the test exchange volume 'should be $1100mls/m^2$ body surface area' (Alexander et al. 1997, p S26).

3.4 Complications

Problems related to peritoneal dialysis in children

With the exception of nutritional factors, the complications of peritoneal dialysis in children are similar to those in adults. Nutritional management of children on peritoneal dialysis is important because growth retardation, low energy, low protein intake and biochemical manifestations of malnutrition are often found in children treated with long term peritoneal dialysis. Adequate nutritional assessment, good dietary review and specialised counselling often overcome the pitfalls of malnutrition and growth (Salusky & Nelson 1993, p 364–365).

Because protein losses to the dialysate are greater in children than in adults, protein intake is considered a vital factor in ensuring adequate growth of children on peritoneal dialysis. Alexander (1996, p 1349) recommends that an additional protein intake of 0.3g/kg/day should be added to the recommended daily allowance (RDA) for height-age. Daily energy intake is augmented by the absorption of between 8 and 20 kcals from the dialysate (Alexander 1996, p 1349). Babies who are falling behind their expected growth rate can have their diet supplemented and occasionally totally replaced by enteral feeds.

Even though children undergoing peritoneal dialysis have an unrestricted diet, especially in terms of protein intake and receive a constant supply of carbohydrate calories from their dialysate, achieving normal growth remains difficult. The use of subcutaneous recombinant human growth hormone (rHuGH) over the last decade has demonstrated significant improvements in growth velocity of children with chronic renal failure (Scharer & Gilli 1992, p 603).

As well as the reasons for post catheter insertion leaks seen in adults, dialysate leaks in children can also be the result of poor wound healing related to malnutrition, tissue oedema or the long term use of steroids (Bunchman and Maxvold 2000, p 643).

Caring for the child on peritoneal dialysis remains an ongoing challenge for the renal multidisciplinary team. The time and resources invested in these children and their families will no doubt optimise therapy and minimise complications in the long term.

References

In text references

Alexander, S., 1996, 'Peritoneal dialysis', in *Replacement of Renal Function by Dialysis,* Jacobs, C., Kjellstrand, C., Koch, K., (eds.), 4th ed., Kluwer Academic Publishers, Boston.

Alexander, S., Harmon, W., Jabs, K., Warady, B., 1999, 'Chronic dialysis in children', in *Principles and Practice of Dialysis,* Henrich, W., (ed.), 2nd ed., William and Wilkins, Maryland.

Alexander, S., Salusky, I., Warady, B., Watkins, S., 1997, 'Peritoneal dialysis modalities', *Peritoneal Dialysis International,* vol. 17, Suppl. 3, pp S25–S 27.

Bloxsum, A., Powell, N., 1948, 'The treatment of acute temporary dysfunction of the kidneys by peritoneal irrigation', *Paediatrics,* vol. 1, pp 52–57.

Bunchman. T., Maxvold, N., 2000, 'Complications of acute and chronic dialysis in children', in *Complications of Dialysis,* Lameire, N., Mehta, R., (eds.), Marcel Dekker, New York.

Debeukelaer, M., Batisky, D., Melber, S., 1999, 'Acute dialysis in children', in *Principles and Practice of Dialysis,* Heinrich, W., (ed.), 2nd ed., Williams and Wilkins, Maryland.

Fine, R., Tejani, A., 1994, 'Dialysis in infants and children', in *Handbook of Dialysis,* Daugirdas, J., Ing, T. (eds.), 2nd ed., Little, Brown and Co. Boston.

Holloway, M., 1993, 'CAPD/CCPD orders in children', in *Dialysis Therapy,* Nissenson, A., Fine, R., (eds), 2nd ed., Hanley and Belfus Inc., Philadelphia.

Mendley, S., Fine, R., Tejani, A., 2001, 'Dialysis in infants and children' in *Handbook of Dialysis*, Daugirdas, J., Blake, P., Ing, T., (eds.), 3rd ed., Lippincott Williams and Wilkins, Philadelphia.

Salusky, I., Nelson, P., 1993, 'Nutritional management of children on peritoneal dialysis' in *Dialysis Therapy*, Nissenson, A., Fine, R., (eds)., 2nd ed., Hanley and Belfus Inc., Philadelphia.

Swan, H., Gordon, H., 'Peritoneal lavage in the treatment of anuria in children', *Paediatrics*, 1949, Vol. 4, pp 586–597.

Tank, E., Tank, J., Corneil, A., 1993, 'Peritoneal Access in Children' in *Dialysis Therapy*, Nissenson, A., Fine, R., (eds)., 2nd ed., Hanley and Belfus Inc., Philadelphia.

Warchol, S., Roszkowska-Blaim, M., Sieniawska, M., 1988, 'Swan neck presternal peritoneal dialysis catheter: five year experience in children', *Peritoneal Dialysis International*, vol 18 no 2 pp 183–187.

CHAPTER FOUR

Paediatric renal transplantation

Introduction

Although renal transplantation has been conducted successfully since 1954, children were not considered suitable candidates for transplantation until the early 1960's (Fine et al., 1987). Physiological, social and psychological difficulties for the child, the side effects of immunosuppression and technical difficulties with the surgical procedure slowed acceptance of transplantation for the following decade. As these difficulties were successfully addressed, transplantation became increasingly accepted as a treatment option. It is now universally accepted that transplantation provides the child with the maximum opportunity for normal growth and development and is most likely to give them the best quality of life (Al-Akash & Ettenger 2001, p332).

4.1 Donor selection

The choice between living and cadaveric donor

A living related donor is preferred for the paediatric recipient because they offer a number of advantages. The use of such a donor allows transplantation to be planned to coincide with optimal health for donor and child, and to take place at a time suitable for both. Other family members suitable to be donors include grandparents, uncles and aunts. Transplants from living donors have a better short and long term survival rate for all paediatric age groups. Survival rates for one, three and five years are 10%–20% better than when cadaveric kidneys are used, and approach 30% at five years for very young patients (Al-Akash & Ettenger 2001, p336). The use of a living donor also allows an immune conditioning regimen to be commenced during the pretransplant week e.g., with mycophenolate mofetil and prednisolone and for a final cross match to be performed (Al-Akash & Ettenger 2001, p348).

If a related donor is not available, the child is placed on the cadaveric transplant waiting list. The pretransplant work up for both living and cadaveric recipients is similar to that which occurs in adults with the exception of a renewed interest in pretransplant blood transfusion. These blood transfusions are now administered with concomitant cyclosporine cover and initial results for both living and cadaveric transplants at one and five years are encouraging compared to similar graft survival rates without blood transfusion (Niaudet et al. 2000, p 456). One-year graft survival in cadaveric transplants is 83%, and seven-year survival is 59% (Al-Akash 2001, p 336). It is recognised that the survival figures will improve when units that perform large numbers of transplants are compared with those for smaller units (Al-Akash 2001, p 339).

Transplantation before or after dialysis?

Pre-emptive transplantation—transplantation that occurs prior to dialysis, is preferred for children (Al-Akash & Ettenger 2001, p 335, Neumann 1997, p 516). The advantages include the prevention of uraemia and optimizing normal growth and development. However, the failure of a transplant can cause serious drawbacks for the child, because dialysis usually needs to be commenced immediately and the child may not be psychologically prepared (Neumann 1997, p 516). Graft survival appears to be higher with pre-emptive transplantation, for unknown reasons. It has been suggested that noncompliance could be higher in this group, possibly because they have never experienced dialytic forms of renal replacement therapy, therefore, careful psychological assessment needs to be undertaken prior to the procedure (Al-Akash & Ettenger 2001, p 335).

4.2 Surgical technique

Practical considerations

The most practical approach to transplantation would be to match the recipient with an appropriately sized cadaver kidney, as this would overcome many of the technical and physiological challenges associated with using adult kidneys. However this is seldom the case, because it is rare to receive appropriately sized paediatric cadaveric kidneys and the success rate using kidneys from very young donors is low, due to the increased incidence of vascular thrombosis. Sibling donors of a similar size would be suitable, but as many have not reached the legal age for consent, they are a seldom used option (Allen & Chapman 1994, p 258). Anencephalic donors have been used in the past for both paediatric and adult recipients (Fine & Ettenger 1987, p 829). The current use of these infants as organ donors is controversial, primarily because of the difficulties associated with establishing brain death (Allen & Chapman 1994, p 258).

Anaesthetic considerations

When transplantation is being undertaken, a number of anaesthetic precautions need to be observed. As with adults, these precautions include avoiding anaesthetic agents that are excreted by the kidney as well as those that have active metabolites that are renally excreted (Mauer et al.1992, p 949).

A paediatric anaesthetist should always be in attendance during the procedure, and is responsible for the volume status of the child as well as for the anaesthesia. A multilumen central venous catheter is inserted, usually in the operating theatre after the child has been anaesthetised, in order to maintain adequate filling. A central venous pressure between 12 to 15 mm Hg [16.3 to 20.4 cm H_2O] should be achieved prior to releasing the vascular clamps. A higher pressure is desirable in a small child receiving an adult kidney (Al-Akash & Ettenger 2001, p348).

Surgical considerations

The surgical placement of the kidney in a small child differs from that of an older child or adult. For children weighing 20 kg or more the kidney is placed extraperitoneally. An intraperitoneal approach is required for those weighing less than 20 kg and receiving an adult kidney, (Neumann, 1997, p 516). The technique is much the same for a small child receiving a small kidney with modifications to the anastomoses of the aorta and vena cava to prevent thrombosis (Martin & Noseworthy 1984, p 462). If the donor is aged less than two years, the kidneys are usually transplanted 'en-block', together with the donor aorta and vena cava.

The surgeon will determine whether the kidneys should be transplanted together or separately in donors aged between two and five years (Gritch & Rosenthal 2001, p 151). Other surgical considerations include the technique of ureteroneocystostomy that is similar to that used in adults where a large sized urethral catheter is used. A large suprapubic catheter placed at the time of transplantation is preferred for the small child. When the recipient is to receive a kidney of an appropriate anatomical size, the technique is similar to that conducted in the adult (Allen & Chapman 1994, p 259).

Many surgeons prefer to remove the appendix at the time of transplantation because it can be difficult to differentiate between appendicitis and the tenderness that accompanies acute rejection (Allen & Chapman 1994, p 260–261).

Physiological considerations

Revascularisation of a cold adult kidney provides a major stress for the young recipient and requires careful intraoperative fluid management to compensate for the required increase in cardiac output. If an adult kidney is placed into a small child, perfusion of the kidney can cause hypovolaemia, hypotension and vascular thrombosis. It is usual to transfuse whole blood (Allen & Chapman 1994, p 260), or packed cells (Al-Akash & Ettenger 2001, p 348), prior to release of the vascular clamps. A dopamine infusion of 2-3 µg/kg/min is usually commenced to facilitate adequate renal perfusion (Al-Akash & Ettenger 2001, p 348).

Loss of body heat as the kidney is perfused is a further cause of physiological stress. Authors differ in their opinions as to the value of warming the kidney prior to reperfusion. Some authorities consider that such warming leads to tubular damage produced by warm ischaemia (Allen & Chapman 1994, p 258–260), others recommend that it be undertaken following anastomosis and prior to revascularisation (Mauer et al. 1992, p 949). The risk of hypothermia can be reduced if the operating room is kept warm and heating blankets are used. Warm moist packs can be used to minimise exposure of bowel and warm saline abdominal lavage can be used if required.

Early diuresis can be assisted with mannitol 0.25gm/kg and lasix 1mg/kg at the time of revascularisation (Allen & Chapman 1994, p 258–260).

4.3 Nursing management

Nursing management in the immediate postoperative period is similar to that of any child who has undergone major surgery (Neumann 1997, p 516). The main postoperative focus is on achieving graft function and early mobilisation without the difficulties that accompany rejection, infection, fluid overload and technical mishap. To achieve this, the child has to be monitored closely for the first few days with precise attention to fluid and electrolyte replacement (Allen & Chapman 1994, p 263). Remember that normal renal function in the child reflects different biochemistry from that of the adult, and take care to use paediatric values appropriate for the age of the child to assess graft function.

Post operatively the child will return with a central venous catheter for fluid replacement and central venous pressure measurement, an arterial line for blood pressure monitoring and blood taking, an indwelling catheter to measure urine output and drain tube(s) to collect leakage from the vascular and ureteric anastomoses. Routine monitoring includes vital signs, central venous pressure and urine output (Allen & Chapman 1994, pp 263–264). Meticulous fluid balance and maintaining sufficient central venous pressure to ensure appropriate renal perfusion is vital to a successful outcome. Children can become hypotensive despite fluid overload and apparently adequate central venous pressure. This is due to the 'relative preponderance of right ventricular failure' and the presence of 'large capacitance veins in the adult donor kidney', and can result in thrombosis and subsequent loss of the kidney (Allen & Chapman 1994, pp 264).

Urine output is measured frequently; often quarter hourly during the immediate postoperative period and intravenous fluids are given to match the output. An additional allowance is added to compensate for insensible fluid loss. Close observation in the early postoperative period is necessary to identify poor graft function, but also because a large adult kidney is able to produce 'an hourly urine output [that is] equivalent to an infant's blood volume' (Freeman & Wels 1991, p 157). Antibiotic and immunosuppressive therapy is administered in accordance with individual hospital procedure. Protocols for the type of immunosupressive therapy to be used, antibiotic use and fluid replacement varies between institutions and in accordance with the biochemical status of the child.

Drugs used to achieve immunosuppression and as prophylaxis against viruses such as cytomegalovirus, are the same as those used in adults.

Postoperative complications are also similar with urinary leaks and vascular thrombosis occurring most commonly when kidneys from young donors are used and occurs irrespective of whether an 'en-block' or separate approach is taken (Gritch and Rosenthal 2001, p 151). There is some evidence to suggest that failure to take immunosuppressive drugs is higher in this group of patients (Palmer and Slook 1992, p 377). This applies particularly to older girls and adolescents, where the visible side effects of some immunosuppressive drugs often result in noncompliance. In an American journal, noncompliance after three to six months is second only to graft rejection as a cause for transplant failure (Nuemann 1997, p 522).

Occasionally ventilatory support is required if an adult kidney has been used in a small child because the increase in intra-abdominal pressure causes respiratory difficulties.

References

In text references

Al-Akash, S., Ettenger, R., 2001, 'Kidney transplantation in children', in *Handbook of Kidney Transplantation*, Danovitch, G., (ed) 3rd ed., Lippincott, William and Wilkins, Sydney.

Allen, R., Chapman, J., 1994, *Paediatric Renal Transplantation*, Edward Arnold, Melbourne.

Fine, R., Ettenger, R., 1987 'Renal Transplantation' in Holliday, M., Barratt, T., Vernier, R., (eds.) *Paediatric Nephrology,* 2nd edn, Williams and Wilkins, Baltimore.

Fine, R., Salusky, I., Ettenger, R., 1987, 'A therapeutic approach to the infant, child, and adolescent with end stage renal disease', *Pediatric Clinics of North America,* no. 34, pp 789–801.

Freeman, J., Wels, J., 1991, 'Anaesthesia for organ transplantation', in *The Handbook of Transplant Management*, Makowka, L., (ed.), Landes, Austin.

Gritch, H., Rosenthal, T., 2001, 'The transplant operation and its surgical complications', in *Handbook of Kidney Transplantation*, Danovitch, G., (ed) 3rd ed., Lippincott, Williams and Wilkins, Sydney.

Martin, L., Noseworthy, J., 1984, 'Surgical aspects of transplantation: technique and complications', in *End Stage Renal Disease in Children,* Fine, R., Gruskin, A., (eds.), W. B. Saunders, Sydney

Mauer, M., Nevins, T., Ascher, N., 1992, 'Renal transplant in children, in *Paediatric Kidney Disease*, Edelmann, C., (ed.), 2nd ed., Little Brown and Co., London.

Neumann, M., 1997, 'Evaluation of the pediatric renal transplant recipient', *ANNA Journal*, vol. 25, no. 5, pp515–523, 538.

Niaudet, P., Dudley, J., Charbit, M., Gagnadoux, M., Macleay, K., 2000, 'Pre transplant blood transfusions with cyclosporine in pediatric renal transplantation' *Pediatric Nephrology*, vol. 14, no. 6., pp 451–456.

Palmer, J., Slook, P., 1992, 'Successful use of Orthoclone OKT3 for steroid resistant acute rejection in pediatric renal allograft recipients', *ANNA Journal*, vol. 19, no. 4, pp375–377.

Recommended reading

Shaben, T., 1993, 'Psychosocial issues in kidney transplanted children and adolescents: literature review', *ANNA Journal*, vol. 20, no. 6, pp 663–668.

Physical and psychological consequences of renal disease in children

Introduction

Factors that determine the physical and psychological impact of chronic illness are not intrinsic to any particular disease category. Chronically ill children share many features that are common across disease categories and the factors that determine ultimate function tend to be demographic, psychosocial and developmental. When chronic disease occurs in children, the chronological age and the developmental age are two quite distinct categories. Each has specific requirements that need to be catered for if the child is to achieve their maximum potential. Recognition of the importance of the developmental characteristics specific for a given time in a child's life has led to a much more relaxed atmosphere in hospitals. Parents and significant others in the child's life are now encouraged to participate as fully as is practical in the treatment program. Hospital environments are made as friendly and colourful as possible, outings are encouraged and specially qualified teachers attend schooling where possible.

This chapter has been included to introduce some of the physical and psychological hurdles that the child with renal failure must endure and serves as a reminder that renal disease affects much more than just the kidney.

5.1 Physical complications of end stage renal disease

Anaemia

According to Mendley et al. (2001, p 577) anaemia is more severe in children than adults. The severity of anaemia is directly proportional to the degree of renal failure. The low haemoglobin level is proportional to the low haematocrit level and the appearance of the erythrocyte is usually normocytic, normochromic and hypoproliferative with a low erythropoietin level. Children on haemodialysis tend to be more prone to anaemia due to a greater amount of blood loss from the extracorporeal circuit. Recombinant human erythropoietin (rHuEPO) has proven to be an effective therapy in correcting anaemia in the paediatric population. Blood transfusion is warranted when the haemoglobin level ranges between 5 and 6 gm/decilitre and signs of fatigue, anorexia, reduced exercise tolerance, increased heart failure and chest pain are present (Gruskin et al.1992, pp 884–885).

Growth

Growth retardation is one of the most significant manifestations of end stage renal failure in children and can occur before there is a significant reduction in glomerular function (Scharer & Gilli 1992, p 593). Trained personnel with knowledge of the normal growth process should evaluate and assess growth. These normal processes can be divided into three stages:

1. A period with a high but rapidly declining growth rate from birth to the age of 3 or 4 years.

2. A period with steady growth between 6 and 7 cm/year until the onset of puberty, around a mean age of 11 years in girls and 13 years in boys.

3. Final growth occurs in the pubertal period, with a growth spurt reaching a peak of 7cm/year in girls and 9cm/yr in boys at a mean age of 12 and 14 years respectively (Scharer & Gilli 1992).

These same authors recommend using chronological age for plotting growth data. The relationship of weight to height can be expressed by comparing the standard deviation scores (SDS) for weight and height or by indicating both weight and height as a fraction of the 50th centile for age. Bone age films of the left hand and wrist are also useful in assessing skeletal maturity. Growth retardation can be avoided by close monitoring of height and weight, early intervention with nutritional supplements by oral, enteral or parenteral means to provide the nutrients required for growth and development especially in the early years. The use of subcutaneous injections of recombinant human growth hormone (rHuGH) in recent years has demonstrated significant improvements in growth velocity (Scharer & Gilli 1992, p 603).

Renal osteodystrophy

The incidence of renal osteodystrophy in children is greater than in adults (Gruskin et al.1992, p 878). It is caused by disorders of mineral metabolism and is related to disturbances in calcium and phosphorous regulation, alterations in vitamin D hydroxylation, and changes in parathormone production. Other factors that influence the development of renal osteodystrophy are the prolonged uraemic state, restricted food intake and exposure to aluminium (Gruskin et al.1992, p 878). The mechanism of osteodystrophy development is similar to that for adults, but the impact differs in some aspects because the bones of children are not fully developed. The four forms of renal osteodystrophy found in children receiving maintenance dialysis are osteitis fibrosa cystica (hyperparathyroid bone disease), osteomalacia (rickets), osteopenia and aluminium-related osteomalacia (Gruskin et al. 1992, p 878). The most common form seen in children is a combination of osteitis and rickets. Stunted growth, enlargement of the wrists and ankles and 'knocked knees' are common clinical signs of bone disease in children. In these children, activity can be restricted, and if they complain of continuous pain, it could be the sign of a fracture or epiphyseal slipping. Epiphyseal slipping is age-related and tends to occur late in the course of uraemia, with the incidence decreasing after dialysis commences (Gruskin et al. 1992, p 878).

Acid base regulation

The acidosis of end stage renal failure is caused by the inability of the kidney to excrete excess hydrogen ions. Acid retention is detrimental in children due to their metabolic growth requirements. Therefore, it is paramount that the decreasing pH be neutralised and buffered as early as possible (Linshaw 1992, p 640). The standard therapy to correct acidosis is the administration of sodium bicarbonate or sodium citrate. This treatment should be used cautiously in children who are oedematous and hypertensive. To minimise the effects of sodium load and maintain sodium balance, sodium bicarbonate supplements should be accompanied by sodium chloride restrictions (Linshaw 1992, p 40).

Nutrition

The growth rate of healthy children is greatly influenced by their nutritional status, especially during the first two years (Scharer & Gilli 1992, p 602–603). Therefore, the main aim of nutritional management of the child is to provide a regime to minimise the biochemical consequences of uraemia, improve nutritional status and maximise growth. This goal appears simple, but it is often difficult to achieve. Adequate nutritional management of a child requires precise clinical assessments by a paediatric nephrologist and a paediatric renal dietitian using a combination of assessment tools and parameters. The assessment should include anthropometric measurements, dietary history evaluating energy intake and protein stores, biochemical parameters, and evaluation of water balance and prescribed medications. Anthropometric measurements of weight, length or height and head circumference in children younger than 2 years provides information that is a good indication of the child's growth and muscle and fat stores.

Nutritional management of infants, children and adolescents is based on the same principles. However, appropriate dietary modifications are necessary for the different age groups. Infants require special formulas fortified with additives to increase caloric and protein intake. They should be introduced gradually to allow the infant's gastrointestinal tract to adjust to the changes. Older children and adolescents tend to have specific likes and dislikes and can find it difficult to adhere to the recommended dietary regime.

The alteration in the taste sensation experienced by uraemic children can lead to anorexia. Therefore, creative methods have to be used to increase food intake. The establishment of a close relationship between the child, parents, paediatric nephrologist, renal dietitian and renal nurse is very important. Charts, games and pictures as well as written information all help the family retain the information given to them. Dietary plans should also be flexible and accommodate some favourite foods and eating habits. Parents should establish consistent guidelines to govern their child's eating habits.

5.2 Psychological complications of chronic illness

Just as there are physical complications of paediatric renal failure, there are psychological complications specific to the paediatric population. A team effort by the nephrologist, nurses, dietitians, social workers, play therapists, teachers and psychologists is essential in the care of children with end stage renal disease. The psychosocial challenges of chronic illness in children differ from those facing adult patients (Gruskin et al.1992 p 893). Treatment with dialysis creates many stressors for both children and families and continues for an indefinite period of time. Dialysis, fluid and dietary restrictions, pain, growth retardation and frequent hospital admissions, present major obstacles to these children. The stress on the family is enormous, especially at the time of diagnosis and initiation of dialysis.

Anxiety and fear are common. Irritability and mood swings, withdrawal from social contacts, dependence on parents and hospital staff and aggression are some of the characteristic behaviours of these children. Anxiety among children on haemodialysis is commonly related to the insertion of needles and the necessary hospital attendance three times a week for treatment. Separation from family and friends, disruption of schoolwork and interruption of leisure time can cause further anxieties. A great deal can be done to help overcome these fears and anxieties if staff and family members take the time to explain procedures slowly, with several pauses at each step to allow time for the child's anxiety to dissipate. A teacher can be organised in hospital to liaise with the school to continue schoolwork while the child is on haemodialysis, or during periods of prolonged hospitalisation. Children should be encouraged to participate in the sports of their choice to help them achieve their own level and stay in contact with their peers.

Due to their illness these children experience pain on an intermittent but regular basis. Children on haemodialysis experience pain when their fistula is cannulated and children on either modality experience pain when they receive their daily or second daily injections of recombinant human growth hormone and recombinant human erythropoietin. Pain can often be alleviated with a local anaesthetic cream and the fears associated with the discomfort of treatment can be minimised by relaxation therapy and guided imagery.

The family's routine can be significantly altered when a child has a chronic illness. The family structure as well as all the variables affecting the family must be considered when trying to offer assistance to cope with the situation. Families have to adapt to a new lifestyle, dietary modifications and changed social relationships, employment and holidays. They often have to make sacrifices on behalf of their children. In spite of the stress that the family endures, they can experience positive outcomes if given the correct support. Often siblings suffer a loss of attention when parents tend to focus on the chronically ill child. They can manifest excessive jealousy and inappropriate behaviour in an attempt to attract parental attention. Therefore, they need special help and counselling to cope with their feelings. This can be achieved by encouraging families to participate in support groups organised by nursing staff, medical staff and social workers. Comprehensive, consistent and systematic education of the families in the care of these children can increase the family's capacity to cope with chronic illness (Gruskin et al., 1992, pp 893–894).

Despite the fact that children with end stage renal failure who have received a transplant have to make additional adjustments they do not appear to have any greater personality or psychological disorders than other children with chronic illness. Studies have shown that where obvious personality disturbance is present, it was detectable before the transplant, on personality testing (Mauer et al. 1992, p 973). Although tools to study the psychological impact of transplantation on children are limited and specific research is rare, some common crisis points have been identified. The major stressor during the early transplant period is returning to school, primarily because of the alterations in physical appearance that occur due to immunosuppression. During the 'middle' transplant period, four to eleven months, problems emerge between the child and the adult donor if a cadaveric kidney was not used. These difficulties typically arise when the adult attempts to control the behaviour of the child and uses the donated organ as a means of manipulation.

The 'late' transplant period involves further problems. If the kidney is rejected, the child frequently experiences extreme depression followed by difficulty accepting the need for further dialysis. If the kidney continues to function well, memories of the surgery and dialysis fade, and the child begin to neglect medication, out patient appointments and general 'transplant specific' self-care (Mauer et al. 1992, p 973). A 1993 study by Shaben acknowledged the dearth of understanding surrounding the psychological issues relating to transplantation in children. This study recommended that the paediatric and adolescent populations be divided, to ensure that the different needs of each group are determined. The findings also suggest that qualitative studies intended to identify the needs of both groups be followed by quantitative studies designed to test the findings of these studies.

References

In text references

Gruskin, A., Baluarte, H., Dabbagh, S., 1992. 'Haemodialysis and peritoneal dialysis, in *Pediatric Kidney Disease*, Edelmann, C., (ed), 2nd ed., Little Brown and Co., Boston.

Linshaw, M., 1992, 'Acid-Base Disturbances', in *Paediatric Kidney Disease*, Edelman, C., (ed), 2nd ed., Little Brown and Co., Boston.

Mauer, M., Nevins, T., Ascher, N., 1992, 'Renal transplant in children', in *Paediatric Kidney Disease*, Edelmann, C., (ed.), 2nd ed., Little Brown and Co., London.

Mendley, S., Fine, R., Tejani, A., 2001, 'Dialysis in infants and children' in *Handbook of Dialysis*, Daugirdas, J., Blake, P., Ing, T., (eds.), 3rd ed., Lippincott Williams and Wilkins, Philadelphia.

Shaben, T., 1993, 'Psychosocial issues in kidney transplanted children and adolescents: literature review', *ANNA Journal*, vol. 20, no. 6, pp 663–668.

Scharer, K., Gilli, G., 1992, 'Growth retardation in kidney disease', in *Pediatric Kidney Disease*, Edelmann, C., (ed), 2nd ed., Little Brown and Co., Boston.

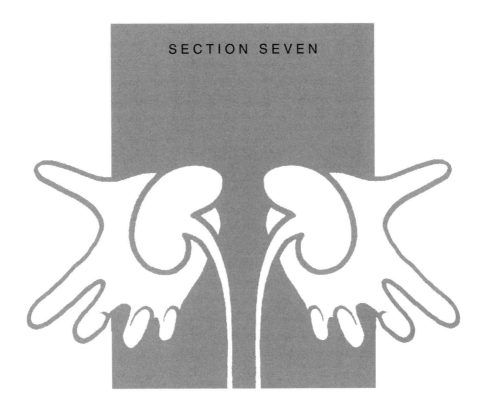

SECTION SEVEN

Use of complementary therapies and alternative medicine in renal disease

Introduction

The use of herbal remedies, dietary supplements, and 'alternative' or 'complementary' forms of medicine is becoming increasingly popular among the general population. Many people believe that they play an important role in the maintenance of health and general well being. The reasons given include the belief that herbal remedies are a 'more natural' form of treatment and that Eastern cultures approach the provision of health care in a holistic way that is uncommon among Western health care providers (Vanherweghem 2000, 330).

Some people with renal failure believe that the use of herbal medicines and dietary supplements will slow the progress of their disease and reduce the symptoms of the associated comorbidities and their use by this patient population is of increasing concern to health care providers (Dahl 2001, p186, p 190). Of principle concern is the dearth of reliable information available about the composition of many of these substances, their pharmacokinetics, and possible drug interactions (Dahl 2001, p186, p189). Production regulation may vary in different countries, therefore it is important that patients travelling to areas that do not have such regulatory processes in place do not inadvertently use preparations that are nephrotoxic, or bring them home for later use.

Many people do not view herbal preparations as 'drugs' and are unaware of, or do not consider, the problems associated with taking them from one country to another. Contamination with pesticides, poisons and heavy metals has been documented and the inclusion of hormonal or glandular extracts of animal origin in some of these products has the potential to transmit infectious agents (Dahl 2001, p186, p189). There are also several documented cases of acute renal failure occurring following the ingestion of traditional Asian medicines (Abt, et al. 1995, pp 211–2; Seedat 1993, pp 801; Lee, et al. 1999, pp 227–230; Vanherweghem 1998, pp 9–13; Hilepo, et al. 1997, p 361).

Several herbal remedies in common use have known adverse effects that could impair residual renal function. They are shown in table 7.1.1.

Table 7.1.1: **Commonly used herbal preparations and the adverse events relevant to renal disease associated with their use.**

Herb	Adverse effect
Aloe (*barbadensis/vera capensis*)	Severe electrolyte disturbance, especially hypokalaemia.
Aristolochic acid	Used to promote weight loss and associated with chronic interstitial fibrosis and tubular atrophy.
Asparagus root (*Asparagi rhizoma*)	Promotes diuresis *without* accompanying sodium loss and is therefore not suitable for the treatment of oedema or hypertension.
Buckthorn bark/cherry (*Rhamus cathartica*) (*Frangulae cortex/ Rhamni cathartici fructus*)	Severe electrolyte disturbance, especially hypokalaemia.
Bromeliad (*Bromelainum*)	Potentiates the action of oral anticoagulants.
Cascara sagrada bark (*Rhamni purshianae cortex*)	Severe electrolyte disturbance, especially hypokalaemia, albuminuria, and haematuria.
Cat's claw (*Uncaria tomentose*)	Acute allergic interstitial nephritis.
Cinchona bark (*Cinchonae cortex*)	Potentiates the action of oral anticoagulants.
Cianidanol	ARF, Disseminated Intravascular Coagulation, haemolysis, autoimmune and allergic reactions.
Danshen (*Salvia miltiorrhiza*)	Potentiates the action of oral anticoagulants.
Ephedra (*Ephedrae sinica/ anevadensis*)	Hypertension, arrhythmia.
Echinacea (*Echinacea angustifolia/ purpurea/pallida*)	Used as an 'immune stimulant' and may oppose the immunosuppressive medications used to prevent tissue rejection. Can worsen autoimmune disease including type 1 diabetes.

Feverfew (*Tanacetum parthenium*)	Mouth ulcers, tachycardia.
Garlic (*Allium satvum*)	Potentiates the action of oral anticoagulants. Gastritis.
Ginseng (*Panax ginseng/quinquefolium*)	Opposes the action of oral anticoagulants. Can cause hypertension, anxiety, insomnia and asthma attacks
Green tea (*Camellia sinensis*)	As above.
Goldenseal (*Hydrastis Canadensis*)	As above.
Ginkgo biloba	Potentiates the action of oral anticoagulants.
Juniper berry (*Juniperus communis*)	Promotes diuresis *without* accompanying sodium loss, and is therefore not suitable for the treatment of oedema or hypertension.
Horseradish (*Armoracia rusticana*)	As above.
Liquorice (*Glycyrrhiza glabra*)	Pseudoaldosteronism and subsequent sodium retention and potassium loss, headache, hypertension and CCF.
Lovage root (*Levisticum officinale/radix*)	Promotes diuresis *without* accompanying sodium loss and is therefore not suitable for the treatment of oedema or hypertension.
Noni juice (*Morinda citrifolia*)	Hyperkalaemia.
Rhubarb root (*Rhei radix*)	Severe electrolyte disturbance, especially hypokalaemia.
St. Johns Wort (*Hypericum perforatum*)	Reduces cyclosporine levels and may potentiate rejection in transplant recipients. Should not be taken with psychoactive drugs.
Senna leaf/pod (*Sennae folium/fructus*)	Severe electrolyte disturbance, especially hypokalaemia.
Water cress (*Nasturtium officinale*)	Promotes diuresis *without* accompanying sodium loss and is therefore not suitable for the treatment of oedema or hypertension.
White Sandalwood (*Santalum lignum album*)	As above.

(Dahl 2001, pp 189–190, Myhre 2000, pp 475–476, Geraghty 2000 p 13).

The impact on residual renal function in patients with renal impairment who use essential oils or aromatherapy is not well documented. Those observed include hypotension (personal experience) and the precipitation of a 'renal crisis' in a patient with

Scleroderma (Orion and Brenner 1998, p 230). Such side effects are unusual where essential oils are used topically or in a vapouriser and at the correct dose. Doses of essential oils should be modified for people with renal disease, the young and the elderly. Renal damage is possible if essential oils are used orally because they are metabolised in the liver and largely excreted by the kidney. If the kidney is not functioning the essential oils could accumulate in the blood. This is usually not the case with aromatherapy as it is practiced in many countries, but it is possible in countries such as France where essential oils are used orally.

There are numerous other therapies that are used as alternatives to, or in conjunction with conventional medicine. These therapies include Therapeutic Touch, reiki, various counselling strategies, visualisation, massage, play therapy and music. Play therapy is especially useful for young children who require repeated and distressing painful procedures. They can all help improve a person's quality of life and by promoting positive thinking they can be of real assistance in helping people cope with a chronic disease. Many complementary therapies also provide enormous spiritual benefits.

To reduce the possible adverse effects of alternative therapies in patients with renal disease it is recommended that health care professionals include the following when discussing care with their patients.

1. Use questions specifically designed to ascertain the use of herbal or dietary supplements

    e.g. *'Are you taking any special vitamin or herbal preparations?'* or
    'Are you being treated by any natural therapy practitioners?'

2. Avoid negative comments about these therapies. Use phrases such as:

    'Lots of people take tablets/herbs/mixtures like these. Let's check and see how they mix with the tablets you doctor has asked you to take.' instead of 'These can be really harmful, I don't think that you should use them any more. Best to throw them away.'

3. If patients wish to continue using their supplement, despite being given good reasons and evidence why it could be undesirable, suggest that they discuss a 'trial of use' with their nephrologist.

4. Always recommend they use properly labelled products with detailed information about the contents, and that are purchased from countries where regulated standards for production exist and are enforced.

(Dahl 2001, 190–191).

References

Abt , A., Oh, J., Huntington, R., Burkhart, K., 1995, 'Chinese herbal medicine induced acute renal failure', *Arch Intern Med,* vol. 155, no. 2, pp 211–212.

Dahl, N., 2001, 'Herbs and supplements in dialysis patients: panacea or poison?', *Seminars in Dialysis,* vol. 14, no. 3, pp186–192.

Gerghty, M., 2000, 'Herbal supplements for renal patients: what do we know?' *Nephrology News and Issues.* March pp 12–13, 42–44, 54.

Hilepo, J., Bellucci, A., Mossey, R., 1997, 'Acute renal failure caused by "cat's claw" herbal remedy in a patient with systemic lupus erythematosus, *Nephron,* no. 77, p 361).

Lee, C., Wu, M., Luand, K., Hsu, K., 1999, 'Renal tubular acidosis, hypokalemic paralysis, rhabdomyolysis, and acute renal failure—a rare presentation pf Chinese herbal nephropathy', *Renal Failure,* vol.21, no. 2, pp 227–230.

Myhre, M., 2000, 'Herbal remedies, nephropathies and renal disease', *Nephrology Nursing Journal,* vol. 27, no. 5, pp 473–478.

Orion, E., Brenner, S., 1998, 'Sclerodermas renal crisis in a association with essential oils' *Acta Derm Venereol,* vol 73, no. 3, p 230.

Seedat, Y., 1993, 'Acute renal failure in the black population of South Africa', *Int. Journal of Artificial Organs,* vol.16, no. 12, pp 801–802.

Vanherweghem, J., 1998, ' Misuse of herbal remedies: the case of an outbreak of terminal renal failure in Belgium', *Journal of Altern Complement Med.,* vol. 4, no 1, pp 9–13.

Vanherweghem J., 2000, 'Nephropathy and herbal medicine', *American Journal of Kidney Disease,* vol. 35, no. 2, pp 330–332.

Recommended reading

McCabe, P., 2001, 'Complementary Therapies in Nursing and Midwifery: from Vision to Practice.' Ausmed Publications, Melbourne.

Appendix 'A'

Appendix 'A'

CARE PLAN	PERFECT MAINTAIN	GOOD REVIEW/MAINTAIN	EQUIVOCAL REVISE CARE PLAN	ACUTE INFECTION <4 WEEKS REVISE CARE PLAN	CHRONIC INFECTION >4 WEEKS
PAIN/TENDERNESS	None	None	None	Only if exacerbation	May be present over cuff
COLOR	Natural, pale pink, or dark	Natural, pale pink, purplish or dark, bright, pink <13mm	Bright pink or red < 13 mm	Bright pink or red > 13mm only if exacerbation	Natural, pale pink, purplish or dark, bright pink < 13mm
CRUST	None or small, easily detached or specks of crust on dressing	None or small, easily detached or specks of crust on dressing	Present, may be large and difficult to detach	Present	Present, may be difficult to detach
SCAB	None	None	None	May be present	May be present
DRAINAGE (EXTERNAL)	None	None	None even with pressure on sinus; dried exudate on dressing	Purulent or bloody, spontaneous or after pressure on sinus; wet exudate on dressing	Purulent or bloody, wet exudate on dressing
GRANULATION TISSUE (EXTERNAL)	None	None	Plain or slightly exuberant	Slightly exuberant or "proud flesh" may be present	"Proud flesh" or slightly exuberant typically visible
SWELLING	None	None	None	May be present	May be present
DRAINAGE (SINUS)	None or barely visible, Clear or thick	None or barely visible, Clear or thick	Purulent or bloody, sometimes clear	Purulent or bloody	Purulent or bloody
GRANULATION TISSUE (SINUS)	None	Plain beyond epithelium	Slightly exuberant	Slightly exuberant or "proud flesh"	"Proud flesh" or slightly exuberant
EPITHELIUM	Strong, mature. Covers visible sinus	Strong, mature at rim. Fragile or mucosal deeper	Absent or covers part of sinus	Absent or covers only part of sinus	Absent or covers only part of sinus
MUST BE ABSENT FOR UNINFECTED CATEGORIES	Any visible granulation tissue or fragile epithelium Red, bright pink, or purplish color, any diameter Difficult to remove crust	Any external drainage Purulent or bloody drainage in sinus Exuberant granulation tissue Pain, swelling Red color	Purulent or bloody external drainage Distinctly exuberant granulation tissue Erythema > 13mm Pain, swelling	**INDICATIONS OFTEN SEEN WITH TRAUMA:** Pain, bleeding, scab, deterioration of exit appearance. Exit appearance will depend on intensity of trauma and length of time before evaluation.	

Adapted in part from: Twardowski ZJ. and Prowant. Bf. Classification of Normal and Diseased Exit Sites, *Peritoneal Dialysis International,* Vol. 16, Supplement 3, 1996.

372

Index